without condoms

without condoms

unprotected sex, gay men & barebacking

Michael Shernoff

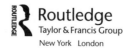

Routledge
Taylor & Francis Group
New York   London

Published in 2006 by
Routledge
Taylor & Francis Group
270 Madison Avenue
New York, NY 10016

Published in Great Britain by
Routledge
Taylor & Francis Group
2 Park Square
Milton Park, Abingdon
Oxon OX14 4RN

© 2006 by Taylor & Francis Group, LLC
Routledge is an imprint of Taylor & Francis Group

Printed in the United States of America on acid-free paper
10 9 8 7 6 5 4 3 2 1

International Standard Book Number-10: 0-415-95024-4 (Softcover)
International Standard Book Number-13: 978-0-415-95024-4 (Softcover)
Library of Congress Card Number 2005012244

Library of Congress Cataloging-in-Publication Data

Shernoff, Michael, 1951-
    Without condoms : unprotected sex, gay men & barebacking / Michael Shernoff.
        p. cm.
    Includes bibliographical references and index.
    ISBN 0-415-95024-4 (pb : alk. paper)
    1. Gay men--Sexual behavior. 2. Safe sex in AIDS prevention. 3. Risk-taking (Psychology) I. Title.

HQ76.S48 2005
613.9'5--dc22   2005012244

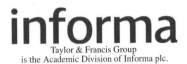

Taylor & Francis Group
is the Academic Division of Informa plc.

Visit the Taylor & Francis Web site at
http://www.taylorandfrancis.com

and the Routledge Web site at
http://www.routledge-ny.com

To John,
whose love and support enrich each day
and whose challenges to think more critically
improved this book.

CONTENTS

ACKNOWLEDGMENTS

This book has had a long gestation period. Its roots were planted when my friend and colleague, psychologist and researcher Perry Halkitis, asked me to contribute a chapter on psychotherapy with gay men who bareback for a special issue of *The Journal of Gay and Lesbian Psychotherapy* that was simultaneously published as a book entitled *Barebacking: Psychosocial and Public Health Approaches.* As I began to look at the extensive research on barebacking and to formulate a framework of clinical issues pertaining to barebacking, my original draft for that chapter grew to be twice as long as space allowed. Several colleagues to whom I showed that manuscript suggested that what I had written was in fact an outline for a book of my own on the topic of barebacking. I started what became a three year journey to learn about and understand (as best any of us are able to) this fascinating and sometimes disturbing topic. I am deeply indebted to Perry for agreeing to write the foreword to this book and consider him one of the godfathers of this work.

The following individuals, in no particular order, on both sides of the Atlantic, were extremely generous in reading sections of my evolving manuscript and providing enormously insightful and helpful feedback about how to improve and clarify my thoughts and words: Greg Cason, Dominic Davies, Steve Cadwell, Craig Hutchinson, Michael Bettinger, Gareth Hagger-Johnson, Charles Isola, Robert Remien, Alex Carballo-Dieguez, Ariel Shidlo, Petros Levounis, Jack Drescher, Gil Tunnel,

Leo Wilton, Michael Ross, Christian Grov, Margaret Nichols, Jeffrey Guss, David Ostrow, William Meyerhofer, and Esther Perel.

A special note of thanks goes to my dear friends and valued colleagues Edith Springer and Donald McVinney. They introduced me to the concepts of harm reduction and motivational interviewing, which have transformed how I think about and practice psychotherapy. They taught me everything I know about these two modalities and were always available to answer questions about theories or practice issues related to these two innovative approaches to working with people.

Steven Dillon and Patrick Dalton were generous in answering medical questions as well as offering insights from their own medical practices.

The following people most generously helped me track down references and in some cases obtained articles for me: Steven Palmer, Tim Horn, and Connie Von Tobel.

David Acosta, Barry Callis, and Michael Siever very generously shared with me the innovative work that they are doing in this area.

There is no way that I could have managed to search the literature and access articles so easily had it not been for the kindness of Alysse Jordon, social work librarian at Columbia University, who took the time to teach me how to conduct online literature searches, and to whom I am eternally grateful for her patience when I was a slow learner or came to a stumbling block.

My friend Laura Markowitz took on the daunting task of agreeing to edit the manuscript chapter by chapter. Her encouragement, excitement about the evolving project, exquisite intelligence, insights, editorial skills, and most of all patience with my all-too-often convoluted initial drafts were invaluable in shaping, refining, and polishing some very rough drafts into what I can only hope is a coherent and easily read finished product.

At Routledge, Dana Bliss was a welcome, friendly, intelligent, and ever-helpful presence, who eased my anxieties about being editorless during the writing after the woman who was the initial editor left the press to have her first child. Jay Whitney took on the daunting task of joining this project as editor after the initial draft had already been completed. He brought an energy, fresh insights, intelligence, creative ideas, professionalism, and a much-appreciated sense of humor to this project at precisely the moment when I needed such an infusion. I am most grateful to him for his contributions in helping this book come to life.

Most of all, I want to acknowledge and sincerely thank all the men who agreed to speak to me about their experiences, thoughts, and feelings on this issue and who allowed me to include their stories in this book.

FOREWORD

We find ourselves at an interesting time in the lives of gay men in the United States. Some 20 years after the initial diagnosis of AIDS in our community, many have died and a new generation of gay men has emerged in the shadow of this epidemic — at a time when the social and political climate toward gay men is both better and worse than it was 20 years ago.

Certainly we have made strides in demanding equal treatment under the law, and yet the battle persists regarding our rights to marriage. The entertainment industry has taken notice, portraying gay characters, albeit stereotypical ones; the advertising world, acknowledging the level of wealth in our community, now gears products and product placement to gay couples and singles, although this is certainly not altruistically motivated. Yet, even in light of what some may consider progress in our society with regard to the lives of gay men, one constant remains — a cloud that darkens our existence.

The AIDS virus is the constant with which every gay man lives. While arguments have been made in the literature and in the press regarding the spread of this epidemic to other communities of our country, the fact remains that gay men as a group are disproportionately affected by this disease. Per person, we as a community have suffered the greatest impact of this epidemic. This is not to minimize the suffering and losses of other communities upon which the epidemic has wreaked havoc, but as a whole in the United States and Western Europe, gay men have suffered the greatest blow from this virus.

Yet one wonders why after millions of dollars spent on education and prevention, gay men continue to place themselves at risk. Recent epidemiological trends indicate spikes in new seroconversions after a period of leveling in the early 1990s, and new infections have been noted among those who were, at the time of their infections, well aware of HIV transmission risks. This is a puzzling reality with which to grapple. One can certainly understand how a 20-year-old gay man became infected in 1981 when no one was aware that the virus even existed, but what is the explanation of the 20-year-old who seroconverts in 2001? If we posit that the majority of new infections among gay men in our country are the result of unprotected sexual intercourse — condomless sex — then why does this phenomenon continue to exist if gay men are well aware that such behavior places their health at risk?

As a species, we often seek simple explanations for matters that are complex and multifaceted, as if there is a simple magical "x" factor that will help explain a human behavior. Throughout the course of the AIDS epidemic, we have sought these simple explanations — men do not know how to use condoms and thus they are taking risks, men do not have the knowledge of how HIV is transmitted and thus they are taking risks, men are using too much alcohol and thus they are taking risks, men lack the efficacy and skills to use condoms and thus they are taking risks, men are depressed and thus they are taking risks, gay men as a community suffer from posttraumatic stress disorder and thus they take risks, men are optimistic after the development of highly active antiretroviral therapy (HAART) and thus they are taking risks, and certainly the most popular hypothesis at the moment — gay men are using crystal methamphetamine and searching for sex on the Internet and thus they are taking risks. Certainly, each of these elements holds some truth, but in and of themselves they are insufficient to explain the condomless sex phenomenon. Being able to identify that simple factor to explain this behavior would make our lives easy. Manipulate the "x," modify this factor, and the "y" will automatically change, just like adding food to the center of a maze will make a mouse more efficiently learn how to navigate that maze. Perhaps, therein lies one answer to our misunderstanding. The mouse has a motivation to run through that maze quickly — what motivation do we as gay men have for using condoms during sex?

Second, unless we understand the complexity and the interaction of all elements working together we will never truly be able to understand why gay men take sexual risks. To this end, our efforts must be driven by holistic understandings of gay men as human beings, for whom psychological, sociological, and biological elements interact to affect our decision making. I have written, in my own work, that we have been guilty of treating sex as a rational, cognitive act. In a volume that I coedited, *HIV + Sex: The Psychological and Interpersonal Dynamics of the Gay Men's Sex Lives*, we consider the shortcoming of such thinking, suggesting that sex is more than a rational act, and that for HIV-positive men specifically, the sexual act is one that transgresses the logical and encompasses numerous domains including the social, the emotional, and the spiritual, in addition to the cognitive. Developmental psychologists have long considered the interplay of all of these domains, yet somehow we have missed this important understanding in dealing with the HIV epidemic.

Then how does this all speak to the topic at hand — barebacking? First, let me suggest my own understanding of this phenomenon. In 1998, when I first started thinking and writing about barebacking, I was certain what the expression meant. Years later, I am more uncertain of what barebacking is, perhaps because of the multitude of meanings it holds for gay men. In the academic literature, some, including myself, have suggested that barebacking is simply intentional unprotected sex, although we as researchers have not even been consistent in our definitions. For example, is it only anal sex? Does ejaculate have to be shared? Is it barebacking when a condom is used for part of the experience? And why is oral sex excluded? Second, if barebacking truly implies intentions toward unprotected sex (let us assume anal sex), then when does the intention have to be present to constitute a barebacking act — 5 minutes before the act, 5 hours before, or 5 days before? And to this end what do we mean by intent? Third, is the act of barebacking different from one's identity as a barebacker? I have argued that these in fact are two very different conditions. Barebacking as a behavior and barebacking as an identity are not synonymous expressions, and if this in fact holds some truth, then why do we simply group all those who have sex without condoms as barebackers? Finally, if we believe that heterosexuals also have condomless sex, including condomless vaginal intercourse, then does the term barebacking exclude them? The bottom line here is that condomless sex, be it called barebacking or any other term that is in vogue at the moment, holds serious health implications for the gay community as a whole. What we call this behavior does not really matter; the outcome of such behavior is what is important.

In February 2005, the New York City Department of Health announced the identification of a gay man who had seroconverted with a version of the HIV virus that is resistant to treatment by three main classes of antiviral medications. By no means a surprise to me or any of my colleagues who had long predicted such an occurrence, the announcement reignited the discussion about the risks that gay men appear to be taking. Simultaneously, a schism emerged in the community itself about the veracity of this finding. I am not certain how anyone can deny the severity of this biological event. Even a most basic understanding of virology and epidemiology would suggest that this occurrence potentially holds grave consequences for those engaging in risk-taking behaviors. But perhaps what is troubling to some in this announcement is the "overly simplistic" link that was made between the use of crystal methamphetamine and this seroconversion, as if the use of the drug itself was solely responsible for the behavior of this individual. Once again, we sought a simple explanation for why this event had occurred, separate from the contexts, emotions, and logic that led this particular man to place himself at risk by having condomless sex.

Thus, it is this type of simplistic thinking that needs to be avoided when we consider the barebacking phenomenon. First, some gay men will choose to have condomless sex based on clear, well-considered information. For example, why should a confirmed seroconcordant HIV-negative couple who do not have sex outside the relationship not engage in barebacking? Would we require a recently married heterosexual couple to have sex with condoms throughout the duration of their relationship? A similar argument could be made for a seroconcordant HIV-positive couple, in light of no compelling clinical evidence about reinfection. The point here is that barebacking is not always a faulty decision as some might lead us to think. There are circumstances in which condomless sex is based on sound reasoning and carries minimal risk. For other men, however, the vast majority, barebacking will carry risk associated with potential seroconversions or acquisition of other sexually transmitted infections. Thus, consideration must be given to the context and the circumstances through which gay men choose to engage in condomless sex.

Second, for men who do place themselves at risk through barebacking there are no simple explanations for why they choose to behave in this manner. There are clearly numerous factors at play that lead men to make these decisions, and consideration must be given to the emotional, social, contextual, and biological determinants for this decision making. If we are truly concerned about the health of gay men and the gay community as a whole, then holistic understandings toward behavior must be the approach.

I have been asked numerous times by the press why I believe that current prevention efforts are failing with regard to gay men. My answer is always twofold. First, the HIV epidemic and treatments for the epidemic have evolved much more rapidly than our thinking about how to further curtail the spread of the disease. (I point anyone interested to the shortsighted and somewhat antiquated efforts undertaken by our most prominent AIDS service organizations.) Second, I believe that we will not solve these "problems" if we remain focused on the behavior itself and not on the roots that drive the development of these behaviors. Providing information about the consequences of barebacking on one's health is not in and of itself harmful but is rather a band-aid to the problem. Efforts on the parts of all working with the community must be directed to the individual-level processes that drive men to take risks. Unless we work from within the person to understand why it is that he chooses to behave in the manner in which he does, and thus implement change on that level, we will never truly be able to fully understand and address the behavior of concern.

It is this type of thinking that my colleague Michael Shernoff brings to the topic at hand. A well-established clinician in the field, Michael has worked with many gay men who grapple with the reality of condomless sex and understands these intrapsychic and dynamic processes that may lead some men to take risks. Thus, in the pages that follow, Michael sheds insight into the inner workings of some gay men, and provides a critical eye in helping us to decipher the phenomenon we have come to know as barebacking. Perhaps what is most refreshing in this approach is Michael's stance that in considering the barebacking phenomenon, we are left with questions to ponder for which there are no simple answers. In other words, simple print campaigns and community forums will not do the trick. This is a lesson to which our colleagues in our departments of health should pay close attention as they hand out hundreds of thousands of dollars for fancy posters that are not based on the vast knowledge garnered from social science research and that pay no attention to inner processes that lead to risk behaviors.

Indeed, we as gay men find ourselves at an interesting time. Recent efforts have emerged from within our community to try to help unite us in our battle against HIV and the numerous other factors that have brought us to what some have labeled a "second wave" of the AIDS epidemic. I am reminded of the early days of AIDS, when community-driven efforts led by leaders such as Larry Kramer and Michael Hirsch and writers such as Richard Goldstein and Robert Massa sought to unite us as a community in which the common enemy was the disease itself. I miss those days in which there was a new zeitgeist that created a community of gay men united for a common cause and take offense to newer efforts, which in their attempt to unite serve rather to stigmatize, demonize, and alienate gay men rather than combating the disease itself. Understanding where we are as a community and why we take risks through condomless sex will lead us to a newer zeitgeist of which we are so dearly in need. Thus, the reader is asked to carefully consider the words of the author and the men whom the author interviewed — listen to their voices, and let their statements lead us.

Perry N. Halkitis, Ph.D.
Professor of Applied Psychology
Director, Center for Health, Identity, Behavior, and Prevention
Studies (CHIBPS)
New York University

PREFACE

In July 1981, an article in the *New York Times* heralded the arrival of what would become the greatest modern public health disaster—AIDS. A "perfect storm" of circumstances made it possible for the virus to gain a foothold in the gay population, whence the epidemic emerged full-force. Among the enabling factors were the rise of visible gay communities, the commercialization of venues for casual sex, an increase in the number of gay men assuming both passive and active roles in anal sex, and a dramatic rise in the use of recreational drugs. The epidemic was abetted by a fatal combination of government inaction and community denial. A unified and expeditiously implemented national HIV-prevention program would have slowed the spread of the virus. But a combination of disgust on the part of a conservative Republican administration and disbelief by many gay men that there could be anything ominous about the way they were exercising their newly won sexual freedoms diverted attention from the real threat: HIV transmission through unprotected anal sex. As I write, we are beset by a similar deadlock. On the one hand, a renewed sexual abandon among some gay men has led to a decrease in their use of condoms. On the other hand, an increasingly militant conservative ideology is resolutely advancing a social and political agenda that is at odds with a proactive common sense approach to HIV prevention.

One often gets the sense from reports in the popular press that the phenomenon of barebacking is something new, but I recall that, even in the earliest days of the epidemic, friends as well as clients in my psychotherapy practice discussed their not always using condoms for anal intercourse, despite full knowledge of the risks this entailed. As a person who loves sex and loves life, also as a person who has contracted HIV, I am in equal parts fascinated by and concerned about what compels some men to take sexual risks. Being a sexually active gay man, my interest in sex without condoms is personal and immediate; but it is also civic-minded, humanist, and professional. Increasing numbers of men in the community that has nurtured me, and that I love, are becoming infected with this deadly virus. Because I live with HIV, and have survived with it for more than two decades while so many others have not, I am not naive about the risks these men take. I don't just mean HIV-negative men. All men who have sex without condoms are exposing themselves not only to HIV but also to the host of other sexually transmitted diseases that are on the rise among sexually active gay men. The AIDS epidemic is not over. The current treatments are not a cure for AIDS, nor are they without seriously debilitating side effects. The stakes remain very high for men who choose to forego condoms, for themselves, for the gay community, and for society at large.

This book is geared toward three audiences, each with its own interest in the topic (despite frequent overlaps): gay men and those who love them, health care and mental health professionals who work with gay men, and professors and students of human sexuality. Readers from each of these groups will find much in the following pages that will interest and challenge them: not only about the phenomenon that is the book's focus, but also, more generally, about the lives and sexualities of gay men and male couples in the contemporary Western world. Inevitably, my gay readership will include men who have barebacked; of these, some will be proud of it, others, ambivalent about it or worried that this behavior may indicate that something is wrong with them. In every instance, they will find their stories reflected here, via case studies and research. Readers of all kinds will likely find that, to some degree, their prior judgments and preconceived notions about gay men and gay sex are upset by my open-minded approach to the material. Clearly, barebacking lends itself to rhetoric that is sensationalistic and alarmist, not to say titillating. I have done my best to avoid these pitfalls, but

I should say from the outset: the subject demands frankness, and I have not shied away from it.

Obviously AIDS prevention issues affect a broad population world-wide. The prevention of heterosexual and woman-to-woman transmission of HIV are critical concerns, but they are outside the scope of this book. I believe that the topic of condomless sex by men who have sex with men is sufficiently important to warrant book-length treatment on its own.

Finally, a word about the book's voice — or better, its voices. It seemed to me that the best way to acknowledge the complex, multi-layered nature of the topic, as well as the variety of pertinent expertises and target readerships, was to make use of several authorial voices, shifting from one to another as required by the unfolding argument. One of them is of course my voice as a professional psychotherapist, but I also write, when the occasion demands, from the vantage of a social historian, a social science researcher, a sexologist, and a folksy storyteller. It is my hope that this multiplicity of viewpoints enriches the book, weaving a compelling narrative that will interest a variety of readers.

Several acronyms are used frequently in the coming pages. Though each is defined the first time that it appears, I thought it would be helpful if they were listed here and defined for the sake of simplicity.

UAI   unprotected anal intercourse
MSM   men who have sex with men
STD   sexually transmitted disease
STI   sexually transmitted infection

Michael Shernoff

ABOUT THE AUTHOR

Michael Shernoff received his MSW from SUNY Stony Brook in 1977. He has been a psychotherapist in private practice in Manhattan since 1983. From 1991 until Spring 2001 he was adjunct faculty at Hunter College Graduate School of Social Work. He currently teaches at Columbia University School of Social Work.

For seven years he was the online mental health expert for TheBody.com, the largest HIV/AIDS Web site in the world. He is a prolific author and editor who has written extensively on mental health issues of gay men, male couples, gay sexuality, and HIV/AIDS.

He can be reached via his Web site at: www.gaypsychotherapy.com.

ON A MORE PERSONAL NOTE

I have always been fascinated by sex, and by the incredible variety of human erotic pleasures and practices. I grew up in a household where there were almost no intergenerational discussions about sex or sexuality, not even the perfunctory father–son talk about "the birds and the bees." But the domestic atmosphere was such that I emerged from it, blessedly, without an iota of sexual shame. I remember stacks of *Playboy* magazines in my older brothers' bedroom, that I was never discouraged from reading. Always prone to push the envelope, I boldly asked my father, just before leaving for college, to pick up a box of Trojans for me from my uncle's pharmacy. He smiled and brought them home. I also had the good fortune to come of age at a time when the sexual revolution and the gay liberation movement converged, opening up endless possibilities for me to explore my burgeoning sexual desires — with men as well as women, with an ease and frequency that now, from the far side of 50, astounds me. Where did I find the energy to pursue so much sex and still complete college and two graduate degrees?

Neither of my parents was proud of my being gay, but they never sought to instill either guilt or shame in me after I came out to them. They eventually came to accept my being gay, and always welcomed me, my friends, and my partners into their home and family gatherings.

My fascination with sex turned into a commitment as a mental health professional to help others develop their own abilities to live sex-positive lives regardless of their sexual orientation. Often, this necessitated helping them dismantle sexual shame. I became a serious student of human sexuality, psychology, and social work, and my life as a psychotherapist has largely been devoted to the care of sexual minority individuals.

From the onset of the AIDS epidemic, my personal interests and professional responsibilities took on a new and dire urgency. As I watched hundreds of loved ones — friends, clients, neighbors, acquaintances — sicken and die, I was at the forefront of developing interventions to help gay and bisexual men to change their sexual practices in ways that, hopefully, would minimize transmission of the virus. With my late best friend and colleague at Chelsea Psychotherapy Associates, Luis Palacios-Jimenez, I developed one of the first AIDS prevention efforts that was unapologetically gay and sex-positive. Luis and I conducted a workshop for more than 15,000 men across North America. We also trained other professionals and volunteers to run it and eventually, under the auspices of Gay Men's Health Crisis in Manhattan, we wrote a teacher's manual enabling others to do so. The book that you hold in your hands is a culminating expression of my lifelong commitment to sexual health and sexual well-being for all people, and of my dedication to public health issues.

Part One

GAY MEN, SEX, AND
CONDOMS: AN OVERVIEW

CHAPTER ONE

Introduction and Overview

Is there any such thing as safe sex? Since the beginning of time, the consequences of sex have been dangerous — even deadly. Sex has been responsible for the spread of debilitating and sometimes lethal diseases, such as hepatitis, syphilis, and gonorrhea, and has often led to unplanned parenthood and back-alley abortions, as well as possible death of mother and child. Sex has never been safe, but most contemporary, Western gay men only consciously began to think about the mortal risks of sex after the onset of AIDS. When it became common knowledge that one way HIV spread was through the exchange of bodily fluids, sexual encounters took on a whole new ominous possibility. While other STDs could be treated if caught in time, AIDS still has no cure. The disease often progresses with ferocious speed and always with devastating impact. Having sex with an infected partner, or taking precautions for safer sex and having them fail, could literally kill you.

Of course, long before the onset of HIV, gay men were aware of the physical as well as emotional dangers of sex. Sexual encounters with other men, not to mention openly expressing romantic feelings of love for members of the same sex, carried serious consequences including discrimination, job loss, exile from family and friends, harassment, gay bashing and other physical abuse, and even murder. It is still true today that being gay can get a man crucified on a fence in the middle of Wyoming.

Although diverse societies throughout the ages have shown varying degrees of acceptance and intolerance toward men who had sex with other men, or same-sex romantic couples, the first half of the twentieth century was a particularly difficult time. Gay men were routinely put in prison or sent to mental institutions where they were subjected to barbaric attempts to forcibly change their sexual orientation, although their only crime was their sexual desire or love for other men. The Nazi regime attempted mass extermination of its gay population. Gay men tried for the most part to make themselves invisible to mainstream society, gathering in secret to socialize and keeping their secret from families, friends, and coworkers. Mainstream society condemned gay men as "perverts" and "freaks." Until 1973, homosexuality was classified as a mental illness by the standards of psychiatric diagnoses created by the American Psychiatric Association.

GETTING ORIENTED

Many people think that the gay health care movement began in response to AIDS, when in fact it was preceded by 15 years of groundbreaking work by gay and lesbian activists, health care workers, students, and social service providers who raised consciousness about the special needs of the gay and lesbian population, challenged heterosexism and homophobia in their professions, and advanced knowledge and understanding of how to serve lesbian and gay clients. This was the platform that allowed the community to respond quickly and professionally when AIDS began its deadly progress.

It is relevant and necessary to begin an exploration of barebacking with a little history. Sex without condoms has never stopped happening, even when AIDS was at its most lethal. Chapter 1 of this book offers a brief history of gay social activism, the way sexual liberation and gay liberation became inextricably linked in the 1970s, and how the gay cultural norms around uninhibited, nonmonogamous sex came to define gay male culture. I then describe how AIDS changed the sexual and social landscape for gay men. While the new rules of sex in the time of AIDS were largely defined by the public health campaigns to promote safer sex, many gay men still engaged in unprotected sex. What was new was that every man had to figure out for himself what risk he felt was acceptable to take. Of course, peer censure plays a part in the shaping of gay culture, and so I will briefly recap some of the gay community's controversial conversations about unsafe sex. As barebackers came out of the closet, public health workers and therapists started to become more alarmed. Researchers began to measure the prevalence of the behavior, and I will review some of those findings. The main question of this book is, how should barebacking be viewed? Is it deviance? Is it an understandable response to a hostile, uncertain world? Or is it an understandable behavior for a variety of reasons and rationales?

EARLY HOMOSEXUAL ACTIVISM IN THE UNITED STATES

The first effort to organize homosexuals in the United States was an attempt in 1950 to resist police harassment, led by Harry Hay, founder of the Mattachine Society in Los Angeles. This marked the birth of the homophile movement. As historian David Carter (2004) explains, "The founders of the Mattachine Society used the word homophile because they believed that this new term, with its incorporation of the Greek word for love, could help counter the stereotype of homosexuals obsessed with sex" (p. 18).

By the 1960s, the Mattachine Society, with chapters in cities around the United States, was not the only predecessor to the contemporary gay liberation movement. In San Francisco, the League for Civil Education (LCE) was formed by the openly gay drag queen Jose Sarria, the first person to run for elected office as an openly gay person in the country. In 1962, San Francisco bar owners and employees formed the Tavern Guild, which retained an attorney and bail bondsman for any person arrested in or near a gay bar. Soon afterwards, also in San Francisco, the Society for Individual Rights was founded "with a more open and democratic approach than that used by LCE or California's Mattachine organization 'to create a community feeling that will bring a Homophile Movement into being'" (Carter, 2004, p. 105).

These organizations provided the foundations upon which gay men began to actively become more open and public about their homosexuality. It was also in the late 1960s that increasing numbers of gay men began to rebel against the limited view of masculinity and against heterosexism in general and began to venture out of their private clubs and private lives and go public. The climate, at least in major urban areas like San Francisco and New York, made them feel a degree of safety, largely because there was a critical mass of gay men congregated in one area, and there is some strength in numbers. Following the 1969 riots that occurred after what the police expected to be just another routine raid on a Manhattan gay bar — the Stonewall — the Gay Liberation Front was born (Carter, 2004). Soon afterward, the movement for increased visibility of and acceptance for gay people who refused to act like second-class citizens took off. It happened in conjunction with a decade of social upheaval including the civil rights movement, the Vietnam War protests, women's liberation, and the sexual revolution.

By 1979, gay men had established a visible, distinct culture in urban areas. Gay consciousness continued to evolve as more men proudly began to live their lives openly, out of the suffocating constraints of the closet. They created gay-friendly spaces and communities in certain neighborhoods, which propelled momentous political gains for gay civil rights. As gay people started to come out of the shadows and defy social expectations of heterosexuality by holding hands and kissing in public, gay people began to feel a sense of solidarity. Gay-friendly cities such as San Francisco and New York became Meccas for gay men in pursuit of open and liberated lives.

Central to the new, open gay culture was a celebration of sex. Although they might still struggle inside themselves with feelings of shame or torment about their same-sex desires, more and more gay men were eager to explore their sexuality. They began to celebrate and flaunt those desires and sought creative ways to fulfill them. Bathhouses, bars, and discos for gay men, as well as other venues for men to meet and have sexual encounters, flourished. In the 1970s, in America's largest cities, gay men no longer had to be furtive about their same-sex desires. Whether or not they identified as homosexual or bisexual, men who had sex with other men could find willing and abundant sexual partners, and plenty of establishments catered to helping them hook up with one another. There appeared to be no limit to the erotic possibilities. Men had sexual adventures with other men with reckless abandon. Beyond worries about not contracting the usual STDs, getting gay bashed, or finding that a partner was closeted, the majority of gay men did not worry about permanent, negative consequences of their sexual partying. Gay bathhouses, sex clubs, backrooms, and orgies were plentiful and popular. An entire generation of gay men came out in a gay subculture that encouraged men to have sex with strangers as casually as they might shake hands with a new acquaintance.

THE CONVERGENCE OF SEXUAL LIBERATION AND GAY LIBERATION

Because sexual freedom was synonymous with gay liberation, a steady supply of sex with unknown partners was a rite of passage for many "liberated" urban gay men. It was not uncommon to find men who prided themselves on their long lists of sexual encounters and partners and their variety of sexual escapades. After a lifetime of learning that their same-sex desires were wrong, sinful, or perverted, throngs of gay men embraced their open pursuit of sexual satisfaction. No more repression, no more guilt and shame, no more hiding. It seemed that many gay men interpreted "out and proud" to mean hooking up as often as possible. Men cruised for sex all over the United States, from the piers and Central Park in New York to Griffith Park in Los Angeles, and in truck stops, gyms, YMCAs, and public restrooms and other locales around the country.

GAY SEXUAL HEALTH BEFORE AIDS

What was the impact of this sexual explosion on the budding gay culture? For one thing, uninhibited sex came to define what "pride" and "healthy" meant to hordes of gay men. In the gay community of the 1970s and early 1980s, monogamous couples were a distinct minority. Gay community norms were founded on an ideology of promiscuity that even today largely defines for many gay men what it means to be gay. As the late AIDS activist Michael Callen (1990) explained: "Seventies gay liberationist rhetoric proclaimed that sex was inherently liberating; by a curiously naive calculus, it seemed to follow that more sex was more liberating" (p. 4).

But even back in the 1970s, a decade before AIDS, sex was not altogether safe. There were undiagnosed STDs that could become debilitating. But while these diseases were inconvenient, most men were confident that the treatment was easy and cure was often assured: a matter of an injection or of a course of prescribed pills. A few illnesses — herpes simplex, anal condyloma (genital warts), and intestinal parasites, to name a few — were rapidly growing nuisances, but not killers. A slowly growing awareness regarding hepatitis was the first inkling many gay men had that certain STDs could prove fatal.

One of the first individuals who attempted to sound an alarm about the health risks attached to having lots of casual and often anonymous sex was (openly gay) Manhattan physician Dan William. In 1978, by which time he was already a prominent figure in the gay community in New York City, William was profiled in an article in *Christopher Street*, a then-popular national gay magazine. In a sidebar to the article, entitled "V.D. at the Tubs: A Modest Proposal" (Stein, 1978), he expressed grave concern about the public health implications of the huge increase in rates of intestinal parasites he was treating, as well as increased numbers of cases of hepatitis, along with other STDs, in his gay male patients. He observed that these diseases were being spread frequently and widely. His primary concern was men who returned to sex venues such as bathhouses and backrooms after being diagnosed with an STD who had not yet completed their courses of treatment or confirmed that they were no longer infectious, thus passing on whatever disease they had. The article had no discernible effect on gay men's sexual behavior either in New York or anywhere else. It would take more than one article for scores of gay men to allow sexual health concerns to impact recreational sex.

THE IMPACT OF AIDS ON GAY MEN'S SEXUALITY

The gay sexual free-for-all provided the perfect environment for HIV to proliferate in the gay community. The intimate acts between gay men, and the sheer number of men engaging in them with one another, allowed the virus to spread from man to man like wildfire. As gay activist Gabriel Rotello (1997), former editor of the one-time major New York City gay newspaper *Outweek*, explained in his controversial book *Sexual*

Ecology, "Sexual versatility (one's willingness to take both insertive and receptive roles in anal sex) became valorized and widespread in gay subculture beginning only in the 1970s; it contributed significantly to epidemic amplification (of HIV) because viral transmission occurs primarily unidirectionally in anal sex, from the insertive to the receptive partner. In mathematical terms, sexual versatility compounds the rate of viral transmission to epidemic proportions" (pp. 77–78). Thus the convergence of the explosion of gay men acting on their sexual desires combined with the development of large numbers of men engaging in anal sex with versatility allowed HIV to spread and flourish.

There was no way at the time that gay men could wrap their minds around the possibility of a lethal sexually transmitted epidemic such as HIV. But the news of a mysterious disease that was killing gay men sent shock waves though the entire community. Some refused to stop playing, but eventually they could not ignore the fact that they were playing with their lives every time they had sex with another man. The rules of the sexual playground changed.

In the early days of the AIDS crisis, writer Larry Kramer (1983a, b, c) began to raise the alarm in ways that stirred controversy. Using language worthy of an Old Testament prophet, he said it was incumbent upon gay men to change the way they were having sex so as to prevent the spread of the virus. His opponents struck back in kind, calling him "antisex" and "homophobic," a "reactionary" and a self-loathing gay man. The virulent intensity of the exchange cannot be understood without taking into account the long-standing Puritanism of American culture, and the pervasive sense among gay people, after the Stonewall riots of 1969, that this same Puritanism was the foundation stone of the closet. Kramer's preachy and patronizing tone was deliberately provocative, and the anger it provoked was intensified by the moralism of his notorious earlier novel, *Faggots* (1978). But despite all of this, Kramer was clearly being targeted as the bearer of bad news. It was difficult for many to believe that their hard-won sexual freedom could have negative consequences. Large numbers of gay men dismissed Kramer's passionate exhortations. To many, they smacked of a kind of antigay rhetoric the gay community was used to hearing from queer-hating conservatives — that gays would pay for their "sins." In fact, leaders on the right wing of America's political spectrum blamed the AIDS epidemic on gay men's "immoral behavior" and claimed it was God's punishment for their perversions. These messages activated some gay men's own internalized homophobia[1] and they came to believe, or at least question, whether God really had sent a plague to smite modern-day Sodomites. Some gay men refused to apologize for their sexual revolution and would not hear anything that smacked of "preachiness" or moralizing. Activist and writer Eric Rofes (1996) suggests that from the onset of the earliest AIDS prevention messages, both the tone and content of the "safe sex" campaign turned off a sizable number of people in the community. Kramer's sometimes shrill, but nonetheless prophetic, warnings were an early example of the failure to reach the targeted audience of sexually active gay men in a way that helped them reevaluate the risks of recreational sex.

As the era of unrestrained sexual expression came to an end and the time of funerals and memorial services began, sex became more dangerous and frightening than ever. Gay men learned to fear bodily fluids and to shun sexual encounters altogether. In the early days of the AIDS epidemic, many sexually active gay men were consumed with fear that they might have already contracted the disease, and if somehow they had not they were desperate to avoid becoming infected. Faced with a disease that had few treatments and no cure, the health care and AIDS activist communities developed campaigns to try to prevent HIV and other STD infections. Beginning in the 1980s, programs were developed to help gay men eroticize safer sex (Palacios-Jimenez & Shernoff, 1986; Shernoff & Palacios-Jimenez, 1988; Shernoff & Bloom, 1991). This sex-positive approach (which is described in more detail in the next chapter) was one of the programs that was successful in stopping the sexual transmission of HIV. For many years, rates of STDs and new HIV infections among gay men dramatically fell (McKusick, Horstman, & Coates, 1985; McKusick et al., 1985; Martin, 1987).

THE AGE OF SAFER SEX

As information began to filter out into the community about how HIV was spread, many gay men were open to hearing about "safer sex." But what exactly was "safer sex"? Confusion ensued. Some were saying that anal intercourse with a condom was "safer" sex; others limited "safer" to mutual masturbation. Social conservatives espoused that the only truly "safe" sex was abstaining from it altogether.[2]

In the first decade of the epidemic, the main incentive propelling gay men toward the practice of safer sex was fear. McKusick, Horstman, and Coates (1985) found that gay men who had been face-to-face with someone in the advanced stages of AIDS, and who thus could access vivid images of this person, were more likely than others to reduce their number of sexual partners.[3] In the mid-to-late 1980s, sexually active gay men made significant changes in their sexual practices. They had fewer sex partners, and they began to use condoms during anal intercourse (McKusick, Horstman, & Coates, 1985; McKusick et al., 1985; Martin, 1987). This was a confusing time for gay men. From the vantage of a psychosexual identity that was always already stigmatized, and thus potentially unstable, gay men now had to negotiate a perplexing landscape of information and misinformation. Even after determining what pertinent "facts" were trustworthy, it was not always easy for them to know whether a particular sexual practice was safe or unsafe.

The terminology current at the time only added to the confusion. At first, AIDS prevention campaigns opted for the phrase "safe sex," but this was soon replaced with "safer sex," to acknowledge the hard reality that none of the prevention techniques in question was fail-safe. More than 20 years later, it remains difficult for gay men to figure out what their personal "sexual safety" limit ought to be. The debate over what is and is not "high-risk" sex continues, notably around fellatio. A handful of such transmissions have been documented (Vittinghoff, Douglas, & Judson, 1999), but not many, and even these are not uncontroversial, a circumstance that raises the quandary of quality-of-life versus public health concerns with a particular acuity. It is now freely admitted that even "safer sex" is not without its risks: a welcome development, insofar as this is a baseline reality. But in making sense of this, we must remember that sex has never been free of risk, and acknowledge that, however one may feel about such a prospect, it never will be.

RIDING "BAREBACK": THE HISTORY OF THE CONTROVERSY

Experts agree that the riskiest form of sex for transmitting HIV is unprotected anal intercourse (UAI) (Vittinghoff, Douglas, & Judson, 1999). UAI, now known as "barebacking," has also been called "raw sex," "natural sex," and "uninhibited sex." Since the onset of the AIDS epidemic, there have always been some gay men who refused to practice safer sex, though aware that condoms could mitigate the risk of contracting HIV through anal sex (Gauthier & Forsyth, 1999; Goodroad, Kirksey, & Butensky, 2000; Halkitis, 2000; Halkitis & Parsons, 2003; Halkitis, Wilton, Parsons, & Hoff, 2004; Mansergh et al., 2002; Suarez & Miller, 2001). Some chose to disbelieve that HIV causes AIDS. Others were unwilling to sacrifice their sexual pleasure for possible longevity, and others deliberately sought to place themselves in harm's way. Some of the men today who are having unprotected sex are the same people who always had sex in this manner.

It is important to understand that men were barebacking even during the earliest days of the AIDS epidemic, though the term was not used in print until 1997, and that the behavior has never completely stopped. As early as 1990, research conducted in San Francisco indicated that 18 percent of men who identified themselves as exclusively gay had engaged in the practice of UAI (Bartolomeo, 1990) at least once in the past year. Chuck Frutchey (1988), then education director of the San Francisco AIDS Foundation, stated that "this finding indicated that helping gay men to resist the temptation to slip back to unsafe sex practices was (even then) more of a problem than getting them to adopt safe-sex habits initially. Clearly, where we need to put a lot of effort now is in maintenance programs. We do not have to teach gay men how to have safer sex — they know that already. What we have to do is have programs that encourage them to maintain safe-sex behavior."

It seems as if little has changed in the years since Frutchey made this dire prediction. But one thing that has evolved is the variety of ways that sex without condoms is now viewed, interpreted, and understood 30 years into the AIDS epidemic. For many gay men in the 21st century, there is not the same strong community norm about having safer sex as existed during the height of the AIDS epidemic. How has this change come about? Is it an understandable and normal evolution as well as possibly dangerous and maladaptive? What role does gay-affirmative psychotherapy have in answering these tough questions and working effectively with gay men who bareback who want to examine this aspect of their behavior? And what would make a gay man become ambivalent about taking precautions not to contract or spread an incurable disease?

The rise in unsafe sex has been discussed within the gay community for more than a decade. The mainstream media began covering the issue in 1994, when the *New York Times* magazine ran a first-person account by a gay HIV-positive Generation X-er who did not describe unsafe sex but did announce himself as part of the "second wave" of gay seroconversions (going from HIV negative to HIV positive). He wrote, "At this point, let's face it, we're the least innocent of 'victims' — we have no excuse, the barrage of safe sex information, the free condoms, blah, blah, blah. . ." (Beachy, 1994, pp. 52–53). When gay journalist Michelangelo Signorile (1994) and prominent queer theorist Michael Warner (1995) both wrote about their own unsafe sexual encounters, these public revelations highlighted the extent to which safer-sex education programs were failing. Warner's description in *The Village Voice* of anal sex without a condom illustrated the degree to which intellectual sophistication and an openly gay identity did not guarantee consistency regarding safer sex practices. The problem of gay men having sex without condoms entered mainstream national consciousness in 1996, when a *New York Times* magazine cover story (Greene, 1996) featured Mark Ebenhoch, a white gay man in his thirties, who became HIV-positive due to his having intentionally had unsafe sex. Most of the letters occasioned by these articles expressed shock and outrage, while a minority were relieved to finally have this issue aired publicly.

Other people were addressing the issue of barebacking even before the term first appeared in print. Prominent porn star and author Scott O'Hara publicly extolled the virtues of having unsafe sex. In 1995, O'Hara wrote an editorial entitled "Exit the Rubberman" in *Steam*, a journal he published that was devoted to sex in public spaces. He wrote: "I'm tired of using condoms, and I won't" (O'Hara, 1995). The letters from readers — admittedly self-identified as people into sexual adventurism — were overwhelmingly favorable. O'Hara, who has since died of AIDS, and other HIV-positive men restated their positions in magazines such as *POZ* and *The Advocate*. Letters to the editor against the anticondom statements voiced by O'Hara and others revealed the frustration, fury, and sadness of gay men who had worked tirelessly since the start of the AIDS epidemic to reduce infection rates and who had buried friends and lovers. They were appalled that the attitude of O'Hara and others who shared his ideas about barebacking might result in a return to those terrible times of death and grief. Another group of readers voiced relief that this difficult issue was at last being brought into the public discourse. The term "barebacking" first appeared in print in *POZ,* in an article entitled "My Turn: Riding Bareback," in which the late AIDS activist and writer Stephen Gendin (1997) described the thrill of not using condoms during anal sex with other HIV-positive men. Gendin explained that "barebacking," which traditionally refers to riding horseback without a saddle, was the vernacular term for UAI. After his article appeared, *POZ* was flooded with letters, the majority of which condemned Gendin for glamorizing a behavior that would lead men to court death.

In 1997 porn star Tony Valenzuela inadvertently took on a public role as the poster boy of unsafe sex. The event that propelled Valenzuela into national notoriety occurred at that year's Creating Change Conference in San Diego. Creating Change is the National Gay and Lesbian Task Force's annual conference for leaders of the gay movement as well as for community activists. In an impromptu speech at a community town hall meeting, convened to discuss recent attacks on public sex and promiscuity by gay conservatives, Valenzuela spoke of his work in the sex industry as an escort and as the first openly HIV-positive porn actor in the U.S. The furor was caused by this remark: "The level of erotic charge and intimacy I feel when a man comes inside me is transformational, especially in a climate which so completely disregards its importance." Few who heard Valenzuela speak seemed to pay attention to his cautionary caveat: "When I talk about having unprotected sex, I am speaking for myself, and not as a proponent of condomless sex for all." Yet as Stephen Gendin (1999a) reported in an article entitled "They Shoot Barebackers, Don't They?" Valenzuela's clearly stated position about not advocating condomless sex for all was undercut by his defiant assertions:

"I am a sex gourmet in a community serving sexual TV dinners . . . and I have placed myself in the middle of HIV anarchy." His speech to a room of 2000 gay and lesbian leaders created an immediate uproar that degenerated into a shouting match, as Valenzuela's few defenders tried to articulate responses to the almost universal outrage and condemnation. This was but an early salvo fired in the ensuing debates around barebacking that have been taking place ever since.

The debate reappeared in the mainstream with a 1997 *Newsweek* article called "A Deadly Dance" (Peyser, 1997), which discussed the phenomenon of gay men not using condoms. Barebacking "arrived" when it made it into a 1998 episode of the television series *ER*. The story involved a gay sex worker describing how customers paid him a higher fee for bareback sex. That same year, former Miss America Kate Shindle weighed in on the issue in an *Advocate* article entitled "Barebacking? Brainless!" She predicted that funding for AIDS prevention would cease if gay men's flagrant disregard for safer sex practices came to the attention of government agencies. It was too late; by then barebacking was already a part of public discourse. Then, Vice President Al Gore referred to barebacking in a conversation with the president's AIDS Advisory Council (Scarce, 1999a).

The print controversy about barebacking continued in 1999, when *POZ* published an article by San Francisco AIDS activist Michael Scarce (1999b) called "Safer Barebacking Considerations," in which he developed strategies for helping reduce the harm associated with barebacking, which he explicitly stated were not a set of HIV guidelines and were "intended only for gay men who have already decided not to use condoms for anal sex." In his opening column in that issue of *POZ*, publisher Sean Strub acknowledged that Scarce's article was controversial, but also wrote that "safer barebacking comes out of a grassroots, *Our Bodies, Ourselves*, tradition of taking charge of one's own health" (p. 2; referring to the title of the first feminist book published about women's health). As Carballo-Dieguez and Bauermeister (2004) note: "Since then, barebacking has generated heated controversy in gay circles. Some gay writers have strongly condemned the behavior (Lenius, 1999; Ricks, 1999; Signorile, 1997, 1998, 1999, 2001). Others have seen in it an expected reaction to absolutist HIV prevention messages (e.g., 'Use a condom every time') and have been somewhat more accepting of it" (Gendin, 1997; Mallinger, 1998; Gendin, 1999b; Mirken, 1999; National Sex Panic Summit, 1997; Rofes, 1999; Salyer, 1999; Scarce, 1998; Sheon & Plant, 1997).

Never one to shy away from controversy, Stephen Gendin (1999b), in another column for *POZ*, discussed how he and his boyfriend, Kyle "Hush" McDowell, had been barebacking and that it ultimately resulted in Hush's becoming infected. In a companion article, Hush (McDowell, 1999) described that his wanting to "desperately hold Stephen's interest" was the major rationale why he allowed himself to have "raw sex within hours of meeting," which resulted in his seroconversion. Hush had come out as a gay man after the advent of HIV. He knew all about safer sex.

In January of 2003, *Rolling Stone* published an article entitled "Bug Chasers: The Men Who Long to Be HIV+" (Freeman, 2003), which chronicled the story of men who reportedly sought unsafe sex with the explicit intention of becoming infected. The story created another uproar, with the rhetoric about barebacking becoming highly polarized. Those who oppose barebacking labeled barebackers as "dangerous sex fiends" (Scarce, 1999a), and barebackers called their detractors "condom Nazis" (Scarce, 1999a). (I will revisit this article in Chapter 5.)

In defense of condomless sex, O'Hara (1997) wrote, "I may die at a younger age than my gay brothers who are more cautious, who limit the number of their sexual contacts, and than my straight brothers who, presumably, are rigidly monogamous. And you know something? I decided a long time ago that it is worth it" (p. 36). O'Hara in fact died on February 18, 1998, at age 36, from AIDS-related lymphoma.

A few years later, in 2000, Tim Dean wrote an indirect response to O'Hara: "Unfortunately, this kind of implicit cost-benefit analysis completely misses the point that unsafe sex is a social activity as well as a question of individual decision making. This is in fact perhaps *the* key point regarding barebacking. It does not merely affect an individual, but also the men he is sexually active with as well as the community within which he lives. Unlike other risky behaviors such as smoking, drinking, and substance abuse (which arguably can be indulged as solitary pursuits), unsafe sex always directly involves somebody else" (Dean, 2000, p. 140).

Dean's comments speak to the concept of "sexual ecology" formulated in the context of AIDS by Rotello (1997), and maintain that there is the need to examine barebacking using an ecological or holistic framework that looks at the individual as well as the social and communal relationships within which he is living.

DEFINING THE TERMS: WHAT IS BAREBACKING?

Some pathologize those who take sexual risks as being self-destructive, suicidal, damaged individuals. Savage (1999) suggested that "for some gay men, danger is a permanent fetish" (p. 62). Others condemn the judgmental culture as once again wanting to cast gay desire and gay sexuality as sick and perverse. One of the goals of this book is to provide a well-balanced view of men who have sex without condoms and to explore barebackers' motivations to have intentional, unprotected sex and risk contracting an incurable disease.

At this point it will be useful to clarify some terms. Many people use the phrases "unprotected" and "unsafe" sex interchangeably. This is inaccurate and confusing. Unsafe sex refers to when an HIV-negative man has UAI with either a partner of unknown HIV status or with a partner he knows to be HIV-positive, thus opening the possibility of HIV transmission and new infection. Unprotected sex is anal intercourse without a condom between two HIV-negative men. Monogamous male–male relationships where both partners know that they are HIV-negative are not at risk for transmission of HIV even if they do not use condoms, provided that they have sex only with each other or only have safer sex with any outside sexual partners. "If there is no virus or other pathogen to transmit, the sex is not unsafe" (Blechner, 2002, p. 31). These men obviously trust each other to sustain sexual fidelity. The "if" of "if they have sex only with each other" is a very big one, as will be discussed in Chapter 7.

Originally, social scientists (Sheon & Plant, 1997; Nary, 1998; Gauthier & Forsyth, 1999) used the term "barebackers" to refer to men who intentionally seek out condomless anal sex, as distinct from men who have UAI due to poor planning or accidents. Some (Goodroad, Kirksey, & Butensky, 2000; Carballo-Dieguez, 2001; Suarez &

Miller, 2001) write that for a behavior to be barebacking two crucial criteria must be met: intentionality, and the potential for the risk of viral transmission. Researchers often hear people say that there are many situations in which sex without condoms is not barebacking. If people in a monogamous couple where both are HIV-negative do not use condoms, most do not describe this as barebacking. Similarly, people who get caught in a moment of passion and once in a blue moon have unintentional unprotected sex, or who have sex with condoms but they break, or people who were drunk one night and did not use a condom are not said by the above researchers to engage in bareback sex.

As barebacking has become more prevalent in the gay community, the perception and definition of it has evolved. "Whereas the term originally was used to describe engaging in premeditated, consciously chosen unprotected anal sex, it has now been incorporated into colloquial discussions to describe the unintentional, unprotected 'slip-ups' that occur" (Morin et al., 2003, p. 357). Halkitis, Greene, and Mourgues (2005) discuss that among a sample of New York gay men there is a wide variety of meanings given to and understandings of the ways that the term barebacking is used. Mansergh and colleagues (2002) propose defining the term "barebacking" (for both HIV-negative and HIV-positive men who have sex with men [MSM]) as "intentional anal sex without a condom with men who are not a primary partner (that is, not someone the individual lives with or sees often and to whom the individual feels a special emotional commitment)" (p. 653). This will be the definition used throughout this book.

There is evidence that sex without condoms is the relatively infrequent act of a relatively large number of gay men (rather than the very frequent act of a few) and that it is often moderated by relationship status as well as HIV status (Coxon & McManus, 2000). Despite the risks — or perhaps because of the risks — it holds a certain mystique in some segments of a community that had to learn to be afraid of sex all over again. One does not have to look very hard to find Internet sites devoted to the glorification of barebacking. A walk through a gay sex club may reveal men openly engaging in barebacking. But as will be discussed in Chapters 6 through 9, large numbers of men in committed partnerships are not using condoms every time they have anal sex.

It is important to state and to reiterate, that even anal sex with a condom is not 100 percent risk free for preventing HIV transmission. Condoms may have a tear or hole in them; they are often incorrectly used and can break.

COMBINATION THERAPY AND SAFER-SEX FATIGUE

Perhaps it is not coincidental that the trend toward an increase in sex without condoms coincides with the time when combination anti-retroviral therapy, also known as HAART[4] (highly active antiretroviral therapy), became widely available (Ekstrand, Stall, Paul, Osmond, & Coates, 1999; Wolitski, Valdiserri, Denning, & Levine, 2001). A common rationale gay men give for risking HIV infection is that HIV is no longer the death sentence it once was. Mansergh and colleagues (2002) report that barebackers in their study stated that knowing that fewer people are currently developing AIDS, even after contracting HIV, contributes to their having more unsafe sexual behavior. Opting to have high-risk sex is sometimes connected to the advent of combination HIV antiretroviral therapy (Kelly, Hoffman, & Rompa, 1998; Remien & Smith, 2000; Vanable, Ostrow, McKirnan, Taywaditep, & Hope, 2000; Ostrow et al., 2002; Morin et al., 2003). In Mansergh's research, barebackers reported that improved treatments had caused them to have more unsafe sex. New drug therapies provide gay men with a misplaced sense of complacency. Many believe that contracting HIV is not a risk to life. For the young — who still tacitly believe in their immortality — this logic is not far-fetched. As noted earlier, in the early days of the AIDS epidemic, fear helped propel men to change how they had sex. Everywhere one looked there was a gay man dying of AIDS, another memorial service to attend, and pages of obituaries to scan for familiar names.

Some barebackers believe that HIV-positive men who are on HAART and who have low viral levels or viral levels that are beneath the level of detectability are less capable of transmitting HIV to others and therefore safer as sexual partners (Kalichman, Nachimson, Cherry, & Williams, 1998; Suarez et al., 2001). As Suarez and Miller (2001) state, "The belief that HAART might reduce infectivity may not be totally erroneous" (p. 290). Pinkerton and Holtgrave (1999) maintain that there is limited evidence that HAART reduces the risk that HIV can be transmitted. But the question of HAART's correlation with a lowered risk of HIV transmission during unprotected sex remains open. Not everyone with an undetectable viral load in his blood also has a corresponding undetectable viral load in his semen (Suarez & Miller, 2001).

Catalan and Thorley (2001) suggest that one contributing factor to the resurgence of unsafe sex is the de facto erasure among many gay men of the distinction between HIV as a chronic illness and as a severe illness. "Describing HIV as a chronic illness implies that it is a less severe condition, a manageable if not altogether curable condition" (Catalan, 2001, p. 2). Thus, from the perspective of a young gay man, today in his mid-twenties, the prospect of chronic or even terminal illness 20 years later can appear so remote as to offer no deterrent to unsafe sex. On this point, Tim Dean writes: "In view of American culture's emphasis on youthfulness, which gay subculture reinforces, the prospect of not having to endure middle age thanks to AIDS may positively encourage sexual recklessness" (p. 140).

Today, thanks to HAART and improved prophylaxis, which prevents most of the AIDS-related opportunistic infections that once were invariably fatal — along with weight training combined with testosterone, human growth hormone, and steroids — people with HIV and AIDS are often imposing, muscled hunks (Halkitis, 2000; Shernoff, 2002). Suarez and Miller (2001) discuss "the eroticization of HIV" and suggest that this may play a large role in changing the community perception of AIDS, which may then lead to increased risk-taking. "Gone are references to AIDS as the grim reaper. Today's images of persons living with HIV are of healthy, virile, and physically fit individuals" (p. 290). For the past several years, advertisements run by the pharmaceutical companies for antiretroviral drugs always picture young men (and women) looking robust and buff and engaged in strenuous physical activity like climbing mountains or sailing. These visual representations of people with HIV and AIDS reinforce the mistaken notion that HIV is no longer a serious or even life-threatening condition. One study conducted in San Francisco of 997 men seeking services at a municipal STD clinic showed that 76 percent had seen HIV drug advertisements that portrayed men who are healthy, handsome, and strong either daily or weekly. Within this subset, those men who were HIV-positive believed that HIV was a less serious disease. The same participants believed that seeing these advertisements influenced their decision to have unprotected sex (Klausner, Kim, & Kent, 2002). Declines in safer sex also have been correlated to the reduced visibility of AIDS and a sense that the crisis has passed (Rosengarten, Race, & Kippax, 2000). Without visual reminders of how devastating AIDS can still be, intelligent men who are well-informed about HIV and how it is transmitted are more likely to take sexual risks.

Manhattan psychologist Mark Blechner (2002) writes: "Young gay men today may be lucky not to have lived through the terrible times of the early days of the AIDS epidemic, but consequently, many such people do not share the great sense of relief that the previous generation felt at being able to stay alive by mere condom use. Some instead feel resentment and deprivation at the constraints of safer sex" (p. 29). He suggests further that it is easy for older people who have enjoyed condomless sex and survived the epidemic to be condescending as they try to convince younger gay men about how the tradeoff between condom use and safety is obviously worth it. For younger people, who in any case often feel invincible, the subjective valuation of condoms, risk, health, and pleasure may be different (Blechner, 2002). Gay men of the generations that came out into a world where AIDS was already a reality grew up knowing they had missed the halcyon days of gay men's sexuality. They feel left behind and envious of what they missed. They may also consciously or unconsciously measure their sex lives against the now-mythic time of the 1970s and feel frustrated and resentful of the precautions they must take to avoid HIV infection.

Research by New York psychologist Alex Carballo-Dieguez (2001) documents the existence of men who are well-informed about HIV transmission and the means to prevent it, and who had managed to avoid unprotected sex for many years. But his data also indicate that for various reasons, they progressively relaxed their safer-sex standards and started to experiment with condomless sex. These are not only younger men who engage in barebacking. Middle-aged gay men who were sexually active prior to the onset of the AIDS crisis, and who lived through those terrible years that decimated the gay community, are now engaging in sex without condoms (Bonnel, Weatherburn, & Hickson, 2000).

There are those who have been practicing safer sex for years and even decades who report experiencing safer-sex fatigue or burnout, and who cite this as one rationale for their returning to sex without condoms (Halkitis, Parsons, & Wilton, 2003). Ostrow and colleagues (2002) confirmed these findings when they found that burnout from years of exposure to prevention messages and trying to maintain safer-sex practices was an independent predictor of UAI among HIV-positive men in four U.S. cities. As for younger gay men, in-school sex education, increased availability of condoms, and increased knowledge of HIV risk and safer sex practices helped educate them about how to avoid HIV infection and other STDs. While it is true that these programs have done much to decrease the amount of unsafe sex (Rotheram-Borus, 2001), HIV infection in this young population remains at one of the highest rates in all age groups (Koblin et al., 2000; Valleroy et al., 2000; CDC, 2003).

HOW MANY ARE BAREBACKING?

We still do not know, with any degree of precision, the extent of male–male sex without condoms in the United States. Goodroad and colleagues (2000) state that, at the time of their writing, "The phenomenon of barebacking was noticeably absent from the scientific literature" (p. 31), whereas there were many articles addressing the failure to use condoms and the reasons for such behavior. Carballo-Dieguez and Bauermeister (2004) report that a literature review conducted by them in mid-June 2002, using four search engines (Medline, PsycInfo, EbscoHost, and ProQuest), yielded only three articles in scientific journals containing the word "barebacking," as opposed to dozens otherwise addressing unsafe male–male sexual behavior. Another review, conducted by myself three years later, in August 2004, using the same search engines netted 43 articles containing the term "barebacking." This is a clear indication that, in the interim, awareness of the phenomenon, and interest in it, had grown significantly.

At the 2003 National HIV Prevention Conference in Atlanta, hosted by the Centers for Disease Control and Prevention (CDC), the

CDC released data that showed that the number of gay and bisexual men diagnosed with HIV climbed for the third consecutive year in the United States in 2002, fueling fears that the disease might be poised for a major comeback in these high-risk groups. HIV diagnoses among men who have sex with men surged 7.1 percent in 2001, according to data collected by the CDC. New diagnoses in MSM have increased 17.7 percent since 1999, while remaining stable in other vulnerable communities (CDC, 2003b; Simao, 2003). This research exposes an alarming trend, but is it merely speculative to blame the resurgence of HIV infection in the gay and bisexual community on barebacking? Perhaps there is a correlation: according to the CDC researchers, between 1994 and 1999, the number of gay men who reported not using condoms as well as having multiple sex partners rose from 24 to 45 percent (CDC, 1999a, 2002, 2003a).

In the mid-1980s, reports of increased condom use and reduced high-risk sexual practices accompanied dramatic decreases in rectal gonorrhea and syphilis in MSM (Fox, 1998; CDC, 1998). Today, data from around the country show that both syphilis and gonorrhea cases are surging in the gay community. Several recent studies have pointed to comparatively high, and increasingly higher, levels of STDs among MSM from all racial and ethnic groups (CDC, 1999, 2000, 2002; Fox et al., 2001; Avery et al., 2001, Wolitski et al., 2001). Since skin-to-skin contact is necessary to transmit STDs, the rise in the rates of these STDs among gay men is seen as statistical evidence suggesting an increase in barebacking (Bonnel et al., 2000). It therefore can be concluded that barebacking also correlates with the surge in new HIV infections.

In fact, researchers have found that an increase in syphilis is often followed by a wave of new HIV infections. Syphilis can be detected sooner and so acts as an early warning signal for new behavioral trends. One 26-city study conducted between 1994 and 1999 revealed that during that period, the proportion of gonorrhea cases among MSM more than doubled from 6 to 13 percent (CDC, 1999). One STD clinic in Washington, D.C., reported that gonorrhea cases increased 93 percent from 1993 to 1996, with 82 percent of these cases diagnosed in MSM (Simao, 2003). These statistics point to a sea change in sexual practices: a dramatic increase in skin-to-skin contact during sex. There is no doubt that barebacking is more prevalent in the gay community than at any time since before AIDS, and it is on the rise.

But it is not an either/or equation. Some gay men are still using condoms, but others do not or do not use them regularly. A 2003 survey conducted in New York City found that MSM were more likely than either heterosexual men or women to use condoms. Yet this study also showed that men with a higher number of sexual partners with whom they had anal sex did not report regularly using condoms with their various partners during the year preceding the survey. Of those surveyed, 55 percent said that they had not used a condom the last time they had sex (NYC Department of Health and Mental Health, 2003). This study seems to strongly suggest that among sexually active men who have anal sex with multiple partners, a majority are not regularly using condoms.

Some practitioners of UAI mistakenly believe that they are immune to HIV infection. Others are well aware of the risks entailed by this behavior but engage in it anyway. But what public health officials, health and mental health practitioners, and community activists alike find even more alarming is the existence of "bug chasers": HIV-negative men who actively seek to be infected with the virus. This is the extreme edge of the phenomenon, and the aspect of it that people tend to find most unsettling. I discuss this behavior below (in Chapter 5), but a few preliminary remarks about it are appropriate here. Its prevalence in the United States has not yet been documented, but the anecdotal evidence of its existence is irrefutable. Even if it is relatively rare (which seems likely), it raises uncomfortable questions that are central to the project of this book. What are the ethical considerations it is incumbent upon gay men to consider when they negotiate condom use — or nonuse. More provocatively: Is there something inherently sexy about high-risk sex? If so can any safer-sex campaigns ever hope to prevail over such an allure? Most provocatively: Do all men who have sex without condoms seek, whether consciously or unconsciously, to become infected with HIV?

A look at other Western cultures reveals that condomless sex is not limited to the United States. In a survey of more than 14,000 gay men conducted throughout Great Britain in 2003, 56 percent of the respondents reported having been penetrated by a partner without a condom and over 58 percent reported having penetrated a partner without a condom (Sigma Research, 2004). In Amsterdam, a several-year study of MSM under age 35 found that unsafe sexual behavior with both steady and casual partners among HIV-negative men occurred significantly more often after 1996 (Dukers et al., 2001). Studies in Melbourne, Sydney, Budapest, Russia, and London document recent increases in barebacking between casual male partners (Ridge, Plummer, & Minichiello, 1994; Elford, Bolding, & Sherr, 2002: Van de Ven & Crawford, 1998; Van de Ven et al., 1998a; b; Van de Ven, Rawstorne, Crawford, & Kippax, 2002; Amirkhanian et al., 2001; Csepe, Amirkhanian, Kelly, McAuliffe, & Mosonoki, 2002). For whatever reasons (and they are varied and complex, as we will see), gay men in the Western world are less likely to use condoms than they were a decade ago.

One thing is clear: gay men are not foregoing condoms because condoms do not work to prevent STD transmission. In fact, as the AIDS pandemic continues to unfold, the efficacy of using condoms during anal intercourse to prevent transmission of HIV and other STDs has held up over time. Yet, ignorance and confusion about how STDs are transmitted may still be underlying factors here. Some barebackers believe that in unprotected anal intercourse, HIV cannot be transmitted from the "bottom"[5] to the "top." But as Vittinghoff et al. (1999) have noted, there is now empirical evidence that this is a mistaken assumption. Manhattan physician Stephen Dillon (personal communication, August 24, 2004) describes seeing increasing numbers of gay men who have recently become HIV-positive as a direct result of their ignorance of these data, and of the ensuing need to protect themselves by using a condom regardless of their partner's HIV status.

"BAREBACKER" BECOMES A SEXUAL IDENTITY

Gay culture is well known for its rich diversity of sexual practices and proclivities. Often, a part of gay male identity is centered on sexual preferences. Some men identify as "bears"— referring to their abundant body hair and/or weight. They frequent bear bars and belong to online chat groups for bears. Others identify as "tops," referring to their preference to be the penetrating partner in anal intercourse, and advertise in personals ads that they are looking for bottoms. Research conducted by Halkitis (2003) and Wolitski, Parsons, and Gomez (2004) indicates that in recent years there has been an increase in the number of men identifying as "barebackers." Like bears and tops, they claim this identity as a badge of pride, proclaiming their membership in a subset of the gay community. But not all barebackers do this. Some men who admit to engaging in the behavior of having anal sex without condoms do not claim the identity (Halkitis, 2003; Halkitis et al., 2005c). One of the primary differences between the two groups is that self-identifying barebackers actively seek out condomless sex, while men in the other group do not, but are nonetheless willing to participate in it. Should we differentiate between these two subsets of barebackers?

Two studies of HIV-positive gay men in San Francisco and New York City[6] found that about one quarter of the participants laid claim to the barebacker identity. Those who did so were at considerable risk of transmitting HIV to their sexual partners,[7] for the men who identified as barebackers reported both a higher incidence of UAI, as well as high rates of being both the insertive as well as the receptive partner (Wolitski et al., 2004).

PEER PRESSURE

It is easy to condemn men who bareback as mentally ill or lacking in conscience, but what is the *de facto* role of the gay community in fostering such behavior? Recent research (Morin et al., 2003) finds that men who forego using condoms feel there has been a decrease in social support for staying safe as well as a shift in community norms toward increased acceptability of unsafe sex. It would seem that, to some degree and in some quarters, there is now peer pressure to bareback.

We do well to remember that, while it is true that most people who engage in sex in pursuit of pleasure, it is also true that, in most if not all instances, pleasure alone is not their sole aim. According to Crossley (2002), expressing sexual freedom, rebellion, or empowerment, or all of the above may figure prominently in the predisposition toward barebacking. To quote Mark Blechner (2002): "If we problemize one extreme but not the other, we may lose perspectives on how decisions of risk are made. Risk of HIV infection is serious. But the risk of loss of pleasure and intimacy is also serious" (p. 30). Thus, the varieties of roles that pleasure assumes for gay men in particular as it pertains to sex, and to bareback sex specifically, will be explored in subsequent chapters. The other needs that gay men try to address through sex, and how condomless sex comes to be perceived by some of these men as a viable means of satisfying those needs, will also be examined.

BAREBACKING AS DEVIANCE?

It is important in this context to note that heterosexuals as well as homosexuals and bisexuals engage in sexual intercourse without condoms. Gauthier and Forsyth (1999) point out that "barebacking is considered to be a form a sexual deviance only in certain contexts" (p. 87). They suggest that the way it is viewed changes with the circumstances and populations in question. If the individuals who are engaged in it are married heterosexuals, there is little or no stigma attached, whether the intercourse is vaginal or anal. When the partners are unmarried but romantically involved heterosexuals, there is more social censure, but in the United States it is relatively mild. When the parties are unmarried heterosexuals who are not romantically involved, there is more social censure and disapproval, even when the woman is employing other methods of birth control.

According to these researchers, disapproval of barebacking is most extreme when it occurs between gay men. Their article does not discuss the levels of social censure or stigma both within and from outside the gay community that relate to HIV and relationship status, but their findings reveal mainstream society's biases around gay barebacking as a category and without any regard to the relationship status or circumstances. I suggest that the categories of gay men (regarding condomless sex) in order of least to most social disapproval are as follows:

- HIV-negative men who do not use condoms within the context of a committed, monogamous relationship
- HIV-negative men in a committed but nonmonogamous relationship who do not use condoms with each other but have only safer sex with outside partners

- HIV-negative men within the context of a committed but non-monogamous relationship who do not have safer sex with outside partners
- HIV-positive men in a committed monogamous relationship who bareback only with each other
- Men in an HIV-serodiscordant committed relationship
- HIV-positive men in a committed nonmonogamous relationship
- Single HIV-negative men who do not use condoms with men who represent themselves as uninfected
- HIV-negative men who bareback with men who either do not know their HIV status or who identify as HIV-positive
- HIV-positive men who bareback with men who either do not know their HIV status or who self-identify as HIV-negative

In other words, "What is considered serious deviance often depends on the context in which a behavior occurs more than on the actual content of the acts that comprise that behavior" (Gauthier & Forsyth, 1999, p. 87). Or, as West (1987) puts it: "Many deviant behaviors are merely exaggerated versions of familiar components of ordinary sexuality" (p. 75). This provides us with a useful vantage from which to examine barebacking among gay men.

Throughout the book, I try to reveal the complexity of the longings that gay men seek to assuage through condomless sex. In part, I do this in the hope of expanding the therapeutic treatment options for gay men, for it is my view that without an understanding of this complexity, we will never be able to design intervention strategies that are both sensitive and successful that work, on whatever scale. Many readers will think that my only legitimate purpose here can be to stem the rising tide of barebacking. This is indeed one of my aims, but not the only one. Some aspects of my take on the phenomenon will likely cause surprise. I argue, for example, that, even in the age of AIDS, male–male sex without condoms is sometimes normal, adaptive, understandable, explainable, and probably unstoppable as well as ethically defensible. But this is secondary to my main argument, which is that, even from a public health perspective, and especially when the behavior is ethically indefensible, it is key that we grasp the extent to which that behavior is rooted in a longing for emotional or physical intimacy through sex. Such longings are entirely human, and, in themselves, hardly call for condemnation. This should go without saying, of course, but given the pervasively homophobic culture in which we live, it cannot, as regards same-sex interactions, be repeated too often. So I call upon readers of all sexual persuasions and ethical mind-sets to undertake a thought experiment. As you work your way through the following pages, try to project yourself imaginatively into the skin of men weighing the option of sex without condoms. It is my belief that, to the extent that you succeed in doing so, both your human and your ethical horizons will be expanded in ways that can only lead to clearer, more effective thinking about this potentially explosive topic.

By bringing together relevant history, research, and my own clinical experience, I hope to offer a balanced view of the barebacking controversy. Having said that, I should also say that, to some degree, my views have been shaped by the limits of my firsthand clinical experience. Case examples reflect my therapy practice, which is made up largely of white, urban, economically successful, gay men who are out of the closet and who are covered by health insurance. Clinical work with other segments of the gay population for example, bisexuals, working-class men, or men of color, may look quite different from what I describe here. Clearly, the complications of gay men taking sexual risks cut across all races, classes, and economic levels, but men who are economically disadvantaged may face realities that compound their risk-taking. For instance, a sex worker who chooses to bareback is often motivated by financial rewards because barebacking commands more money than sex with a condom. The research studies I discuss in this book reflect the behaviors and attitudes of men across a wide spectrum of economic, geographical, racial, and age lines.

CHAPTER TWO

Gay Men's Sexuality and Psychotherapy: From Cure to Affirmation

If sex always stuck to the rules, the missionary position would not have become a byword for a lack of imagination.

Clark, 2001, p. 32

ROBERT, A RELATIVELY RECENT BAREBACKER

In discussing his first forays into unprotected sex after years of using condoms assiduously, a patient of mine, Robert,[1] explained: "For many years I was good, really rigorous about always using a condom. After all, I had lost so many friends and lovers to this damn thing, that the least I could do was to keep myself uninfected and healthy. But increasingly, men who I was topping explicitly asked me not to use a condom, and eventually I began to comply. At first this made me uneasy, even though I never did this with someone I just met, no matter what he told me about his HIV status. After a few months of this, when one of my regular sex partners who told me he was HIV-negative asked to top me without a condom, I let him. I was surprised that afterward I was not more nervous. But sex in general is such a life-affirming act, and playing without condoms brought with it such a sense of freedom and reclaiming of many feelings I used to have on a regular basis about myself, and the sex I used to have, that with men who I can trust, I no longer use condoms, and rarely give it a second thought."

As a therapist who works with men who bareback, I have had to find a way to quiet any feelings of alarm or even judgments about this behavior, while also staying respectful and connected to clients no matter what choices they make. I am aware of how important it is to help my clients develop positive feelings about themselves and how they express themselves sexually. Of course, those therapists who still believe that being gay is a mental illness or manifestation of immature or incomplete psychosexual development surely have no qualms about categorizing barebacking as further proof of gay men's psychological immaturity. But for therapists like me, no matter how open-minded and nonjudgmental we strive to be, we still may harbor beliefs that anyone who knowingly places himself at risk for contracting HIV has some serious emotional or mental problems. What role possible psychopathology plays in a man's barebacking will be explored in this chapter.

CHAPTER OVERVIEW

This chapter poses a difficult question: Could unprotected anal intercourse (UAI) be a normal and even understandable development at this point in the AIDS epidemic? Or is it simply pathological? Are men like Robert who bareback "sexually liberated," or are they "sexually compulsive?" Or might they just be making what for them is a rational adaptation to being sexually active gay men with complex emotional needs? Is the potential of risking one's life for sexual pleasure a possibly rational choice, or a sign of mental imbalance — suicidal even? These are some of the overarching questions that haunt the research, discussions, and debates about barebacking, as well as therapy with men who engage in barebacking.

In this chapter, we will begin to explore the psychology of barebacking, including the role of the AIDS epidemic in shaping some gay men's decisions to take risks with their health. We will consider various arguments and debates about the ways that grief, loss, mourning, and even depression play into the picture. While we seek answers to why some gay men bareback, we will also look at how the mental health professions have changed in the last few decades vis-à-vis their attitudes toward gay people, including a brief look at the emergence of gay-affirmative counseling. This chapter — indeed, this book — will draw attention to ways gay-affirmative work with barebackers can be effective.

The last section of this chapter will focus on safer-sex efforts during and since the first days of the AIDS epidemic. How did eroticizing safer sex change gay male sexual culture? Is "survivor guilt" a factor in barebacking? We will also look at both the limits of therapy and the usefulness of using an ecological lens in understanding the barebacking phenomenon.

SEX, SHAME, AND BAREBACKING

Before feminism, efforts to prevent pregnancy out of wedlock among heterosexuals involved a campaign of guilt and shame, primarily directed against women. From an early age, girls were taught to feel ashamed of their sexual urges and to feel guilty if they acted on them. Similarly, gay men have been shamed and guilted into denying their sexual feelings for other men, and social censorship, which we often refer to as "homophobia," has served to keep gay men confused, ashamed, and disconnected from an intrinsic aspect of themselves in an attempt to suppress homosexual behavior. Walt Odets (1994) believes that relying on shame and guilt to ensure that gay men practice safer sex is doomed to failure because those same psychological armaments have rarely been effective in keeping gay men from homosexual behavior and "have never been effective in changing feelings." He writes: "This exploitation is equally unlikely to keep gay men from having unprotected sex, or thinking about it, or having complex feelings about it" (p. 428).

What about gay men who were not on the front lines of the AIDS epidemic? Do they also feel shame about barebacking? Their attitudes toward unsafe sex are addressed by author and activist Patrick Moore, who believes that younger gay men have also suffered losses as a result of AIDS, even if those losses were not of lovers and friends. "For men of my generation [those who came of age sexually after the onset of AIDS], there was the double bitterness of living constantly with death without having enjoyed an earlier era when sex was less associated with guilt and shame" (2004, p. xxvi). Moore reminds us that it is not healthy for the gay community to designate pre-AIDS as a time of "good gay sex" and our current era as a time of "bad gay sex." In fact, for the gay community to have a healthy understanding of itself, the task is to reclaim "both the gay sexual past and AIDS as vital but separate histories" (p. xxvi). While Moore feels that it is essential that individual gay men as well as gay culture not feel any shame about the sexual culture that predated AIDS, he suggests that the shame about this history is still impacting gay men in terms of how they regard their own sexual desires and behaviors. For many, the freedoms, joys, and other benefits of the gay sexual culture that predated AIDS were overshadowed and even negated once the reality that AIDS was sexually transmitted became apparent. This resulted in many men trying to distance themselves from any associations with the rich pre-AIDS sexual culture, even at the cost of being embarrassed by and ashamed of their own attraction to aspects of it whether they lived it or not.

One young man illustrates the connections between barebacking and shame in an interview with Manhattan psychologist Alex Carballo-Dieguez (2001):

> I do understand the importance of barebacking in that it takes back a sense of personal freedom. It moves the sex you are having from the onus of shame and fear that an epidemic caused (fear of getting something, shame that society has put on us for having gotten diseases this way). Not using the condom steps toward that earlier time when we were enjoying each other's intimacy and shared physicality. (p. 230)

THE TALKING "CURE"

The therapy room was not always a safe place for gay men. In fact, gay men have a long and checkered history vis-à-vis the mental health professions. The role psychotherapy plays in men's decisions about barebacking is extremely complex and is a result of how the professions have evolved since the 1960s. As we examine the evolution of the relationship between therapy and gay men over the past few decades, what emerges is a picture of how society's understanding about same-sex love and

desire has quickly and dramatically shifted. Mental health professionals still struggle to understand the diversity of human sexual desire and
behavior. There is still contention and confusion on the part of some
professionals about how their own values and judgments, discomforts
and personal choices come to bear on their treatment of clients dealing
with sexual nonconformity, with barebacking being the most recent and
poignant example. Being conscious of how therapists' attitudes toward
gay men and gay male sexuality have changed is important to com-
prehending the variety of options available to therapists working with
gay men who are exploring their curiosity about, desire for, or history
of barebacking.

Attitudes toward homosexuality have shifted over the course of
the last century — both internally within gay individuals, as well as
in society as a whole. As Hartmann (1996) notes, this evolution has
occurred "not in a pure, linear, smooth, or universal shift, but rather in
a powerful general direction from sin, to crime, to illness, to difference"
(p. xxxi). There have been notable generation gaps within the gay community, resulting in vastly different experiences for gay men that were
related to which decade they came out to themselves and, if ever, to
others. For example, the period in which a gay man came of age greatly
determined how he might feel about his attractions to other men, and
his feelings about acting on those attractions and desires. The era in
which a gay man came of age would certainly have made a difference in
how he was treated by a mental health professional. Herdt and Boxer
(1993) describe four age groupings of gay men that correlate to specific
historical periods in the last century:

1. Those who came of age after World War I.
2. Those who came of age during and after World War II.
3. Those who came of age after Stonewall and the period of gay
   activism around it.
4. Those who came of age in the era of AIDS.

Of course, there were enormous variations within each time period.
But in general, gay men shared similar experiences with those in their
age cohort with regard to mental health services. Those who came out
before Stonewall were almost guaranteed to have encountered therapists

who, although well-meaning, believed that it was in the best interests of their gay patients to attempt to "cure" them of their homosexuality. That is not to say that there were not some therapists who were benign and compassionate and helpful to their gay patients. But all too often, therapy was ultimately damaging, as historian Martin Duberman (1991) illustrates in his memoir, *Cures: A Gay Man's Odyssey*. This book recounts, among other things, Duberman's harrowing and painful history of trying to change his sexual orientation. In one section, he describes how his therapist did nothing to intervene during a therapy group in which Duberman was physically assaulted for being homosexual by another member of the group.

The mental health professions might never have changed their practice of treating homosexuality as a mental illness if not for the efforts of gay, lesbian, and heterosexual-ally activists within the ranks of the various professions. Their efforts culminated in a remarkable event that occurred on December 15, 1973. On that day, the Board of Trustees of the American Psychiatric Association (APA) voted to remove homosexuality as an "illness" in *The Diagnostic and Statistical Manual III* (*DSM*). This definitive guide to mental illnesses continues to shape the nature of diagnosis and treatment among all who practice therapy. This was a moment of great triumph for all those in the mental health fields who had lobbied hard to remove homosexuality from the ranks of pathology. Proponents of the change persuasively argued that the mental health world should be removing the stigma attached to homosexuality in order to promote mental wellness rather than adding to the stigma by continuing to diagnose it as abnormal development, sexual perversion, or any other number of unflattering, demeaning, and shaming conditions.

Before the change in the *DSM*, any gay man who consulted with a mental health professional could expect psychotherapy to focus on trying to change his sexual orientation, even if the individual did not desire such a change. Manhattan psychiatrist and psychoanalyst Jack Drescher (2001) provides a concise summary of the history of "reparative therapies," which is another name for sexual conversion therapies. Psychoanalysis was the branch of the mental health field that was most virulently entrenched in its belief that homosexual behavior was aberrant and doomed a gay person to a life of loneliness, depression, and ultimately suicide. That profession posited that a successful analysis of a homosexual was one in which his or her sexual orientation became heterosexual.

Charles Silverstein (1997), a Manhattan psychologist who was active in the effort to get the APA to depathologize homosexuality, describes what it was like for gay men seeking therapy before the gay liberation movement. Silverstein recounts that prior to the 1970s, there were no established alternative treatment options to sexual conversion therapy for gay people who wanted professional help for the depression and loneliness that were the probable cause of higher-than-average suicide rates among gays that Bell and Weinberg (1978) reported. And while treatment options were lacking, it was also true that before 1973, it was professionally dangerous for gay and lesbian therapists to be open to their colleagues or clients about their sexual orientation. An openly gay individual risked losing his or her credibility with colleagues, which could be professional suicide. Suddenly, referrals would dry up, and the therapist would be denied admittance to psychoanalytic training programs and might even lose his or her license to practice. A few brave souls were openly gay and lesbian, and some worked behind the scenes, along with heterosexual allies, to get the APA to change the *DSM*. When a small, but key, number of courageous mental health professionals began to emerge from their professional closets, they became role models for other gays and lesbians, including their colleagues, patients, clients, students, and supervisees. Out professionals offered hope to others who had not yet come out that it was possible to have dignified and fulfilling professional and personal lives without the shame and secrecy of the closet. They also helped to educate their straight colleagues, many of whom had assumed they did not know any gay people. Through a combination of professional advocacy and simply being open and honest about who they were, the first generation of out mental health professionals helped transform their professions. The trickle-down effect worked slowly, as the broader society began to confront and dismantle the myths and stereotypes about gay men and lesbians.

Even today antigay prejudices exist among mental health professionals. There are groups like NARTH (National Association for

Research and Therapy of Homosexuals), whose objectives are to train mental health professionals on how to do sexual conversion therapy and to advocate for trying to change a person's homosexual orientation (www.NARTH.COM, 2005); Exodus International, which is an organization of Christian Counseling Groups that help people renounce the "gay lifestyle," and seeks "freedom from homosexuality since 1976" (www.exodus-international.org, 2005); and PATH (Positive Alternatives to Homosexuality), which is a "coalition of organizations that help people with unwanted same-sex attractions to realize their personal goals for change" (www.pathinfo.org, 2005). These organizations continue to thrive despite hard empirical evidence that sexual orientation can not be changed and that attempts to do so result in harm to the individual (American Psychiatric Association, 1998, 2000; Shidlo, Schroeder, & Drescher, 2001; Schroeder & Shidlo, 2001; Shidlo & Schroeder, 2002). Any gay man seeking psychotherapy who is unsure of how prospective therapists view homosexuality should not hesitate to directly ask them their positions on being gay, whether they believe that same-sex love and lovemaking is normal, and whether they ever work to help a client change his sexual orientation? If the therapist hedges his or her answer, or is not completely and unambiguously affirming of the normalcy of a person's homosexuality and does not state that changing sexual orientation is not possible or desirable, then I urge the individual to continue to shop around until he finds a gay-positive therapist.

GAY-AFFIRMATIVE PSYCHOTHERAPY

In radical opposition to the pervasive conversion therapies, gay-affirmative psychotherapy was initially described as a "theoretical position regarding homosexuality as a nonpathological human potential. But while the traditional goal of psychotherapy with homosexual males has been conversion (to heterosexuality), gay-affirmative strategies regard fixed homoerotic predilections as sexual and affectional capacities which are to be valued and facilitated" (Malyon, 1982, p. 62). In practice, this meant that psychotherapy became less emotionally dangerous, punitive, and shaming for gay men, and more positive, hopeful, and affirming. A literature began to emerge that asserted that being homosexual was not intrinsically the cause of a person's unhappiness or problems; rather, society's homophobia (bigotry and intolerance of homosexuals) was the source of much of the suffering experienced by sexual minority people. It was a novel approach to therapy with the gay and lesbian population and reflected the gay rights and gay pride movements that were burgeoning during that era.

It was not just political rhetoric that midwifed the birth of gay-affirmative psychotherapy. Evelyn Hooker's seminal research comparing heterosexual and homosexual men (1957) was the first to demonstrate that objective testing could not identify any differences in the psychological functioning between heterosexual and homosexual men in her sample. As Silverstein (1996) writes, a second source of inspiration for this change was the rise of sex research as a scientific discipline, led by Alfred Kinsey and his colleagues (1948, 1953), who published the first exhaustive studies of sexual behavior in the United States. Kinsey's institute spawned an entire cadre of nonhomophobic sex researchers such as Simon and Gagnon (1967), Sonenschein (1966, 1968), and Bell (1972), Bell and Weinberg (1978), and Bell, Weinberg, and Hammersmith (1981).

GAYS COUNSELING GAYS

In the 1970s and 1980s, a cadre of graduate students and professionals led the charge in challenging established theories and models of mental health treatment for gays and lesbians. These individuals seemed to share two common objectives: to provide compassionate and non-biased counseling services to gay people in emotional crisis, and to work politically to remove the stigma of being gay from society. With regard to the first of these goals, these pioneers knew that many gay people preferred to see a gay-identified therapist rather than a therapist who did not identify as gay or refused to disclose his or her sexual orientation. A growing number of gay clients were suspicious of therapists who might suggest that they should consider changing their sexual orientation. This created a demand for openly gay, or at least openly gay-positive, therapists. "I don't want my homosexuality to become the center of treatment," was an often-heard complaint by gays who sought out psychotherapy (Silverstein, 1997).

The first gay counseling centers started to sprout up around the United States in the early 1970s in cities with large gay communities. They were staffed by people who were either mental health professionals or graduate students, or in the case of peer counseling centers, by individuals who were trained and supervised by professionals. Many were walk-in centers staffed by volunteers and were housed in other community institutions, offering services only a few hours a week. The first full-time, gay-affirmative counseling center to open its doors in the country was the Homophile Community Health Center in Boston. Soon after, the Homosexual Community Counseling Center and the Institute for Human Identity opened in Manhattan, where gay and lesbian therapists volunteered their time to provide high-quality psychotherapy. In the years that followed, other gay-affirmative counseling centers opened in Minneapolis, Seattle, Los Angeles, Philadelphia, and Pittsburgh (Silverstein, 1997). As Silverstein (1996) writes: "These gay community centers provided a place where gay professionals could learn more about the emotional problems of gay people and meet other gay professionals. Many gay psychiatrists, psychologists, and social workers who worked in these centers authored the new literature on gay-affirmative psychotherapy" (p. 5). The foundations laid in those early years of creating the genre of gay-affirmative psychotherapy proved invaluable, enhancing the quality of life for gay people and even saving the lives of many who came to therapy hating themselves for being gay.

GAY LIBERATION AS GOOD MENTAL HEALTH

As gay communities coalesced, and members felt more of a sense of belonging to a community of people with similar social, romantic, sexual, and political interests, there was a spate of organizing. People formed groups to fight antigay oppression and founded organizations whose aims were specifically to foster opportunities to socialize with people like themselves — a process that has become known as "homosocialization" (Isay, 1989). Political organizing became, for many, a meaningful opportunity to reduce isolation and loneliness while working for social change. For gay men in particular, another motive for attending gay activist events was the hope of meeting and making social — as well as possibly sexual — contact with the other activists. Positive connections to community were often inextricably bound up in the interconnection of activism and sexual adventures. A lot of emphasis was placed on gay men's right to do whatever they wanted with their bodies. Expressing themselves sexually gradually evolved from something done with furtiveness into a celebratory manifestation that embodied the newly liberated attitudes that "Gay is good" and "Gay sex is healthy."

GAY MEN'S SEXUAL CULTURES

The gay community's norms in the 1970s embraced a high level of sexuality with a variety of partners, both creating and affirming that stereotype about gay men that, to this day, still is a central part of how some gays as well as straights define what it means to be gay. In his provocative book, *Beyond Shame: Reclaiming the Abandoned History of Radical Gay Sexuality* (2004), Patrick Moore writes: "In the 1970s, gay men used sex as the raw material for a social experiment so extreme that I liken it to art" (p. xxiv). Many gay-affirmative therapists worked with gay men to help them ameliorate their internalized homophobia and sexual shame by encouraging them to explore and live out their sexual fantasies and desires. Gay men's sexual desires were normalized and validated during the course of that type of therapy. Of course, there was still plenty of the old-school therapy going on, where therapists viewed any attempt by gay men to express themselves sexually as "gross acting out" and indicative of severe psychopathology.

PSYCHOTHERAPY IN THE TIME OF AIDS

It is hard to imagine what gay culture might have looked like today had it not been so dramatically derailed by the AIDS epidemic. The golden age of sexual adventuresomeness was short lived — maybe a decade long — when AIDS struck. By 1983, informational campaigns within local gay communities in large cities began to disseminate information publicizing the link between certain sexual acts and a new lethal illness afflicting gay men. First known as GRID (Gay Related

Immune Deficiency), what eventually became known as AIDS began to force many gay men to realize that they would have to change their sexual practices dramatically. As these educational efforts proliferated, it became obvious to mental health professionals working with this population, and to public health professionals attempting to help stop the spread of HIV, that many gay men were having great difficulty modifying their sexual behaviors. There were several reasons for this, including initial disbelief that whatever was causing gay men to become ill was sexually transmitted. Additionally, some psychotherapy clients were reporting confusion over the risk-reduction guidelines.

Therapists whose practices were almost or exclusively composed of gay men noticed in their clients increased anxiety, depression, and isolation as well as other signs of emotional disturbance. This was all directly related to the growing health crisis within the gay men's community. As AIDS became less an abstract statistic and took on faces of the sick, the dying, and the dead, it had a pervasive impact on the emotional lives of gay men. Therapists heard client after client describe fears about their own health and the health of friends and lovers. Men of all ages were grappling with grief and mourning as more and more lovers, friends, neighbors, ex-lovers, and acquaintances sickened and died. As the epidemic advanced, grief counseling became a familiar part of the practice of every gay and gay-affirmative therapist during the height of the epidemic. Gay-affirmative psychotherapy in the 1980s increasingly included working with men who were ill and dying as well as with men who were not sick, but were terrified (known as the "worried well"), overwhelmed with caring for sick friends and partners, and at the same time grieving for loved ones who had died. Psychotherapy became an important venue for men to cope with all this stress and to start to understand the broader impact it was having on their inner and communal lives. This was markedly different from the content of sessions before AIDS, when many urban gay men used therapy to discuss sexual self-actualization and sexual exploration, in addition to other issues. Many gay men who, prior to AIDS, had never given serious consideration to entering therapy began to seek out therapists for support, using counseling as a haven where they could unburden themselves.

Among the multiple levels of loss that gay men were struggling to comprehend were a host of losses related to sexual expression. While this might not have been foremost in the minds of someone nursing a partner or close friend through the final, painful stages of AIDS, eventually this issue would emerge as this individual struggled to get his life back together in some way. Even for those who did not directly experience the death of someone close, gay sexual culture — the possibilities it represented and its centrality to so many in that generation of gay men — had been decimated. Therapy became a place for discussing and sharing concerns about sex in the age of AIDS. Gay men sorely needed a therapeutic environment that would not exacerbate any negative feelings they were having as a result of AIDS being sexually transmitted.

There are parallels between Robert's history and how the relationship of gay men and therapy evolved that may help shed light on understanding Robert's beginning to bareback. Initially, gay affirmative therapy began by helping gay people feel good about being gay by providing them with mental health treatment that did not make an issue out of their sexual orientation. After the onset of AIDS it helped men cope with the stress brought on by the epidemic and provided a place to grieve the multiple layers of loss in culturally sensitive ways. Among these losses was the need to mourn the change in gay men's ability to have sex as they had prior to the epidemic. Eventually, therapy became a venue where men wrestled with what level of sexual risk was acceptable to them. Gay-affirmative therapists needed to remain nonjudgmental even in the face of AIDS concerning the importance of anal sex to many gay men. As I validated Robert's losses and urged him to talk about how they impacted him physically, emotionally, and socially as well as sexually, he began to grieve these losses during our work together. Once Robert had mourned his friends as well as the pre-AIDS "life-affirming" role sex had played for him in his life, he began to progressively have sex that was increasingly higher risk.

A BRIEF HISTORY OF AIDS PREVENTION EFFORTS

The first attempts at AIDS prevention consisted solely of brochures, posters, and public lectures that simply stated the facts about risk reduction as they were understood at the time, urging gay and bisexual men to stop higher-risk behaviors. These informational campaigns helped most gay men learn the basic facts about which sexual practices were lower risk and which were not. In therapy or with friends, men might discuss their feelings about changing patterns of their sex lives in response to the AIDS health crisis, but there were no organized venues within the gay community where men could participate in conversations about these changes with their peers.

Most mental health professionals received little or no training in human sexuality or sexuality counseling. Consequently, as a group, psychotherapists were often uncomfortable when discussing sexual matters with clients. The AIDS health crisis challenged all clinicians to learn how to talk candidly and accurately about sexual behavior in general, and specifically to counsel clients on ways to prevent the spread of HIV. Even today, mental health professionals often fail to question clients about areas where they themselves feel uncomfortable or about which they are ignorant or biased. The result is that clients may be engaging in risky sexual behavior that is ignored or overlooked by therapists because of unrecognized countertransference. In my own therapy practice, sessions became opportunities to do safer-sex education. Clients had practical questions that they were sometimes embarrassed to ask. Some wanted to sort through their own feelings about wanting to protect themselves from contracting HIV. They also began to explore their feelings about their desire and/or willingness to take sexual risks, and to consider what kinds of sexual risks they might take and in what circumstances they were likely to take them.

While back in the 1980s most gay men knew the basics — exchanging bodily fluids could spread HIV — the ambiguities implicit in the safer-sex guidelines at that time exacerbated many gay men's anxieties. Safer sex was presented on a risk continuum, with clearly safe sexual behavior at one end and clearly risky sexual behavior at the other (Shernoff, 1988). Individuals were encouraged to decide for themselves the level of risk with which they were comfortable. There were very few clear answers to some of the more pressing questions, especially in the early days of the epidemic. For example, the safety of kissing was much debated. The riskiness of fellatio without a condom was then — and continues to be — a subject of controversy even in the third decade of the epidemic. In the safety of their therapists' offices, clients talked about what level of sexual activity they wished to maintain, and how to make the change to lower-risk sexual behaviors — with all of this happening against the backdrop of the growing sex-negative and antigay attitudes of Ronald Reagan's America.

The fact that therapy could provide gay-positive countermessages to renewed social hostility against gays, as well as supportive and sex-positive messages, was important and probably lifesaving. Gay men had already spent seven decades of the 20th century being battered emotionally and psychologically by shaming, demeaning, and abusive messages about homosexuality. The AIDS epidemic created a new crop of destructive ideas that had a negative effect on gay men's psyches that they needed to fend off. There were prominent mental health professionals who publicized their unrealistic and not-well-founded advice regarding AIDS prevention. For example, Teresa Crenshaw, then a member of the presidential AIDS Commission and president of the American Association of Sex Educators, Counselors, and Therapists, repeatedly stated her opinion "the only absolutely safe sex is celibacy or masturbation, with the next best option being monogamy with a *trustworthy partner* who is not already infected" (italics added, 1987). Her pronouncements received widespread attention. While her statement is true in the abstract, it was extremely unrealistic as well as irresponsible to expect people either to stop having sex or only to masturbate for the rest of their lives. While she might have meant well, she was in fact giving an opinion and claiming it was good for public health. Interestingly, many seronegative gay men are now following Crenshaw's advice in terms of not having safer sex with other uninfected men they deem to be "safe or trustworthy" partners.

PSYCHOLOGICAL ATTACKS ON GAY SEXUAL CULTURE

By the late 1980s, it looked as though the sexual party was over. Most gay men abandoned the sexual bacchanals that had been such a central aspect of gay culture. In the later 1980s and early 1990s, that recreational sexual culture began to be examined by some social commentators and therapists, and the picture they were painting was often not flattering (Quadland & Shattls, 1987). For example, psychologist Patrick Carnes (1983) began to popularize the concept of "sexual compulsivity" or "sexual addiction," which remains a controversial concept because its central premise is based on a heteronormative concept of sexual behavior and frequency. While certainly sex had been a joyful expression of play, self-discovery, and interpersonal connection for many, there had always been those who had used sex as a way to cope with a variety of emotionally distressing realities such as boredom, depression, anxiety, and loneliness. Those men sought sex at least in part to anesthetize themselves against experiencing their uncomfortable feelings. In therapy, these clients struggled with the loss of their self-soothing behavior — sex — and with the abrupt change it had undergone from a source of relief and comfort to a profound source of uncertainty, anxiety, and fear. They wrestled with how to face and cope with feelings that had been intolerable and predated the emergence of AIDS. It didn't help their already existing anxieties that they were now living in a fearful time, with AIDS wiping out large swaths of the urban gay communities across the nation. Some gay men found that their profound anxiety and fears sometimes interfered with their ability to adopt low-risk sexual practices. Some even discussed in therapy sessions how nerve-wracking it was for them not to be able to reduce their number of sexual partners or adopt safer sex precautions, even while knowing that it was precisely the sexual nature of HIV transmission that made them afraid and anxious. When talk therapy alone did not help, a referral to a psychopharmacologist for a prescription of antianxiety or antidepression medication sometimes was appropriate.

Gay men who had used sex as a central way to meet other men often found it difficult to change their patterns of seeking anonymous sex because they did not feel able to learn or comfortable with alternative ways to meet men, to socialize, and have their needs for intimacy and sex met. I reminded those clients that it was not sex with an anonymous partner or even many partners that placed them at risk for spreading HIV, but engaging in high-risk sex acts.

AIDS, SEX, AND MOURNING

Human and sexual loss was followed by anger, another common theme often heard during therapy in response to AIDS. During the height of the epidemic, the seemingly complete disregard by the federal government and by the majority of heterosexual America for the plight of people with HIV and AIDS, as well as discrimination against people with HIV/AIDS and inaction by the Reagan administration — which was clearly rooted in the homophobia of that administration, with its close ties to the religious right wing in America — exacerbated the rage and frustration of the gay community and its allies. Gay men were angry at having lost their carefully built gay families to this plague, at the loss of gay culture, and at the loss of hopefulness and celebration in the gay community.

In a powerful essay entitled "Mourning and Militancy" published in the periodical *October*, queer activist and cultural critic Douglas Crimp (1989) uses Freud's essay, "Mourning and Melancholia" (1917) as a framework for examining various reactions gay men had to AIDS early on. Crimp notes that Freud describes mourning as the reaction not only to the death of a loved one, but also "to the loss of some abstraction which has taken the place of one, such as one's country, liberty, an ideal, and so on" (Freud, 1917, p. 243). Gay-affirmative psychotherapy provided access to sympathetic and understanding professionals with whom men could discuss the multiple losses they needed to acknowledge and grieve as a result of AIDS. As gay men were reeling in response to AIDS, Crimp wrote movingly about how AIDS-related losses affected gay men. Addressing Freud's discussion of mourning, Crimp asks: "Can we be allowed to include, in this 'civilized' list, the ideal of perverse sexual pleasure itself rather than one stemming from its sublimation? Alongside the dismal toll of death, what many of us have lost is a culture of sexual possibility. Sex was everywhere for us, and everything we wanted to venture. Now our untamed impulses are either proscribed once again or shielded from us by latex" (Crimp, 1989, p. 11). If a therapist was not gay affirmative, he or she would most likely not see the value of the sexual culture that gay men had built and now needed to mourn. In my practice I worked with innumerable men who at least initially felt guilty disclosing feelings about the non-death-related losses they were also suffering.

Walt Odets makes a connection between gay men's mourning in response to AIDS-related losses and unsafe sex. "Mourning and the feelings of loss, grief, and emptiness that accompany it are often fended off by an introjection[2] of the dead individual" (Odets, 1994, p. 439). Odets (1994) found that during the height of the epidemic, some gay men had a desire not to survive the epidemic. He believes there were "psychologically comprehensible reasons that some men might not wish to survive the AIDS epidemic," including depression, anxiety, guilt (including guilt about not being infected and guilt about surviving the epidemic and outliving loved ones who had already died), feelings of emptiness and loss, isolation and loneliness, loss of social affiliation and psychological identity, and dreading a future that held more of the same.

What Odets described was confirmed by my own clinical experience with gay men early in the epidemic. Currently, the gay men in my psychotherapy practice no longer report these same intense feelings of hopelessness and despair as a result of AIDS. Odets describes that introjective fantasies are often a normal part of healthy adult experience when, for example, they are one aspect of the power and emotional significance of sexual intercourse, whether it be oral, anal, or vaginal. While introjection is often conceived of as a relatively primitive reaction to loss, identification is considered to be more mature and constructive than introjection. As Odets reminds us, introjection and identification are not always discrete processes. Both, however, work to fend off the experience of separation and loss. Odets gives the example of an uninfected man who has unprotected sex with his lover who is dying of AIDS as one example of literally and figuratively one man's trying to inject his beloved at risk to his own health. As Odets reports in the case cited, a gay man immediately after the death of his lover may feel consciously that he is sick and dying, and that it might not even occur to him that he is not. This is evidence of the power of this particular introjection. For other people, having HIV may be indivisible from being gay and receiving infected semen creates a connection or bond to the gay community, which has become merged in an individual's mind with the community of HIV-infected people.

Yet when talking about the seemingly less tangible losses, many gay men expressed confusion at the intensity of their feelings about the impact of these losses on them and the broader community. They easily understood needing to mourn loved ones who had died. But to quote Crimp again, "To say that we miss uninhibited and unprotected sex as we miss our lovers and friends will hardly solicit solidarity, even tolerance. But tolerance is as Pasolini said, 'always and purely nominal, merely a more refined form of condemnation'" (p. 11). I would add that a crucial aspect of strengthening the therapeutic bond and thus the potential of healing for any gay man expressing feelings about the loss of being able to freely and spontaneously express his sexual desire during the height of the AIDS epidemic was that the therapist be empathic to these concerns. It is only a therapist who values and affirms the intrinsic nature and health of gay sexual expression who is able to do the sophisticated therapeutic work required to help a grief-stricken gay man delve into his complex feelings and reactions that go beyond his grief over the deaths of friends and lovers.

In 1989, when he wrote his essay, Crimp had profound insights into how the memories of sexual pleasures became linked for some gay men to ambivalence about their sexual histories. This has multiple dimensions, which will be explored in the coming pages. For example, sometimes this ambivalence was related to resentment about having to change sexual practices and the need to think in terms of "protection" rather than pleasure. Mental health professionals were on the front lines of these conversations, rants, and laments. Younger gay men who might not have been sexually active before the onset of AIDS and men who were just accepting their own gay identity at that time were disappointed and angry at the lost opportunities to have carefree sex. Crimp (1989) speaks to this: "For men now in their twenties, our sexual ideal is mostly just that — an ideal, the cum never swallowed. Embracing safe sex is for them an act of defiance, and its promotion is perhaps the AIDS activist movement's least inhibited stance" (p. 11). I believe that what Crimp is referring to here when talking about the defiance with which some younger gay men adopted safer sex is a defiance against AIDS and of giving up sex completely.

SEXUAL SHAME, HOMOPHOBIA, AND EROTOPHOBIA

Anger and grief were only two of the side effects of AIDS. The epidemic also triggered shame, internalized homophobia, and even fear of sex for many gay men. Some of the more sexually experienced men reproached themselves for their past sexual pleasures, labeling them "irresponsible behavior" in the wake of AIDS. Crimp states, "When in mourning our ideal, we meet with the same opprobrium as when mourning our dead; we incur a different order of psychic distress, since the memories of our pleasures are already fraught with ambivalence. The abject repudiation of their sexual pasts by many gay men testifies to that ambivalence, even as the widespread adoption of safe sex practices vouches for our ability to work through it" (p. 11). Some men went so far as to adopt a guilt-obsessed celibacy or partial social withdrawal, which in itself created sadness and even depression — all evidence of ambivalence toward their sexual histories.

It was often shame about an individual's sexual history or even desires that contributed to the conclusion that celibacy was the only option for controlling one's sexual behaviors. Those who chose celibacy believed it was the only practical way to protect themselves from AIDS. But this attempted solution came with its own complications — many of the men who retreated into celibacy became even more angry, withdrawn, and depressed. Gay-affirmative therapists spent countless hours attempting to validate their clients' understandable fears while simultaneously trying to help men deconstruct self-blame and internalized negative self-loathing that threatened to undo the hard-earned gains of the gay liberation movement.

Emphasizing abstinence from all sexual activity in an effort to prevent AIDS was never effective and in many cases was counterproductive to the goals of risk reduction. Not surprisingly, as early as 1989, Catania and colleagues (1989) documented that men in San Francisco who attempted monogamy or celibacy in response to AIDS frequently discontinued these practices. Attempts to use abstinence in this way most often led to a "diet/binge" sexual syndrome. During periods of sexual abstinence, men who stopped having sex reported becoming increasingly depressed, anxious, isolated, and lonely. But sex, of course, is a drive; when their frustration reached the inevitable breaking point, they went out and engaged in sex that was usually high risk for spreading HIV. Moreover, these bingers often increased their use of alcohol and drugs (Gochros, 1988), further compromising their ability to follow safer-sex guidelines.

Armed with this knowledge, AIDS-prevention programs began to emphasize that decisions about sexual risk or safer-sex acts are compromised when people are under the influence of alcohol or drugs. A 1985 report prepared for the San Francisco AIDS Foundation found that "sixty-one percent of the men surveyed agree that they were more likely to have unsafe sex when using alcohol or drugs" (Research and Decisions Corp., 1985). Many safer sex programs began to build in a component of helping people learn to recognize and manage the anxiety that arises in social and potentially sexual situations without abusing alcohol or drugs. Alcohol and drug use by gay men is one major factor contributing to barebacking. Recently, attention has been drawn to the alarming growth of abuse of crystal methamphetamine by gay men and how it directly relates to barebacking. (This phenomenon will be discussed in detail in Chapter 4.)

The self-reproach and shame that Crimp and Moore discuss in response to past sexual behaviors could also take the form of a resurgence of internalized homophobia. The onset of AIDS provided an opportunity to bombard gay men with messages from the religious right wing, who were using every opportunity afforded them to sermonize that AIDS was God's punishment being visited upon sinning homosexuals. Simply living in the era of AIDS created numerous additional psychosocial stressors for gay men. But for those who grew up in religious and especially fundamentalist households, these extremist religious messages encouraged a regressive form of internalized homophobia to reemerge. Some gay men who had previously been comfortable with their sexual identity experienced a regression to precoming out emotional states, once again questioning their sexual identity and experiencing doubts and shame concerning their sexual wishes, desires, and behaviors. It required a gay-affirmative therapist to help a man suffering from these thoughts and feelings.

The impact of AIDS upon gay sexual culture and some men's ambivalence about their own desires and past behaviors also elicited "erotophobia," a general fear of sexuality and expressing oneself freely in sexual ways. As writer Michael Bronski (2004) points out, "Nor did we realize — despite our best efforts to pursue a vision of sexual freedom that was both liberating and joyous — that we did not vanquish shame. We just managed to push it to the sidelines. But in the 1980s the shame about sex that we had seemingly maneuvered around came back in full force as shame about AIDS — which was of course, shame squared" (p. xx). When shame and anger are manifested in members of an oppressed minority such as gay men, very often it gets turned against the individual by himself. Some men actually explained their high-risk sexual activities by espousing attitudes that were the equivalent of "fuck it" (the nihilism felt in response to AIDS and the volume of deaths) and "fuck me" ("What's the point of trying to survive this?"). Many of the men who described feeling and behaving this way were exhibiting symptoms of posttraumatic stress syndrome in response to the AIDS epidemic.

MOURNING AND MELANCHOLIA

In "Mourning and Melancholia" (1917), Freud defines and differentiates between the two conditions. He suggests that melancholia (today known as depression), like mourning, can also arise "beyond the clear case of a loss by death ... and include those situations of being slighted, neglected, or disappointed" (p. 251). Crimp (1989) suggests that for men who had been sexually active prior to the onset of AIDS safer sex was embraced less in defiance and more in resignation, making these men's emotional reactions less like mourning and more like Freud's definition of melancholia. He was also careful to suggest that there was nothing pathological about this melancholia. Crimp (1989) notes, "In Freud's analysis, melancholia differs from mourning in a single feature: a fall in self-esteem" (p. 12). It was an exceptional gay man who during the height of the AIDS epidemic did not in the midst of his overall bewilderment and trauma experience some loss of self-esteem. Gay men who experienced a resurgence of internalized homophobia or erotophobia in reaction to AIDS certainly suffered an assault on their self-esteem, one aspect of which is an increase in shame about who they are or what they do, once did, or desire to do. Freud (1917) states that an individual experiencing melancholia suffers from "a delusion of (mainly moral) inferiority" (p. 246). The lowered self-esteem corresponding to the internalized homophobia that was kindled for many gay men in the early days and the height of the AIDS epidemic almost always related to shame either at being gay or for past sexual behaviors, ambivalence about being gay, and/or their sexual history and a questioning of the morality of their sexual orientation and sexual history.

Questioning one's inherent moral goodness and the morality of how one had lived one's life was powerful and potentially depressing, if not emotionally devastating for the men who succumbed to these thoughts. Gay-affirmative therapists were important harbors for men to work through these intense and complex reactions to the plague. This was by no means an uncomplicated therapeutic task, as some even believed the religious fanatics who preached that gay men deserved AIDS as retribution for immoral sexual behaviors. The 1980s was a period of particularly intense vocal and virulent homophobia and sex-negativity.

MOURNING, GRIEF, AND PSYCHIATRIC DIAGNOSES

It is useful to think about men who bareback with contemporary diagnostic criteria in mind pertaining to mourning and depression. Contemporary psychiatric diagnoses concur with points made by Freud in "Mourning and Melancholia." Regarding bereavement, the *DSM-IV* (1994) notes: "As part of their reaction to the loss, some grieving individuals present with symptoms characteristic of a Major Depressive Episode or Post Traumatic Stress Syndrome" (American Psychiatric Association, 1994, p. 299). The *DSM-IV* also states that the bereaved individual typically regards the depressed mood as normal. It was not uncommon for a gay man during the height of the epidemic to be experiencing what became known as "bereavement overload," overwhelmed by the sheer numbers of people who were dying around him. When the *DSM* states that a diagnosis of major depressive disorder is not given unless the symptoms are present two months after the loss, this often had no relevance to gay men deluged by the numbers of deaths they were experiencing, often in close proximity to one another. With the additional losses related to sex and gay culture factored in, it is no wonder that most gay men who lived in big cities were suffering from some degree of depression during the height of the epidemic. Supporting the position taken by Crimp, DSM states that if an individual is experiencing guilt about things other than actions taken or not taken by the survivor at the time of the death and a morbid preoccupation with worthlessness, then it is not characteristic of "normal" grief. Gay men were often wracked by feelings of worthlessness, guilt, shame, and survivor guilt, associated with the rekindled internalized homophobia discussed earlier. For gay men who survived AIDS, it was essential to hold two things to be simultaneously true. Our sexual revolution helped free many of us from suffocating sexual shame and internalized homophobia and yet it also killed off many members of our tribe.

EROTICIZING SAFER SEX

Safer sex was the life preserver thrown to all who were affected by AIDS, but it did not always seem to float quite right. Therapists working in the gay community were attempting to intervene both behaviorally as well as intrapsychically on specific ways of eroticizing safer sex. But this was always an uphill battle. They wanted to take something previously less enjoyable (using condoms) and make it more enjoyable. This was obviously a daunting task. The bigger question was and remains how to take away the appeal of something enjoyable? Will fear of the consequences of UAI always work as a deterrent? Clearly, the answer is it will not work indefinitely but works in the short run. Those involved in AIDS prevention efforts recognized that for men who relished anal sex, preventing barebacking and relapse to occasional UAI was not going to be easy.

Perhaps it was naive to believe that psychotherapy could help stem the tide of new HIV infections. But whenever a gay client talked about sex and his feelings about this central aspect of human life, I seized on it as an opportunity to try to slow the spread of the epidemic. Gay-affirmative therapists scrambled to invent therapeutic approaches that might help change gay men's risk-taking behavior. A colleague of mine, social worker Luis Palacios-Jimenez, and I created a workshop that was conducted under the auspices of community-based AIDS service organizations. It was called "Hot, Horny, and Healthy: Eroticizing Safer Sex (ESS)" (Palacios-Jimenez & Shernoff, 1986). Luis died of AIDS in 1989, but our work hopefully saved other lives.

The workshop was initially developed for the Gay Men's Health Crisis (GMHC) in Manhattan in June 1985. It soon became a center-piece of GMHC's efforts to reach gay men with sex-positive and gay-friendly safer-sex messages. From the mid-1980s until the early 1990s, "Eroticizing Safer Sex" (ESS) was the most widely used AIDS prevention intervention in the world. AIDS service organizations throughout the United States, Canada, England, The Netherlands, Norway, West Germany, Sweden, New Zealand, and Australia all offered the workshop. Luis and I conducted the workshop for more than 15,000 men throughout North America. Because we authored a guide to running the workshop, which was available free of charge through GMHC, people were able to use our outline to customize the workshop to met the needs of their particular communities.

What made our approach unique was that ESS addressed the specific problems of helping gay and bisexual men change their sexual behaviors using a psychosocial and psychoeducational approach that was designed specifically to be a sexual enhancement workshop for gay men — at a time when fear of sex changed their sex lives for the worse. Even during the height of the epidemic, not every gay man used a condom every time he had anal intercourse. Unprotected anal intercourse is still the primary sexual route of transmitting HIV, but instead of being scolding or fear-based, the workshop was generally upbeat and fun. Recognizing how important the exchange of semen was for many men, we consciously began to publicize the concept of "on me, not in me" sex. Inadvertently, since the workshop predated Crimp's 1989 essay, ESS addressed the concerns raised by Crimp when in a large-group setting we asked the men to share what aspects of pre-AIDS sexuality they missed. This was always raucous as well as melancholy. The fact that we stressed that these were real and important losses that needed to be acknowledged and mourned created an important foundation of trust for the men who attended these workshops.

When Luis and I designed ESS, we did not know at the time that the kinds of changes we were encouraging gay men to make in their sex lives would need to be lifelong and multigenerational. Naively, we thought that this was a temporary intervention to help reduce the trauma that AIDS was reaping upon the psyches and erotic desires of gay men until some medical breakthrough occurred that would allow things to return to the way they had been. Perhaps not surprisingly, AIDS prevention workers and mental health professionals like myself who worked so hard to help gay men discover ways to safely enjoy themselves sexually feel somewhat discouraged by the increase in rates of HIV among men who have sex with men (MSM), while at the same time understanding and empathizing with the powerful draw not to always use condoms.

Many of the goals of the workshop were also relevant as therapeutic goals for gay men wrestling with their responses to this new, sexually transmitted, lethal epidemic sweeping through their community. They included:

- Providing individuals with a safe, structured, and supportive environment where they could explore and discuss emotionally laden material about AIDS and sex.
- Helping gay and bisexual men identify negative affective responses induced by the AIDS crisis in relation to their sexuality and sex lives.
- Helping people work through these negative feelings to minimize any impairment in their psychosocial/psychosexual functioning.
- Helping gay and bisexual men change from high-risk to low-risk sexual behavior.
- Helping individuals view many of their reactions to the AIDS health crisis as appropriate responses requiring new crisis management skills.
- Helping men improve levels of sexual health and functioning.
- Encouraging gay men to gain practice in negotiating and contracting around safer sex.
- Increasing individuals' sense of hopefulness regarding their ability to manage the necessary lifestyle changes brought on by the AIDS health crisis.

As mentioned above, as AIDS spread, it became apparent that therapists had to start incorporating questions about HIV and sex into their clinical work. The specific large-group interventions we developed for ESS were easily transposed into questions that could be asked by therapists in either individual or group therapy sessions. Thus the following questions used during the workshop also began to become incorporated into clinical conversations between gay men and their therapists:

- How did you feel when you first heard that you might have to change your sexual pattern in order not to contract HIV?
- How did you feel about the fact that HIV is sexually transmitted?
- When you think about "safer sex," what thoughts and feelings do you have?
- What do you miss about sex?

Even today, many of these questions are relevant for therapists to inquire about in their work with gay men who are taking sexual risks. The process of inviting them to reflect on their behaviors and the feelings associated with these behaviors as well as the desires that inspire the behaviors is still at the heart of clinical work. Yet many clients were not comfortable discussing sex in their therapy and sometimes felt intruded on or angered by such discussions. Often, by initiating frank discussions about AIDS, the therapist was able to confront the client's denial that AIDS could touch him. When this line of questioning elicited anger from the client, it sometimes reflected transference issues that stemmed from the client's perception of the question as a negative parental injunction. Other times clients welcomed this kind of intervention on the part of the therapist, and it was met with acceptance and insight. Yet, both in the early days of the epidemic as well as today, exploring such negative feelings provides a fertile ground for discussions of sex and sexuality as well as of forbidden desires, self-care, self-image, and the consequences of impulsive behavior. After these issues have been broached, clients often express relief that these highly charged issues can finally be discussed openly with the therapist. In the early days of the AIDS epidemic, psychotherapeutic treatment often benefited from eliciting clients' feelings about the sexual behavior changes they needed to make. Having a professional inquire about the specific behaviors clients missed and validating any feelings of sadness, anger, and mourning related to behaviors and a lifestyle no longer available in the same carefree manner were very useful aspects of working therapeutically with gay male patients.

DECONSTRUCTING SHAME

Gay-affirmative therapy has continued to evolve and has become a richer and more complex discipline, although the core aspect has not changed: to help gay and bisexual men to honestly examine their lives; to feel good about themselves, their sexual desires, and how these desires are expressed; and to become as highly functioning as possible. A positive self-image with regard to homosexuality is a foundation upon which gay men build the healthy self-esteem that is central to the development of a well-integrated personality (Weinberg & Williams, 1984). Difficulties with establishing and maintaining such a positive self-image in an essentially homophobic culture certainly predate the special pressures of this epidemic. But while enhancing self-esteem is clearly essential in gay-affirmative therapy, it is particularly relevant with gay clients who bareback and who may or may not feel bad about themselves for doing it. Odets (1994) believes that poor self-esteem supports unsafe sexual activity. As psychologist and researcher Alex Carballo-Dieguez (personal communication, August 9, 2004) notes, "The correlation between high self-esteem and avoiding high-risk sex is one of those things that seems commonsensical and that every researcher tries to test. But I think that few have found a clear and verifiable correlation."

A conflicted or shame-based attitude toward one's own sexuality may be a poor starting point for taking precautions not to be infected or to infect others. People with negative attitudes toward themselves and others like themselves do not usually take good care of themselves and do not usually express caring for people with whom they interact. Low self-esteem, anxiety, and insecurity make it easy for a person to do something that might be regretted afterward. Bad feelings about oneself, whether they are based on one's sexuality or some other aspect of a person's life, are therefore an obstacle to the battle against the spread of HIV. This is another reason it is so important to create the best possible conditions for self-respect and social integration in AIDS prevention efforts. Yet, as the following chapters will illustrate, it is not only gay men with poor or low self-esteem who are no longer using condoms for anal sex. One challenge for therapists is not to prejudge a man who reports barebacking by jumping to conclusions that he is damaged or self-destructive. After careful evaluation, the therapist might or might not determine that these dynamics are present in individuals who bareback. Yet, as will be illustrated in the chapters that follow, for many gay men, barebacking is self-actualizing and represents an attempt to take care of deep and often essential needs they have.

Making good choices requires a sense of self-respect and personal agency. But as the following chapter will investigate, some men who bareback do not suffer from a lack of self-respect or self-esteem. Any sexual act involving more than one person is an interpersonal communication, whether or not words are exchanged. Seen in this way, sexual behavior is just one of the many ways people communicate with one another. The one-night stand is as respectable as lovemaking within a long-term relationship, and the first date as important as a first meeting in a nonsexual friendship. The freedom to have sex also includes the right not to have sex and the freedom to chose the form of sexual activity. It is imperative that all therapists communicate a respect for the spectrum of ways that sexual and affectional needs are expressed within the extremely diverse gay men's community. As Tim Dean writes, "Thinking about AIDS psychoanalytically doesn't involve conceptualizing unsafe sex in individual rather than social terms, or treating the social on the model of the individual, as some critics charge. Instead it requires us to acknowledge that social relations cannot be grasped without taking psychic processes into account and vice versa" (p. 142). Good gay-affirmative psychotherapy is essential for helping barebackers distinguish between what is psychically dangerous to them from what is physically dangerous. This is "a difficult distinction to maintain when one is engaged in an encounter that is, after all, always physical, whatever else it may be" (Dean, 2000, p. 162).

THE LIMITS OF THERAPY

It is naive to assume that psychotherapy, even with the most sophisticated gay-affirmative therapist, could or even should prevent barebacking. Most mental health professionals today recognize that most people's problems as well as potential resolutions are part of a larger interpersonal and social context. Whether it is using the conceptual framework of "systems theory" (Bateson, 1972), or the more modern concept of an environmental or ecological approach developed by social workers Carol Germaine (1978, 1980, 1981) and Alex Gitterman (1976), this perspective is a useful one for approaching clinical work with men who bareback. Germaine and Gitterman describe social work practice as understanding and intervening on both the ecological or environmental level as well as with the individual client, and his or her immediate system. Germaine (1980) explains that "ecology seeks to understand the transactions that take place between environments and living systems and the consequence of these transactions for each." She believes an ecological perspective is a useful lens through which to examine the social context of clinical work. It is also especially useful in trying to sort through the complexities of gay men who bareback, because we can view barebacking — which always involves more than one person — both as an intrapsychic and an interpersonal behavior. Ecological thinking has at its core the belief that a complex web of interdependence links each of us to another and to our environment. Precisely by developing the concept of "sexual ecology" to discuss how HIV was able to emerge within the gay men's community and the impact that continued unsafe sex has upon the community are we able to understand barebacking symbolically in terms of the web of intrapsychic and interpersonal relations that mediate any sex act. As Tim Dean (2000) writes: "To put it slightly differently, ecological thinking consists in grasping the radical limits of individual autonomy, since the ways in which a largely invisible network enmeshes all social inhabitants means that changes in one part of this vast web of interrelationships necessarily affect others" (p. 155). This point seems to speak directly to those barebackers who feel that their individual freedom and autonomy are paramount each time they choose not to use a condom.

BAREBACKING: AN ECOLOGICAL PERSPECTIVE

In his 1997 book *Sexual Ecology,* Gabriel Rotello specifically discusses gay men's sexual culture and barebacking from a systems or ecological perspective. Rotello posits that the problem with barebacking is not only that gay men who bareback fail to act individually in their own interests, but also that they fail to act collectively in the interests of gay men as a group. What Rotello is saying is that in addition to a specific act of sex without a condom potentially spreading HIV to a previously uninfected person, each act of condomless sex also helps break down community norms supporting condom use.

The usefulness of using an ecological or systems lens to approach questions about barebacking is supported by research. Studies both in the United States (Joseph et al., 1987) and in Norway (Prieur, 1990) demonstrate that having "social resources" is one of the most influential factors in practicing safer sex for gay or bisexual men who already are well informed of the risk of semen exchange and the dangers of unprotected anal sex. These social resources include accepting one's sexual identity and leading a stable life with friends. Another way of putting this is that creating one's own family, and including other gay people in it, is an essential part of having the emotional and social resources necessary to buttress one during times of adversity. This "created family" or "family of choice" may or may not include being part of a committed partnership with one or more people bound together romantically. For gay men without close emotional ties to other people, an active sex life may be the only means of experiencing closeness to others (Prieur, 1990). Therefore, one goal of gay-affirmative therapy is to help encourage gay men to create or strengthen their ties to a community of men. Many gay men who bareback report that it is precisely their desire to feel more connected to a community and foster a sense of community that leads them to take sexual risks.

Thinking ecologically is useful for keeping in mind how the issues of mourning and melancholia have come together for individual gay men and for the broader gay community for approximately the past 20 years. How these factors converge with the natural desire for unrestrained sex that has been a central aspect of gay men's culture and community is important when thinking about the rise in barebacking. Patrick Moore's book *Beyond Shame* (2004) offers extensive discussion of why helping men work through their shame is essential to enhancing their self-esteem and changing community norms, which of course is an ecological approach to preventing new cases of AIDS.

I agree with Crimp when he says that we should not minimize the centrality of freely being able to express one's sexual desires and that the strains of not being able to do so takes a profound toll on both individual and communal psyches. I have come to believe that for many who engage in it, barebacking is an understandable reaction to the decades of sadness and mourning, as well as an attempt to create a life-affirming act in an attempt to repudiate shame, the invasiveness of too many deaths, and additional AIDS-related losses. It might be fair to view barebacking as an overcompensation against the horrors and inhibitions imposed by AIDS. For some gay men, barebacking is symptomatic of a compulsive sexuality that they are unable to control. Others find that barebacking is an attempt to recreate the kind of social network that was created out of connecting sexually with other gay men. It is essential to remember that all gay men living under the cloud of AIDS are also members of an oppressed minority with the ever-present specter of homophobia.

Yet a study of 460 gay men in Australia showed that gay men, regardless of HIV status, who had chronic, low-grade symptoms of depression without a current major depression were significantly more likely to report unprotected sex with a casual partner than were men without any symptoms of depression or men who had a major depression (Rogers et al., 2003). The authors comment, "It is not difficult to understand that gay men who have been stigmatized for much of their lives, and who have lived though the devastation of their community by HIV, may sometimes find themselves in a psychological state where they just don't care about protecting themselves or others." They add that "dysthymic disorder may be the diagnostic representation of such a mental state and since the condition is potentially treatable, it warrants careful consideration in the prevention of HIV at individual and population levels" (Rogers et al., 2003, p. 273). The combination of systemic and internalized homophobia and surviving in the age of AIDS creates a powerful nexus that results in many gay men engaging in behaviors that are symptomatic of an attempt to ameliorate their pain and distress. These behaviors include rates of substance abuse higher than the general population (Morales & Graves, 1983; Stall & Wiley, 1988; McKirnan & Peterson, 1989; Cabaj, 1992), isolation, difficulty in achieving and sustaining intimacy, and for some, barebacking.

Ron Stall is a leading AIDS researcher who was formerly the director of the CDC's Prevention Research Branch at the National Center for HIV, STD, and TB Prevention. Speaking about gay men taking sexual risks, Stall identified four significant epidemics co-occurring in the gay men's communities, which are all interacting, making one another worse, and which influence gay men's willingness to take sexual risks. These are depression, partner violence, substance abuse, and HIV. Stall refers to this phenomenon as "syndemics," a syndrome of interacting epidemics. Speaking of the nearly three thousand men in one study, he said: "The higher the number of the epidemics that any particular man experienced, the more likely he was to have risky sex and to test positive for HIV" (quoted in Specter, 2005, p. 44).

As Patrick Moore (2004) reminds us, sexual liberation did not cause the AIDS epidemic but may be the only way to stop it because the only way to fight shame is to return to an earlier vision of sex as liberation and joy. In response to Moore's vision, Bronski feels that "it is imperative to remember that this is not a sentimental project of memorializing how good the old days were, but rather the first step in creating a new culture — not only in the face of the devastation of AIDS, but as a way to combat it" (p. xx). Yet for gay men who are exploring barebacking and talking about it in psychotherapy, it is especially urgent that the therapist with whom they are doing this self-examination be gay affirmative, sex positive, and conversant with the impact of homophobia on gay men's psyches so as not to inadvertently add to or minimize any shame the person may already be experiencing about this proscribed behavior. In the next chapters, we look at what social scientists have uncovered in researching why gay men are having sex without condoms.

CHAPTER THREE

Why Do Men Bareback?
No Easy Answers

"The terrible thing in this world is that everyone has his reasons"

Octave in *The Rules of the Game*, Jean Renoir, 1939.

TOBY, A PASSIVE BAREBACKER

Toby is a white, 35-year-old, HIV-negative gay man who came to see me because of depression and loneliness. A successful and ambitious architect, he worked exceptionally long hours to make partner in his firm. His last relationship ended during his final year of graduate school, after two years, and he had not had another partner in almost 10 years. Because of his intense focus on work, Toby had not taken the time to cultivate deep friendships. He did have a group of people with whom he would go to clubs to dance a few times a month. Typically, during those outings, he would take MDMA (Ecstasy) and smoke marijuana. He said it helped him lose his inhibitions and cut loose on the dance floor. At the end of the night he would usually end up going home with someone he had just met.

Toby did not seek out barebacking, but he allowed it to happen if the other man wanted to do it. He said he never discussed HIV status with the men he went home with unless the other man initiated the discussion. If a sexual partner initiated the use of condoms for anal sex, Toby said he felt relieved and gladly used them. But if the other man did not bring up the topic, Toby wound up going along with whatever the other man wanted to do sexually, even if it meant having unprotected anal intercourse (UAI). Toby almost never made a date to see any of these men a second time. Toby was sexually versatile but preferred to be the top.

On the weekends when Toby stayed home, he either met men in online chat rooms for sexual hookups or went to sex parties. Again, his attitude toward condom use was passive. If the other man wanted to use them, that was fine with him. But if the other fellow never brought up the topic of condoms, neither did Toby. It was clear that he was well informed about HIV transmission and about the risk he took of becoming infected by barebacking. When I explored this passivity toward using condoms, he explained that he worked such long hours and so intensely that when he did have time off it was essential that he be able to stop thinking and just go a bit wild and lose control. Ostrow and Shelby (2000) describe psychotherapy with men like Toby who use drugs to enable them to lose inhibitions and engage in fantasy sex that they might otherwise have difficulty engaging in without guilt or remorse.

Toby was an only child raised in the Midwest by a devout Baptist single mother who had been deserted by Toby's father shortly after Toby's birth. Toby came out to his mother after he finished graduate school and moved to New York. She did not react well to the news, retreating into the condemning language of her church. She told her son that being a homosexual was going to land him in hell unless he repented and changed his ways. She also told him that he was going to get AIDS because he was gay. Toby sounded bleak when he described the Christian literature she regularly sent him about the evils of homosexuality and how gays were being plagued by AIDS as punishment from God.

I asked Toby what he thought about his mother's views of his sexuality. He said he was frightened — what if what she said was true? — and sad that their relationship has become so combative. He said she was relentless about sharing her views on Toby's "sinful affliction," even after Toby asked her not to raise this subject every time they spoke. I was surprised to hear that he continued to speak with her once a week and to visit with her for a week at Christmas. We explored his conflicted feelings about his relationship with his mother. On the one hand, he recognized that the way his mother treats him was damaging to his self-esteem and was deeply painful. On the other hand, as the only child whom she struggled to raise, he felt a strong sense of loyalty and obligation to her.

I shared with Toby my concern that his barebacking activity was putting him at risk for fulfilling his mother's prophecy that he would get AIDS. He said he worried about it at times, and he had no conscious desire to contract HIV, but he was not willing to kill (his exact expression) the spontaneity of his recreational sexual exploits. In the rest of his life, he was responsible and reliable. In this one area of his life, he wanted to be totally free. I wondered if Toby's behavior was an unconscious desire either to prove his mother right or to get sick and die as a hostile "fuck you" to his mother. I did not begin to share any of these possibilities with Toby until many months after our initial consultation. Every few months Toby would get retested for HIV, and as of this writing he remains HIV-negative.

Fifteen or twenty years ago, I would have been appalled and quite judgmental about Toby's behavior and probably gone into overdrive to try to save Toby from his own impulses. With the advantage of 20/20 hindsight, it is now clear that the rescue approach to treating men who bareback is rarely, if ever, effective. Most of the time, these clients just stopped therapy with me. They did not want or need a rescuer, as well-intentioned as I was. Although it still hurt to hear Toby describe the potentially deadly risks he was taking, I had to practice patience, compassion, and empathy. He was the only one who could take himself out of these high-risk situations, and then only if and when he decided that he wanted to.

Along with my protective feelings for this young man, I felt clinical curiosity about what was driving Toby to take sexual risks with such an apparently casual attitude. Researchers have been eager to find out more about the category of barebackers that Toby falls into — men who are not trying, at least consciously, to become infected with HIV, but who are willing to take risks in order to satisfy deep intrapsychic and interpersonal needs.

RATIONALES FOR BAREBACKING: CHAPTER OVERVIEW

This chapter asks a lot of tough questions: Is barebacking pathological? Is it correlated to personality disorder? Is it all about sex, sensation-seeking, and pleasure? Or is it, as paradoxical as this may seem, actually an attempt to take care of oneself and to forge a deeper intimacy, closeness, and even spiritual communion? We will look at how current antiretroviral therapies may affect decisions to have unprotected sex, and how fear and lack of fear about the danger of HIV infection play into the decision to bareback. The question of whether sex without condoms in the age of AIDS can ever be a rational decision will be explored. As the title of this chapter promises, there are no easy answers to why men have sex without condoms.

This chapter offers multiple meanings that men who have sex without condoms themselves attribute to the behavior. The more we can understand the underlying motivations of unprotected and unsafe sex, the better we can have effective community conversations about how to prevent the spread of HIV and other sexually transmitted diseases (STDs). Lest we forget the potential serious consequences of having sex without condoms, I include the latest information about the health risks of condomless sex, discussing the relative safety of HIV-positive men who bareback with other infected men.

WHY MEN ARE TAKING SEXUAL RISKS

There are abundant theories but no definitive answers about why gay men take sexual risks. After more than three decades of safer-sex messages against the backdrop of gay men sickening horribly and then dying, new medical treatments have stemmed the tide of the pandemic and offered real hope for longer-term survival to people with HIV. Gay men want the AIDS epidemic to be over and want to be able to have sex without fear. They want to celebrate their desire without having to worry, negotiate, be fearful, or keep a shield of latex between themselves and their partners. Younger men want to experience pre-AIDS sex. Queer theorist Tim Dean (2000) writes: "In view of statistics on new seroconversions, some AIDS educators have begun to acknowledge that, unlikely though it may seem, remaining HIV-negative in fact poses significant psychological challenges to gay men" (p. 137). To those who have not been working in the gay men's community for the past 25 years, this statement might seem absurd, but it is true that HIV-negative gay men face unique challenges that make it seem almost easier to seroconvert.

San Francisco Bay area psychologist Walt Odets (1995) was one of the first mental health professionals to question why gay men who had thus far escaped becoming infected with HIV were placing themselves at risk for becoming so. Odets described HIV-negative men who struggled in a world and gay community that, however unintentionally, considered their difficulties inconsequential as compared to those of men who were fighting for their lives. These uninfected men's growing invisibility triggered old childhood feelings of being an outsider, and for some, contributed to an acute psychological crisis that often created a confluence of behaviors and thought patterns that placed them at risk for contracting HIV.

Some have suggested that during the 1980s, gay men unconsciously colluded with the general public's equation of a gay identity with an AIDS identity (Odets, 1995; Rofes, 1996). New York social worker Steve Ball (1998) describes how during the height of the AIDS epidemic HIV-negative gay men often found themselves in the role of caregiver, mourner/widower, or outsider, due to their not being infected with HIV. Some of these men felt that they were not entitled to express their deep fears that they might become infected or discuss their loneliness or burnout when so many peers were dying around them. The dynamics described by Odets and Ball are part of the communal and psychosocial realities that early in the epidemic played a role in contributing to the spread of HIV.

In 1988, I wrote about how fear was one large component of what propelled gay men to change how they were having sex (Shernoff & Jimenez, 1988). Should we conclude that safer-sex campaigns have lost their effectiveness today because gay men are no longer afraid? Gay men who were recently surveyed about their failure to use condoms during anal sex repeatedly told researchers that current AIDS prevention messages do not feel relevant to them and do not convey an urgency about why condom use is important (Halkitis, Parsons, & Wilton, 2003; Carballo-Dieguez & Lin, 2003; Morin et al., 2003). For many younger gay men and for newly sexually active gay men, AIDS is associated with the past (Van de Ven, Prestage, Knox, & Kippax, 2000). In the last 20 years, the roar and urgency of HIV prevention campaigns have faded.

British psychologist and researcher Michelle Crossley (2001, 2002) writes that one factor might be a decrease in the effectiveness of the "health promotion" campaign to change gay men's sexual behavior. Gay men who come out today are raised with AIDS awareness and come out to a chorus of safer-sex messages. But Crossley notes that most "health promotion" campaigns — for example, convincing people to stop smoking and lose weight — have only limited long-term success. She wonders if the "safer-sex" messages ever had much effect on gay male sexual behavior. Crossley raises an interesting question that is difficult to quantify. Obviously, there was a confluence of factors in the early days of the epidemic — most prominently fear, the horrors of sickness, and grief of deaths — and these things made safer-sex AIDS education programs more compelling to the target audience. Crossley suggests that it is impossible to evaluate the efficacy of safer-sex messages in and of themselves since concurrent to when they first began appearing, gay men were overwhelmed by the terror that they might be infected by the then-new disease that was rapidly killing their friends and lovers. Though highly unscientific, comments shared with me by men who attended the safer-sex programs I ran in the 1980s reported that they felt that these interventions proved helpful to them for changing how they had sex in response to AIDS. The men who spoke or wrote to me after attending the workshop often described an enormous relief. They spoke of how important and useful it was for them to simply be in a room with other gay men sharing feelings about how sex needed to change. They also appreciated the permission that was given during these workshops to remain sexually active, albeit with some big differences from what they were used to. They reported being thrilled to be able to participate in a process that helped them reclaim the joy and fun of gay sex amidst all of the sex-negativity and sex-equaling-death messages that were inundating them. Thus, participating in this AIDS prevention workshop helped scores of men feel confident of their ability to make the necessary sexual changes and sustain them.

FACTORS THAT LEAD TO SEXUAL RISK-TAKING

There are numerous theories for why gay men engage in unprotected sex, and research has explored a wide variety of possible rationales for the behavior. These include:

- Negative attitudes toward condom use (Odets, 1994; Flowers, Smith, Sheeran, & Beail, 1997; Hays, Kegeles, & Coates, 1997; Kelly & Kalichman, 1998; Van de Ven et al., 1998ab; Appleby, Miller, & Rothspan, 1999).
- How being in a committed compared to a noncommitted couple relationship affects whether a condom is used (Elford, Bolding, McGuire, & Sher, 2001; Vincke, Bolton, & DeVleeschouwer, 2001).
- Strongly identifying with or feeling alienated from the gay community (Hospers & Kok, 1995; Hays et al., 1997; Seal et al., 2000).
- Internalized homophobia (Meyer & Dean, 1998; Canin, Dolcini, & Adler, 1999).
- A sense of the inevitability of becoming infected with HIV as a gay man (Kelly et al., 1990; Kalichman, Kelly, & Rompa, 1997).
- The effects of substance use (Stall, McKusick, Wiley, Coates, & Ostrow, 1986; Stall, Paul, Barrett, Crosby, & Bein, 1991; Leigh & Stall, 1993; Stall & Leigh, 1994; Hospers & Kok, 1995; Woody et al., 1999; Royce, Sena, Cates, & Cohen, 1997; Chesney, Barrett, & Stall, 1998; Ostrow & Shelby, 2000; Halkitis, Parsons, & Stirratt, 2001; Halkitis et al., 2003; Halkitis & Parsons, 2002; Kalichman & Weinhardt, 2001).

There are probably a multitude of other issues at play as well. As psychologist and former researcher at the Centers for Disease Control (CDC), Ron Stall was quoted as saying, in an article in the Manhattan gay newspaper *Gay City News,* "There are studies that demonstrate a variety of psychosocial health issues, including depression, antigay violence, childhood sexual abuse, or substance abuse, can lead gay men to have unsafe sex" (Stall, quoted in Osborne, 2002, p. 1). In my own practice, I have identified several factors that appear to lead to sexual risk-taking: loneliness, being HIV-positive, having unmet intimacy needs, feeling alienated from the gay community, being in love, and a craving for deeper intimacy and trust.

In San Francisco, Morin and colleagues (2003) identified a number of issues that contributed to the decisions gay men make to bareback. These include (p. 356):

- Younger men often deny HIV risk altogether.
- Gay men think it is inevitable that they will become infected with HIV.
- Impulsive sexual behavior impedes the ability or desire to use condoms.

"Commodification" of HIV or the perception, particularly among low-income men, that becoming HIV-positive will entail certain financial and social benefits, occurs. Isolation and loneliness among gay men lead to poor self-esteem and taking risks in an attempt to connect to others sexually. Social power imbalances related to race and class impede equitable sexual negotiations. Drug use among gay men interferes with the ability and desire to practice safer sex.

While a wide spectrum of rationales for barebacking exists, subtle distinctions must be made around the context of the behavior. As Suarez and Miller (2001) write, "The motivation for engaging in UAI with casual and anonymous partners may differ significantly from the motivation for engaging in UAI with regular partners. Whereas UAI between primary partners is heavily influenced by desires to express intimacy, trust, and love, the same behavior between casual/anonymous partners is most probably not affected equally by these same influences" (p. 288). In Toby's case, his barebacking was not related to a desire to feel closer to a beloved partner but rather his desire to connect sexually and socially with other gay men and to feel uninhibited and free. Toby did exhibit symptoms of an ongoing low-grade depression but otherwise presented as an emotionally stable adult but one who was wrestling with unexamined drug dependency issues.

RATIONAL AND IRRATIONAL BAREBACKING

Two researchers at UCLA developed a model of sexual decision making to assess rationales of adults who have unprotected sex. Pinkerton and Abramson (1992) found that "for certain individuals, under certain circumstances, risky sexual behavior may indeed be rational, in the sense that the perceived physical, emotional, and psychological benefits of sex outweigh the threat of acquiring HIV" (p. 561). This seems to be precisely Toby's relationship to barebacking: the benefits gained — shaking off the constraints of a very buttoned-up work life and having satisfying sexual experiences that also fulfilled social and emotional needs — outweighed the potential risk of becoming HIV-positive. These researchers state that they do not mean to imply "that risky behavior is rational in any *objective* sense — only that, given certain sets of values and perceptions, engaging in unsafe behaviors may appear to the individual to be a reasonable gamble" (p. 561). They also stress that what is rational is a highly subjective matter.

Pinkerton and Abramson describe three factors that influence an individual's subjective assessment of the relative risks of various sexual behaviors:

- Fear of AIDS
- Perceived risk
- Sexual fulfillment

In order for an individual to behave rationally while barebacking, his fear of AIDS needs to be relatively small in comparison to the satisfaction derived through unprotected sex. This was exactly how Toby reported feeling early on in therapy. Yet as our work progressed, he began to express a profound ambivalence about becoming infected. Part of him wanted to stay uninfected, and yet part of him felt unsure of whether he would be willing and able to experience what to him seemed like deprivation of his spontaneity if he were to increase his efforts to keep himself HIV-negative. Pinkerton and Abramson conjecture that for many Americans, "fear of AIDS" may be synonymous with "fear of death by AIDS," and that fear of death is not nearly so great as might otherwise be supposed. "Fear of AIDS" is mediated by the subjective probability of perceived risk. Perceived risk is explained as containing three related components: the threat of exposure to HIV, the probability of exposure leading to HIV infection, and the likelihood of AIDS developing from HIV exposure (Pinkerton & Abramson, 1992). Even when gay men possess a sophisticated understanding of how HIV is transmitted and accurate perceptions of how dangerous risky sex can be, many gay men underestimate their vulnerability to HIV infection (McKusick, Horstman, & Coates, 1985; Bauman & Siegel, 1987; Richard et al., 1988).

Grov (2003) also discusses a category of barebackers that he labels irrational risk-takers. "Individuals in this category typically deny their own risk or use nonscientific/irrational information when engaging in barebacking" (p. 333). Suarez and Miller (2001) feel that many gay youth who bareback fall into the category of irrational risk-takers since they may have never known anyone with HIV and hold pessimistic attitudes about the future largely related to their being gay. Suarez and Miller feel that this combination often leads to young gay men (especially young gay men of color) taking sexual risks.

Pinkerton and Abramson offer possible explanations for the tendency to underestimate the personal risk associated with risky sex, even among "high-risk" gay men. First, they cite a study showing that no one sees himself as the "type of person who gets AIDS" (Madake-Tyndall, 1991). They also suggest that the "I'm not the type" fallacy is often extended to sexual partners. As they note, "Thus, the frightening picture that emerges is one in which it is only the other guy who gets AIDS. To the average gay man, it's those gay men who are overly promiscuous; and to the bathhouse participants, it's those who aren't careful" (Pinkerton & Abramson, pp. 564–565). They also discuss that results from cognitive psychology indicate that in general people tend to view themselves as "luckier" than the norm, and that this extends to the belief that they will not be the one to get AIDS.

BAREBACKING AS AN EXAMPLE OF "SENSATION-SEEKING"

Again and again, we return to the poignant question of why a person would put his life in jeopardy for pleasure. Sex is a source of pleasure that encompasses biological, psychological, and sociological realities (Reiss, 1989). Sex is not only about pleasure. It can be about belonging, feeling desired, desiring semen, organizing one's life, and providing meanings to one's life. "People have sexual relations for a variety of reasons: for love and intimacy, for recreation, for fun, for friendship, for money, to avoid loneliness, to be touched. The essence of sexual encounters is bonding, blending, mutual pleasure, and loss of inhibition. HIV lurking in the background places strict boundaries on all of these aspects of sexuality" (Coates, 2005, p. xiv). The equation for evaluating how the benefits of barebacking weigh against the inherent risks is not simple. Tim Dean (2000) writes: "Most people can't comprehend why anyone would risk death for a good fuck. From a certain viewpoint, unsafe sex appears as inconceivably self-destructive behavior. Indeed, while such health-threatening practices as smoking, drinking, and drug abuse must be indulged in repeatedly over a substantial period before they are likely to cause harm, HIV infection can result from a single unprotected encounter. Casual, anonymous sex without a condom seems suicidal" (p. 139). But the long-term effects of HIV infection on health are easily denied when faced with the immediacy of sexual pleasure, particularly if one is using drugs that fog one's judgment.

One lens through which decisions to bareback need to be viewed is the role of pleasure and how the search for erotic pleasure is intimately related to desire. For one thing, sex without condoms feels much better and is vastly more spontaneous than having to stop the action, unwrap a condom, and properly put one on. Many gay men are articulate about how thrilling and intimate it is to the feel of the warmth of a lover's unsheathed penis and the smooth stimulation of skin against skin. Carballo-Dieguez interviewed a small sample of men who identify as barebackers. One man told Carballo-Dieguez (2001, p. 229):

> The pleasure I feel when I'm having sex, especially if I'm stoned, is so amazing . . . . Passion does not call for protection in my mind. Passion is a very raw emotion . . . . It is not easy to feel real passion, because there are so many barriers put up and so many acts that people have in themselves that they want to express during sex, that protection does not fit in the fantasy.

Much as we try to eroticize safer sex, there is no way around the fact that condoms both decrease the sensation of anal intercourse and interrupt the spontaneity of the sexual act. Sexual fulfillment "encompasses a range of physical, emotional, and psychological factors including, but not limited to, physical pleasure and release, emotional intimacy and security, enhanced self-esteem, and actualized sexual identity. These are all highly valued, immediate benefits of sexual expression (in contrast to the distant, rather ethereal threat of contracting AIDS)" (Pinkerton & Abramson, 1992, p. 565). As previously discussed, recreational sex has been identified by at least certain segments of the gay male community as a means of personal fulfillment and an expression of enhanced freedom and self-esteem. An active sex life is seen as an indication of attractiveness and vitality. A gay man who wants to feel liberated, hot, or sexy might view sex without condoms as the best route to fulfilling his desire to feel any of those ways.

"Sensation-seeking" is defined as "the seeking of varied, novel, complex, and intense sensations and experiences, and the willingness to take physical, social, legal, and financial risks for the sake of such experiences" (Zuckerman, 1994, p. 27). Zuckerman (1993) finds that sensation-seeking and impulsivity are not the same thing, though they are related. They looked at how sensation-seeking, and an individual's affect and the ways risk affects the ability to become sexually aroused, contribute to why men have unprotected sex. These factors illustrate how intrapsychic and interpersonal issues converge to influence an individual's likelihood of taking sexual risks. For instance, men who are high sensation-seekers may be more likely not to use condoms since they value the intensity of skin-on-skin contact during anal intercourse. In short, one man's need for a higher degree of sensation can result in his initiating sexual risk-taking, taking his intrapsychic need into the interpersonal sphere.

Numerous researchers have studied the connection between sensation-seeking and men who bareback. Pinkerton and Abramson (1995) and Bancroft et al. (2003) provide evidence suggesting that sensation-seeking impacts on sexual risk-taking in two principal ways: by increasing the preparedness to take risks in order to achieve the desired immediate benefits and by influencing how the individual appraises the risk. An individual who is highly sensation-seeking is more likely to downplay the risks associated with a particular behavior if he has previously engaged in the behavior (in this case UAI) without negative consequences, such as becoming infected with HIV. Thus as Pinkerton and Abramson (1995) point out, men who are high sexual sensation-seekers seem not to be unaware of the risks associated with their behavior but choose instead to accept these risks. Some of these men may be in denial about the potential risks to their health. Others may simply compartmentalize the risk and not have it affect their behavior. Yet other men engage in a form of magical thinking — believing that they are invulnerable to infection. There are also men who know and accept the risks and are willing to factor them into the equation as one potential cost to an otherwise important, pleasurable, and valued behavior pattern.

Scragg and Alcorn (2002) and Miller, Lynam, Zimmerman, Logan, and Clayton (2004) find that both extraversion (being highly outgoing with the ability to easily engage other people socially or flirtatiously) and sensation-seeking are related to the desire for a greater number of sexual partners. This seems to make sense since sex with more than one person is inherently a social activity and requires one or more partners (Miller et al., 2004). Schroth (1996) also demonstrated that in a sample of gay men he studied there was a strong correlation between sensation-seeking and high number of sexual activities and high number of partners. Interestingly, this same study did not find any relationship between sensation-seeking and unsafe sexual behavior in the well-educated men among the sample surveyed. This finding is contradicted by empirical observations of the well-educated men I see as psychotherapy patients who bareback and often exhibit characteristics of sensation-seeking.

Hoyle, Fejfar, and Miller (2000) conducted a quantitative review of the empirical literature on "normal" personality and sexual risk-taking in which sexual risk-taking behaviors were defined as numbers of partners, unprotected sex, and high-risk sexual encounters, including sex with a stranger. Their work found that a high level of sensation-seeking predicts all forms of sexual risk-taking covered in their review. There was a consistent, but not strong, positive association between impulsivity and sexual risk-taking, with these authors noting that there was a problem in the inconsistent ways that impulsivity was defined. Seal and Agostinelli (1994) showed that impulsivity was one important factor among men who had UAI.

SEROSORTING

In discussing what they call "rational risk-takers," Suarez and Miller (2001) note that there is a group of men whose sexual behavior is based on "rational" consideration of the risks of specific sexual acts. Among this group are couples who are not sexually exclusive who have negotiated safety[1] agreements, and HIV-negative men who only are the insertive partners during condomless anal sex. Suarez and Miller describe a phenomenon that some men use as part of their "rational" approach to barebacking as "serosorting." Robert, the client I described in Chapter 2, is an example of someone who made his decisions to bareback based on the other man's HIV status as an attempt to mitigate the risks of barebacking. Serosorting relies on men discussing HIV status with potential partners and only engaging in risky behaviors with those who are believed to be of a similar serostatus. A study conducted in the San Francisco Bay area among a multiethnic sample of MSM (Mansergh et al., 2002) found that a majority of the men surveyed who had engaged in UAI in the prior 2 years reported engaging in barebacking with a man of the same HIV status when he was the receptive partner. This is obviously not a foolproof method for reducing one's risk of contracting HIV insofar as disclosure of HIV status is not always truthful or accurate (Cochran & Mays, 1990; Rowatt, Cunningham, & Druen, 1999), and some individuals honestly do not know that they are infected.

Despite the limitations of serosorting, Suarez and Miller (2001) report that many barebackers employ this strategy. As evidence, they point to the plethora of personal ads on Web sites devoted exclusively to barebacking as well as on Web sites where gay men cruise for sex where men state their own HIV status and the desired status of potential partners. Hort (2000) posits that barebacking itself is a serosorting strategy insofar as barebacking is often a way for HIV-positive men to disclose their status and assume that anyone who is willing to have unsafe sex with them is also already infected. But as will be discussed in Chapter 5, this assumption is incorrect. Suarez and Miller note that many barebacking ads are posted by men who claim to be HIV-negative and state explicitly that they will only bareback with other uninfected men.

BAREBACKING TO FEEL IN CONTROL

Whether or not a man is making a rational choice when he decides to bareback is often difficult for others to assess, even psychotherapists who must contend with their own judgments and feelings about this particular highly charged, high-risk behavior. But for barebackers who are neither actively nor passively suicidal, there is an internal logic that makes sense to them, especially when the behavior occurs within specific contexts. For example, one rationalization for engaging in unsafe sex is the belief that having an HIV infection will alleviate their worry about becoming infected. This dynamic was first reported by psychologist Walt Odets (1994), when he described men who felt that they were not destined to survive the epidemic and therefore had no motivation or reason to practice safer sex. Odets writes that many survivors of the epidemic have a sense of the inevitability of their "catching AIDS." One example of this was my client Jeff, a 44-year-old, Jewish, HIV-negative man who enjoyed dancing at New York clubs and going to an occasional circuit party. Since he almost never used condoms but made every effort to limit his sexual partners to other uninfected men he met, he decided to have "HIV–" tattooed on his left arm since he disliked the necessity of asking about HIV status. Immediately after getting himself tattooed he discussed his feeling that it was only a matter of time until he eventually got infected. "When it happens I can just have the vertical bar added to my tattoo so it will accurately read "HIV+," he told me, pleased with his strategy.

At first, his reasoning seemed as slippery as a child telling himself that he might cheat on the test because he was destined to fail, and getting caught would spare him the misery of bringing home an F. This kind of illogical logic is not uncommon, even in adults. In the early 1990s I remember working with Matthew, a 36-year-old, biracial Wall Street professional who came to see me. He was so worried about whether or not he had become infected during a recent weekend-long sexual orgy that it was interfering with his very demanding job. As he described himself, usually he was conservative about sexual risk-taking to the point that his unwillingness to tongue-kiss brought several promising relationships to an end. Yet, there were certain situations in which he engaged in UAI, though only as the insertive partner, feeling that while this was not completely risk-free, it was relatively safe. During our first therapy session, Matthew commented that since he was a sexually active gay man, it was inevitable that he would become infected with HIV. This gave him some inner permission to take sexual risks. "That way, once it happens I will no longer obsess about whether or not I am infected," he explained, slumped and miserable on my couch.

SEMEN EXCHANGE AND EMOTIONAL CONNECTION

Vincke and colleagues (2001) found that "the incorporation of semen is an important value for many in gay cultures, a means of showing devotion, belonging, and oneness. Unsafe sex can therefore be an expression of positive values and of good feelings" (p. 58). There is something deeply erotic, profoundly connecting and, some feel, even sacred about one person giving his most private and special fluid, semen, to the other as a gift of love and a symbolic joining of two souls. The many levels of meaning and special significance that giving and receiving of semen has for gay men cannot be underestimated as a contributing factor to the rise in barebacking — especially in romantic couples, as will be examined in Section 2 of this book. Early in the second decade of the AIDS epidemic Odets wrote, "Now that a decade of prohibition has made semen exchange relatively unusual and 'special,' it has become all the more powerful and meaningful" (Odets, 1994, p. 432). Obviously, what it means to give or receive semen varies from one gay man to another. Some have described drinking semen as literally ingesting the vitality, strength, manliness, or very essence of the man whose semen they either drank or received anally. There are men who feel that sharing their own or receiving the semen of a lover is a visceral as well as symbolic gift of love or a spiritual communion. There are those who revel in experiencing the esthetic and sensual pleasures in giving or receiving semen. By no means is this a comprehensive list. The meaning of sharing semen between two men is as varied as the men who engage in this act.

THE PSYCHOLOGY OF PEER PRESSURE

Since attempts to satisfy sexual desire that go beyond masturbation necessarily involve interacting with one or more people, attempting to categorize an individual's motivations for barebacking as either being predominantly intrapsychic or predominantly interpersonal creates an artificial distinction that grossly oversimplifies the dynamics at play. As Bancroft et al. (2003) point out: "After a period of focusing on education about safer sex, there is now increasing attention being paid to situational and individually oriented factors that may help to explain high-risk behavior" (p. 555). Bay-area psychologist Stephan Morin writes, "The normalization of the term 'barebacking,' combined with media attention and community-level discussion about it, have contributed to the perception that the behavior is widespread in the community, creating a [new] social pressure to conform" (Morin et al., 2003, p. 357).

Recent research finds that men who forego using condoms feel there has been a decrease in social supports for staying safe as well as a shift in community norms toward increased acceptance of unsafe sex. In effect, they feel some peer pressure to bareback (Morin et al., 2003). The shifting winds of the gay sexual culture have a huge impact on members of a minority group that is partially defined by sex and desire. As I pointed out in the previous chapters, accepting, internalizing, and adopting sexual norms are part of most gay men's core identification as gay men. Thus in the immediate aftermath of the onset of AIDS, the community norms for sexual behavior shifted from the anything-goes realities of a pre-AIDS world to adopting safer sex, which allowed many men to remain sexually active. Safer sex and condom use were viewed as core elements of gay pride and as part of the glue that bound the community together. Currently, with the waning of the most obviously horrific aspects of AIDS, the sexual status quo is once again in transition, but this time away from the standard of safer sex, as the pendulum swings back in the direction it had been moving prior to 1982.

Bancroft et al. (2003) studied the impact of sexual arousal and the relationship between mood and sexuality on sexual risk-taking. They found that the patterns of contact, where people met for sex, and how many partners they had was related to whether or not they took sexual risks. Their findings showed evidence that much "cruising" behavior by men in public places that results in public sex is relatively low-risk because the sexual activity is usually limited to mutual masturbation or oral sex.

IS BAREBACKING SYMPTOMATIC OF MENTAL ILLNESS?

In contrast to the researchers above who have shown that for some gay men barebacking is a rational activity, there are social scientists who have tried to determine whether men who bareback have a documented higher level of mental disorders than do men who do not take sexual risks. Gerrard, Gibbons, and McCoy (1993) have shown that affect can influence judgment and decision making. They found that some depressed, anxious, or sad people take greater sexual risks while others who have the identical affect are more sexually conservative. Thus it seems apparent that affect alone is not the determining factor in why some gay men bareback.

Some researchers investigated whether suffering from an anxiety disorder could increase an individual's risk-taking behaviors. Two studies show an association between sexual risk-taking and the use of sex to reduce tension or cope with stress (Folkman, Chesney, Pollack, & Phillips, 1992; McKusick, Hoff, Stall, & Coates, 1991). Yet neither of these studies demonstrated that a correlation existed between the way the participants used sex and a diagnosable mental disorder. Research by Halkitis and Wilton (2005) on the meanings of sex for HIV-positive gay and bisexual men found that of the 250 men interviewed, most discussed the role of sex as a mood stabilizer, stress reducer, and facilitator of intimacy. Though Halkitis and Wilton were only reporting on HIV-positive men, my clinical experience shows that most gay men, no matter their HIV status, would concur. Clearly, some people use sex to anaesthetize themselves to tense or difficult feelings or situations. This seems to speak directly to at least part of the function that sex in general and sex without condoms served for Toby in coping with his everyday sadness, loneliness, and other non-pathological feelings.

One of the most common symptoms of depression is decreased libido, so it is curious that sex drive, paradoxically, seems to increase in some depressed gay men. Psychologist Thomas Coates, who is on the faculty at the David Geffin School of Medicine at UCLA, suggests two possible explanations: "One possibility is that these men seek out sexual partners to alleviate depression. Another is that depression decreases self-esteem, leading these men to engage in sexual behavior that they might otherwise not find acceptable. Rather than driving away a potential sexual partner by trying to negotiate sexual behavior, these individuals may be willing to accept whatever sexual activities the partners want as a way of achieving relief from depression and isolation" (Coates, 2004, p. 6). Coates also points out that there is now research that seeks to explore what the relationship might be between depression, depressive symptoms, and gay men taking sexual risks. He states, "In particular, studies suggest a complex interplay among a variety of factors that interact with depression and the conditions that increase risk or undermine risk reduction" (Coates, 2004, p. 5). Bancroft et al. (2003) note that negative affect could have different effects on sexual risk-taking in different people, with a tendency for negative affect to increase sexual risk-taking in some individuals and to reduce it in others. This is important for mental health professionals to keep in mind when working with gay men who bareback. It is important that they not assume that an individual's depression or anxiety is by itself the significant contributing factor for why he is having UAI, while it very well may be part of the overall equation contributing to why this individual has high-risk sex.

Regarding the connection between sexual arousal and sexual risk-taking, Canin et al. (1999) noted that sexual arousal and the desire for sexual satisfaction impose a sense of urgency that can distort judgment and result in men taking sexual risks. Bancroft et al. (2003) found a correlation between men with erectile difficulties and engaging in UAI. A man who lacks confidence about his erectile ability is likely to be reluctant to use a condom, which would probably aggravate the erectile difficulty. He may, therefore, be more likely to engage in UAI, either as a "top" or a "bottom" (Bancroft et al., 2003). Bancroft's research was conducted prior to the introduction of Viagra in 1998, which is prescribed to treat erectile dysfunction. Thus medical and mental health providers should inquire about the existence of this particular sexual dysfunction in men reporting barebacking, with the intention to refer them for treatment of this problem. If the erectile difficulty is successfully treated, the person may be more willing to use condoms for anal sex.

When sexual risk-taking is examined within the context of diagnosed personality disorders, there is some correlation between men with an Axis II diagnosis[2] and sexual risk-taking. Jacobsberg, Frances, and Perry (1995) reported on the prevalence of personality disorders among gay men seeking an HIV test. The study subjects who tested HIV-negative had a significantly lower rate of personality disorder (20 percent) than did those who tested HIV-positive (37 percent). The presence of the personality disorder was assessed prior to the individual knowing his HIV status, thus suggesting an association between personality disorder and HIV risk. Ellis, Collins, and King (1995) found that gay men who did not use a condom during anal intercourse with casual partners often met criteria that resulted in their receiving a diagnosis of personality disorder. When they examined this finding they discovered that Antisocial Personality Disorder was the main predictor of sexual risk-taking among the homosexually active men they studied.

TO DIAGNOSE OR NOT TO DIAGNOSE?

What is the usefulness of this information for the therapist working with an individual who reports barebacking? Zucker (1996) raises troubling questions about how the traditional diagnostic interview has a heterosexual bias built into it that results in sexual minority individuals being more likely to receive a diagnosis of personality disorder. The terms "impulsivity" and "sensation-seeking," as used in the social science literature, sound value-neutral, but in fact they may not be. They often contain biases that blur the line between spontaneity and impulsivity. Even though a correlation has been shown to exist between high sensation-seekers and impulsivity, this alone does not necessarily mean that all gay men who are high sexual sensation-seekers exhibit characteristics that would deem them diagnosable as having a personality disorder, though obviously some do.

Impulsivity is one important diagnostic criterion of both antisocial personality disorder and borderline personality disorder. Some barebackers are very impulsive individuals, yet this alone, even when combined with the at-risk sexual behavior, is not sufficient to render a diagnosis of Antisocial Personality Disorder in a man who barebacks. On the other hand, for some barebackers this may indeed be an appropriate diagnosis. An important caution is in order when the presence of a gay man's barebacking behavior, high sensation-seeking, or impulsivity might lead a clinician to diagnose the existence of borderline personality disorder. Labeling an individual or pattern of behavior as sensation-seeking also contains explicit judgments about normal behaviors and what levels of risk are acceptable. Important questions are raised, however, about to whom the risk is acceptable and under what circumstances.

The underlying question we have to grapple with is, what risk-taking do we consider acceptable, healthy, and even laudable, and what risk-taking do we consider unhealthy and unacceptable? For instance, I am an experienced scuba diver with more than 30 years of diving experience. One of my passions is to dive among large ocean-going animals and I am thrilled when I sight sharks. This is obvious sensation-seeking behavior and potentially higher risk than a swim at the shore. Yet this pattern of behavior is far from impulsive, as each dive is carefully planned and done under the close supervision of experienced dive guides. Some might perhaps diagnose this passion of mine as pathological since inherent in it is the possibility of a potentially fatal shark attack. I think of it as a fun and exciting recreational activity that provides enormous pleasure and satisfaction that greatly enhances my life. There is an obvious parallel between my choice to scuba dive in places with a high likelihood of close encounters with potentially dangerous sea critters and men taking what for them are calculated sexual risks. Just because a behavior entails risks does not make it *de facto* pathological and self-destructive.

With the mental health professions' long history of diagnosing gay men as psychologically abnormal and disturbed because of their homosexuality, it is important that the simple fact that a man has high-risk sex does not become the sole criterion for him to be diagnosed as exhibiting psychopathology. Does an individual's desire to behave in ways that may be labeled as either impulsive or sensation-seeking now place him at risk for receiving yet another diagnosis that reflects society's intense negativity toward gay male sexuality? This is where astute diagnostic skills and cultural sensitivity to particular realities in the lives of gay men are required in order to not inappropriately pathologize men who are behaving in a manner that the society or clinician is uncomfortable with or sees as inappropriate, without denying the possibility that for some gay men their sexual risk-taking may be part of a constellation of symptoms that justifies a psychiatric diagnosis.

RISKS FROM BAREBACKING

There are a lot of reasons not to bareback. It is probably safe to say that most gay men who bareback are familiar with a majority of the reasons not to do so. Halkitis et al. (2003) point out for HIV-negative men, initial infection with HIV is the most immediate consequence of barebacking. To make matters worse, they risk the potential for this initial infection to be with a medication-resistant/untreatable variety of HIV (Hecht et al., 1998; Wainberg & Friedland, 1998; Boden et al., 1999; Little et al., 1999; Routey et al., 2000; Hicks et al., 2002). The potential of this risk turned real in February 2005, when the New York City Health Department issued a report about a new, rare, and aggressive form of HIV that had been diagnosed in one man, setting off concerns about a new and more menacing kind of HIV infection (Santora & Altman, 2005). The man contracted HIV while using crystal methamphetamine and had sex with multiple partners. This form of the virus was resistant to three of the four classes of antiretroviral drugs used to treat HIV, and the man who had contracted this strain progressed to full-blown AIDS in approximately 3 months.

In a follow-up report in the *New York Times*, some experts noted "that they had seen the rapid progression of HIV to AIDS and high drug resistance before, though not both in combination. They said that the New York case could indicate more about the vulnerability of the infected man's immune system than about the dangers of the virus in his body" (Perez-Pena & Santora, 2005, p. 39). When questioned about the report of this strain of HIV, many leading AIDS researchers and physicians did not express surprise at the emergence of such a strain of HIV. Dr. Thomas Frieden, the New York City health commissioner, said that "more testing was needed before health officials and scientists could be certain about the extent of the threat. But for now, the responsible reaction was to treat it as a real menace and to alert the public" (quoted in Perez-Pena & Santora, p. 39). Experts counseled caution and the need for further research to be done before determining how potentially serious a threat this new form of the virus posed.

For HIV-positive men, barebacking may lead to "superinfection"[3] (Blackard, Cohen, & Mayer, 2002; Jost et al., 2002) and rapid loss of CD4 cells, especially through continual exposure to ejaculate (Wiley et al., 2000). It also puts them at risk for contracting other STDs that may lead to opportunistic infections such as Kaposi's sarcoma (O'Brien et al., 1999; Rezza et al., 1999), coinfection with hepatitis C (Flichman, Cello, Castano, Campos, & Sookoian, 1999; Mendes-Correa, Baronne, & Guastini, 2001), and immune system deterioration (Gibson, Pendo, & Wohlfeiler, 1999; Bonnel, Weatherburn, & Hickson, 2000), (Halkitis et al., 2003, p. 352).

With all of these medical reasons not to bareback, Tim Dean (1996) writes: "How can we successfully combat AIDS without understanding the appeal of sexual self-immolation and the full range of defensive reactions to that appeal?" (p. 75). Is Dean essentially accusing barebackers of seeking to kill themselves? On some level it would appear so. I certainly understand why this would be the reaction of many people, health care and mental health professionals included, to barebacking. Yet, it has not been my experience from working with and knowing many men who bareback that this is the salient operative dynamic.

LOVE, DESIRE, AND RISK

It seems to me that when a person knowingly places himself at risk for contracting HIV, "sexual self-immolation" cannot be the only motivation or appeal. There have to be strong positive forces at work as well. As will be discussed in Chapter 6 and Chapter 7, love and a desire for a greater degree of intimacy and interpersonal connection are often felt to be strong, positive motivations for barebacking. Scott O'Hara, the writer and former porn star already quoted in Chapter 1, gives the following example of how he evaluated the risks and benefits of barebacking even when he had not found out his own HIV status:

"I would say that the risks are commensurate with the rewards. Bareback sex indicates a level of trust, of cohesion, that I don't think is achievable when both partners are primarily concerned with preventing the exchange of bodily fluids" (1997, p. 9).

How the positive rationales for barebacking measure up against the potential risks once again suggests that using an ecological approach that encompasses unconscious, intrapsychic as well as interpersonal factors has the ability to provide a broad and comprehensive way of trying to understand barebacking for each individual who engages in it and is troubled by this behavior. This also demonstrates the difficulties that AIDS prevention workers are up against in attempting to try to design interventions aimed to encouraging gay men to take fewer sexual risks.

Sex is more than actions and positions. Actions contain meanings stemming from relational and cultural values. Use of a condom, for example, may be associated with a negative message because refusing semen may be perceived to be a rejection with far-reaching emotional implications. Vincke and colleagues (2001) note that "considering that people are in search of meaning, sexual acts constitute an emotional and symbolic language. The meanings that gay men assign to specific sexual acts can make behavioral change difficult" (p. 57). They also discuss how the major finding of research into the symbolic meanings of sexual behavior relates to AIDS prevention. All people construct and assign meanings to their sexual behavior according to the particulars of the setting, partner, and relationship. The meaning that is constructed is integral to an individual's calculations as to whether or not a particular action is rational. This brings us back to the theory espoused by Pinkerton and Abramson (1992). In specific circumstances, risky sexual behavior is thought of as rational insofar as the perceived benefits derived from sex outweigh the possible risk of contracting HIV. Vincke and colleagues found that men who take sexual risks perceive sexual techniques in terms of the inherent gratification and the associated dangers with "pleasure and danger being two independent dimensions used to structure the cognitive domain of sex" (p. 68). It is useful for therapists working with barebackers to remember this and to explore with clients how danger and pleasure are kept apart as well as how these two dynamics overlap.

THE VARIOUS MEANINGS OF BAREBACKING

Carballo-Dieguez (2001) found that among men he interviewed who bareback, sex has multiple meanings. For some, sex meant being liked, desired, and needed; finding company in times of boredom; reaffirming one's personal freedom; shedding a stigma; defying the established order; and/or exploring masculinity. In discussing the multiple meanings and implications of sex, Frost (1994) expands upon Carballo-Dieguez's findings, stating, "For many gay men, sexual behavior is a statement of their sense of being gay, an affirmation of their right to be gay, an expression of love, a vehicle through which to achieve intimacy, and a repudiation of the felt prohibition by the greater society. For other gay men sex is a sport, a means of repairing from narcissistic injury" (p. 166). The points raised by both these authors speak directly to feelings that some barebackers have regarding the intrapsychic as well as interpersonal benefits they derive from barebacking.

Many people of all sexual orientations use sex as an attempt to ameliorate psychic pain or social discomfort. Speaking specifically about gay men, Yep, Lovaas, and Pagonis (2002) suggest that for many gay men the interconnection between the sexual and emotional or psychological aspects of their psyches speaks not only to the reality that some gay men use sex as an attempted "panacea" for their problems but also contributes to active resistance to changing risky sexual behavior. One study conducted during the height of the epidemic found that a majority of men surveyed agreed with the statement, "It is hard to change my sexual behavior because being gay means doing what I want sexually" (Aspinwall, Kemeny, Taylor, Schneider, & Dudley, 1991, p. 433). All therapists working with gay men who bareback must spend considerable time exploring the numerous and layered meanings that sex has for each individual and how sex with and without condoms affects the ability of various sexual opportunities and situations to meet these needs. When Toby describes why he barebacks, he is expressing how the various meanings that sex and beliefs about being gay have for him contribute to his unsafe sexual behaviors.

Considering the variety of risks of barebacking to both HIV-negative and HIV-positive men, it is instructive to hear from gay men who bareback about what they perceive are the benefits that outweigh the risks of barebacking. One of the most prominent and prolific researchers on gay men and barebacking is New York psychologist Perry Halkitis. Halkitis and his colleagues have conducted numerous studies on gay men, barebacking, and drug use and publish their research results in an impressively timely manner. In a survey of 518 gay and bisexual men conducted in Manhattan in 2001, the following were the most-often-cited benefits of barebacking given (Halkitis et al., 2003, p. 353):

- Barebacking increases intimacy between men.
- Barebacking makes sex more romantic and affirms love between men.
- Barebacking is sexier than sex with condoms.
- Barebacking is more "butch" and manly and affirms masculinity.
- Barebacking is "hotter" than sex with condoms.
- There are psychological and emotional benefits to barebacking.

Barebackers' postings on a Web site analyzed by Carballo-Dieguez and Bauermeister (2004) expressed some different attitudes about their behavior than those expressed by the men interviewed by Halkitis. For men who were in favor of barebacking and who acknowledged doing it, the following were their rationales for not using condoms during anal sex (Carballo-Dieguez & Bauermeister, 2004, pp. 7–10):

- Barebacking is enjoyable.
- Barebacking equals freedom.
- Barebackers are well informed about HIV and aware of the risks.
- Barebacking is not too dangerous. (Many respondents believed that most barebackers are already infected with HIV and are having unprotected sex among themselves.)
- Barebacking is a personal responsibility.

BAREBACKING RESEARCH FROM GREAT BRITAIN

Unfortunately, in the United States we have only small-scale studies from which to draw larger conclusions. The federal government has resisted funding any national study of gay men's sexual behaviors even though the findings would be of great interest and use to social scientists in terms of designing effective and targeted AIDS prevention programs that were culturally specific for the various subpopulations of gay men. Social scientists researching AIDS prevention among gay men in the United States have been stymied by conservatives in Congress who, in response to vocal activists of the religious right wing, have blocked all efforts to fund a national survey of gay men's sexual habits by either the National Institutes of Health (NIH) or the National Institute of Mental Health (NIMH).

But in Great Britain, large studies of gay men's sexual behavior have been conducted. Sigma Research evolved from Project SIGMA, which, between 1987 and 1994, carried out a five-phase cohort study of gay and bisexual men funded by the United Kingdom's Medical Research Council and the Department of Health. Sigma Research is a semi-autonomous unit affiliated with the Faculty of Humanities and Social Sciences of the University of Portsmouth; it has undertaken more than 50 research and development projects concerned with the impact of HIV and AIDS on the sexual and social lives of a variety of populations. This work includes needs assessments, evaluations, and service and policy reviews funded from a range of public sources.

The 2003 Gay Men's Sexuality Survey (GMSS) had more than 4000 respondents (Reid et al., 2004), from all racial, cultural, and economic backgrounds. This makes it a reliable cross section of gay men throughout Great Britain. Among the many findings from this extensive study was information about barebacking. A project conducted by SIGMA (Henderson, Keough, Weatherburn, & Reid, 2001) was an attempt to gain insight into how men who did not know their HIV status managed the physical as well as psychological sexual risks that were part of UAI. The majority of men surveyed in this study reported that UAI was momentary and was terminated immediately after penetration. Often the enjoyment was tempered by concerns about HIV risk, which competed with the pleasure derived. A second group of men acknowledged that UAI continued for longer than momentary penetration. Some of the men in this group had problems with initial penetration and used momentary penetration without a condom to enhance their erections in order to put a condom on and then continue until ejaculation. In contrast to this were accounts where some men decided not to use a condom at all but withdrew prior to ejaculation as a risk-reduction strategy (coitus interruptus). There was a third group of men in this study who did not use a condom, and UAI ended with ejaculation inside of the receptive partner. One man who was the insertive partner described his feelings as follows (p. 21):

> (Interviewer) So how was that?
>
> (Interviewee) Brilliant. I mean this was even better because I came inside him.
>
> (Interviewer) Were you concerned at that time? Was it going through your head what you were doing?
>
> (Interviewee) Absolutely, definitely, but it was just so good and I just didn't want to stop. [laugh] But it was good, it was brilliant. He was enjoying it again, I was enjoying it.
>
> (Interviewer) After you finished what happened? Did you talk at all?
>
> (Interviewee) No.
>
> (Interviewer) Did you think about it later?
>
> (Interviewee) Yes again. I thought about it after and I've wanked about it since, you know, the joy of it.

BAREBACKING, INTERNALIZED HOMOPHOBIA, AND TRANSGRESSION

Crossley (2004) suggests that condomless sex may be for some gay men a current manifestation of their need to hold on to transgressional aspects of their outlaw sexuality. She sees this as a consistent feature of gay men's individual and social psyche since the early days of gay liberation. In today's world where the political focus of much of the gay liberation movement has become gay marriage, gays serving openly in the military, and gay parenthood, the goals of organizations fighting for gay rights have shifted from gay men radically transforming American society to now assimilating into it in conservative and heteronormative ways. For men who have relished their identity as "sexual outlaws," barebacking is consciously one way to behave in a transgressive manner that is generally prohibited by mainstream society as well as by many within the gay community. Is there anything "nastier" and more transgressive than going against the expectations of society and literally and metaphorically tasting the forbidden fruit of unbridled, forbidden (queer) passion that is not constrained by the tight covering of latex bondage? As Gauthier and Forsyth (1999) note, "Breaking the rules for some is simply very exciting" (p. 94). "Hard as it may be to understand, some gay men have unsafe sex because they want to . . . skate close to the edge. Danger can be erotic, even the threat of contracting a deadly disease" (Peyser, 1997, p. 77).

In another article, Crossley (2002) sees that for some, bareback sex is not just an act of sensual pleasure or expression of pathology, but an assertion of sexual freedom, rebellion, and empowerment. This seems to mesh perfectly with her previous thesis about bareback sex being related to meeting the need some gay men have to be conspicuous about not being part of the mainstream. Crossley's observation is in keeping with the points made by Crimp (1989), Rofes (1996), and Moore (2004) about how the vibrant and creative sexual culture created by gay men in the 1970s still exerts a powerful pull on the gay psyche and is a highly valued aspect of gay communal memory and history that contributes to why some men bareback. The following quote (Carballo-Dieguez, 2001, p. 229), by another of the men interviewed by Carballo-Dieguez, illustrates the points that Crossley makes about the power of barebacking as a transgressive act.

> It is exhilarating, it is the forbidden thing, it is like a drug, it is what you are not supposed to do, it's getting away with murder.

"When we discuss the issue of sexual risk-taking behaviors — particularly in a marginalized, outlawed group, such as gay men — it is imperative to see the historical and cultural forces at work in shaping dynamic understanding of such behavior," writes Marshall Forstein, MD, professor of psychiatry at Harvard Medical School. "No gay man grows up immune to the insidious and overt messages that his sexual desire is in itself fundamentally wrong and unacceptable" (2002, p. 39). Most gay men grow up in a culture where their desires and even existences are marginalized. Many grow up in families where they are reviled or overtly rejected because of their sexual orientation. All of these factors help to strengthen and reinforce the power of internalized homophobia in an individual's psyche. One of the ways that internalized homophobia may play out is an unconscious sense that the individual is unimportant, undervalued, and not worth very much, thus increasing his sense that he is expendable, and so too are the men with whom he has sex and from whom he seeks love and validation. All of this can help to explain why otherwise seemingly comfortably out and proud gay men are not doing everything possible to prevent themselves from becoming infected and preventing the spread of HIV to their sexual partners. British scholar and cultural critic Jonathan Dolimore addresses these dynamics when he says: "What we have learned from Roland Barthes as from Michel Foucault and Oscar Wilde (albeit differently in each case) is that oppression inheres in those subjected to it as their or our identity, and must eventually be experienced and contested there, and never more so than when this subjection involves desire. Identity for the homosexual is always conflicted: at once ascribed, proscribed, and internalized, it is in terms of identity that self-hatred, violence, mutilation, and death have been suffered" (Dollimore, 1998, pp. 325–326).

RISK-TAKING AND THE UNCONSCIOUS

While researchers have asked gay men to explain why they bareback, very rarely do any of them speak of the deep, unconscious factors and forces that may play a role in increasing their propensity to take sexual risks. In his description of contemporary gay sexual practices, *Sex Between Men*, Los Angeles writer and therapist Douglas Sadownick notes that "sex often is a matter for the unconscious" (p. 5) and "desire is an unconscious manifestation" (p. 216). One of the basic tenets of psychoanalytic theory that Freud (1920) formulated concerns sexuality overlapping with a dimension of negativity. Freud originally called it "the death instinct," but is now commonly referred to as "the death drive." Dean (2000) notes, "AIDS gives ghastly new life to this idea, literalizing longstanding connections (many of them purely mythic) between sex and death" (p. 20). He also suggests that to divorce any account of sexual practices from the unconscious leaves one with merely a commonsensical, conflict-free notion of pleasure and desire. What Dean is most likely speaking to is the reality that the vast majority of safer-sex interventions and programs have all been behaviorally based and have not also tried to address the intrapsychic and unconscious forces that frame our desires and how they potentially become actualized.

Carballo-Dieguez and Bauermeister (2004) remark that the pulls toward and against barebacking can be seen from a psychoanalytic perspective as a battle between the id and superego or, from a philosophical perspective, as a confrontation between hedonists and rationalists. "Supporters of barebacking reported being motivated mainly by what felt good, appealed to their senses, and made them feel free; they used their reasoning to justify their behavior. Opponents of barebacking stressed moral and ethical imperatives and argued that barebacking pleasure-seeking impulses should be suppressed or tamed" (Carballo-Dieguez & Bauermeister, 2004, p. 11). It is only by offering clients opportunities during therapy to delve into their psyches that they can begin to gain deeper understanding of the multiple meanings that sex and, in particular, barebacking has for them on both the manifest and the unconscious levels. Without gaining access to the various meanings that each man who barebacks brings to specific sexual situations and acts, there is no way that each individual can be certain that he is making the kinds of decisions that will leave him feeling good about himself, his sexual partners, and the acts they engage in together.

Mansergh et al. (2002) discuss that some men intentionally put themselves and/or others at risk of HIV and STDs to meet important human needs (for example, physical stimulation, emotional connection). It is obvious, yet crucial to note, that most people who engage in sex are in pursuit of pleasure, though pleasure alone is often not the only reason why anyone may seek sexual encounters.

BAREBACKING AND SELF-CARE

It would be simplistic to adduce a single issue or dynamic as the "rationale" for an individual's engagement in unsafe sex. Usually, a complex combination of factors underlies such behavior, some of which are understandable and adaptive for that particular individual. Theories abound as to the resurgence of unsafe sex among gay men. Cheuvront (2002) wisely cautions: "In marginalizing the risk-taker as a damaged other, anxieties and fears about risk of infection are quelled for patients and clinicians alike. However, when risk-taking behavior is seen as situational, treatment provides a context for inquiry, articulation, and understanding of the patient's unique experiences, feelings, and circumstances" (p. 12). It is all too easy and reductionistic to pathologize sexual risk-takers as self-destructive, suicidal, damaged individuals. Cheuvront seems to agree, writing, "The popular media promote the HIV risk-taker as damaged and resigned to the inevitability of infection" (Cheuvront, 2002, p. 10).

Cheuvront (2002) reminds all mental health professionals working with gay men who bareback that "the meanings of sexual risk-taking are as varied as our patients" (p. 15). He cautions that simplistic explanations and understandings can "assuage the clinician's anxiety by making that which is complex and subject to individual differences appear less mysterious and knowable. Yet, this is not a luxury that clinicians have" (p. 15). It is the task of therapists to help an individual articulate the particular meanings of his high-risk behaviors. Regarding sexual risk-taking, Forstein (2002) asks: "Can care for the soul and care for the psyche always occur in the context of caring for the body?" (p. 38).

Part of the difficulty in finding ways to effectively address sexual risk taking is that many gay men use barebacking as an attempt to find closeness and fulfillment of profound emotional needs. Julian (1997) found that barebacking was a way that some men dealt with personal difficulties and sought emotional relief, breaking out of chronic isolation and connecting socially and intimately with another person. As Prieur (1990) notes for some gay men, "An active sex life may be the only tie to community. All social needs are released there; it is the only means of experiencing closeness to others. For a number of gay men, sex is almost a social amenity" (p. 111). In short, taking the risks associated with barebacking is actually the way some gay men are trying to take care of themselves and meet deep and urgent needs and desires. Cheuvront (2002) suggests that for many gay men self-care may indeed include taking risks, which in the context of barebacking means that the benefits derived from condomless sex in the present vastly outweigh any long-term potential risk to their health. In response to this issue, Forstein (2002) posits that "the question becomes one of understanding the nature of the risk and whether that particular risky behavior alone can attend to the needs inherent in the behavior" (p. 42).

I was reminded of this during a conversation with a colleague of mine who was saying that in order to do effective psychotherapy the clinician must remain close to the client's material and experiences without judging what the client is doing in order to afford the individual the best opportunity for emotional change. My colleague was describing a case where one man's clinical and developmental progress coincided with his getting HIV. During the course of therapy the client and therapist came to see how this individual's sexual risk-taking was a form of finding vitality in a very deadened life. Once he seroconverted, he felt enormous relief and became much better able to attend to self-care. As a result, this therapist understood that for this particular individual as well as for others, on becoming HIV-positive there may be significant meanings and emotional understandings to be derived from this transition which may affirm one's feelings of cohesiveness, capacity to feel understood, and a general sense of participation in the world. "The challenge for the therapist is remaining available to the patient in the wake of these changes" (J. P. Cheuvront, personal communication, March 14, 2005). Analyst Eric Sherman (2005) also poignanatly describes working with a man who was taking sexual risks and became HIV-positive during the course of therapy.

POSTEXPOSURE PROPHYLAXIS

As noted earlier, the advent of combination drug therapies has had a direct impact on some men's perceptions of AIDS, its seriousness and potential lethality. Yet there is another way that combination therapies have a direct relationship with AIDS prevention. Since the late 1990s, one use of combination therapies has been "postexposure prophylaxis" (PEP), also sometimes called "postexposure prevention." As explained by a PEP researcher at the University of California San Francisco, "For HIV-infected persons who are exposed to HIV, there may be a window of opportunity in the first few hours or days after exposure in which these highly active drugs may prevent HIV infection" (DeCarlo & Coates, 1997). PEP with antiretroviral medications is recommended by the U.S. Public Health Service (2001) following occupational exposure to HIV. The effectiveness of PEP in the occupational setting has prompted advocacy for the use of PEP following nonoccupational exposures in humans via sexual contact or injection drug use. Although as Martin et al. (2004) note: "There are sufficient similarities between occupational and nonoccupational exposures to consider extrapolating the biological efficacy of PEP in the occupational setting to nonoccupational exposures, there are critical contextual differences that must be addressed before PEP for nonoccupational exposures can be routinely recommended" (p. 788). There are a number of reasons why health care workers, who have an occupational exposure, are not a comparable group of people to those exposed through sex or shared injection drug-using paraphernalia. Health care workers almost always know whether the patient they are treating has HIV; sexual and drug-use partners do not always know the HIV status of their partners. Health care workers can usually gain access to antiviral drugs within minutes or hours of their injury; individuals exposed through sex or needle sharing probably have to wait at least several hours, if not longer, before they can obtain antiviral drugs (Ostrow, 1999). If postexposure therapy works at all, it works best when administered within 2 to 36 hours of exposure (New York State Department of Health, 2004).

By February 1997, six PEP centers had been established around the United States (Dahir, 1998). As of August 2004, PEP is available through emergency rooms and private physicians throughout the United States, Australia, and Europe. Some professionals worry that if people think PEP works, they will stop practicing safer sex and safer needle use, much as some wanted to block access of women to the "morning after" pill, fearing it would become a substitute for birth control. One important concern is that the availability of PEP following sexual or drug-use exposure could promote increases in high-risk behavior, with repeated requests for PEP (Martin et al., 2004). Margaret Chesney (1997), a co-director of the Center for AIDS Prevention Studies, which is involved with one of the nation's largest PEP clinics at San Francisco General Hospital, stresses, "In addition to the drug therapy, people should be given hours and hours of counseling to help them think about their experience in having gotten exposed, what it means, and how they can keep from repeating it." Martin et al. discuss that for PEP to be a useful intervention for the prevention of HIV infection following sexual or drug-use exposures, it needs to be feasible, safe, and efficacious. They provided risk-reduction education in addition to medication. Martin's research (2004) showed that most individuals do not experience sexual behavior disinhibition after receipt of PEP that includes both antiretroviral medication and risk-reduction counseling.

An informal survey I conducted of five physicians in Manhattan whose practices include large numbers of gay men did not evidence any indications of patients calling these physicians for PEP following a high-risk episode. None of the doctors surveyed reported ever having a patient call immediately after a high-risk sexual exposure to request a prescription for antiretroviral drugs to initiate PEP. One physician described one occurrence when a new patient who had been on PEP three previous times as prescribed by his previous doctors asked if he could have a supply of antiretroviral meds for use "just in case." This physician felt that the man's decision-making process regarding barebacking was partly influenced by PEP availability but did not give this individual the requested prescription. He strongly believed that prescribing the drugs would possibly support increased risk-taking (S. Dillon, personal communication, August 24, 2004).

In a study of how HIV progresses in newly infected individuals, conducted at New York University School of Medicine's Center for AIDS Research, the researchers did not find many study volunteers who have taken PEP. In their opinion, the gay men in this particular study are not very aware that PEP even exists. The men who do know about it seem to have a vague awareness but no specific knowledge. To these researchers it does not seem that the availability of PEP has had a significant impact on risk behavior (M. Marmor, personal communication, August 27, 2004).

CONCLUSION

The rationales for barebacking are as numerous as the men who do it. I have often heard men who bareback as well as my colleagues in the mental health field question whether the behavior is indicative of some underlying mental disorder or at least of unrecognized internalized homophobia. While indeed for some barebackers either or both could be at play, I have also come to learn that, as some of the researchers cited above conclude, in certain situations for certain men what at first appears to be reckless and self-destructive may be adaptive, affirming, and understandable. If we take a step back from the highly fraught and emotionally charged particulars of this issue and attempt to separate what we think is the "right" way to act now that the sexual transmissibility of HIV is a known fact, from moral judgments about the behavior and people who do it, we can begin to understand why barebacking is not always as "crazy" as it may at first appear to be. There are no easy answers to why men bareback or how this tide can be stemmed or even whether it should be stemmed. But at least we can start to ask better questions and open a crucial dialogue.

CHAPTER FOUR

Trips and Slips

PHILLIP, AN EXAMPLE OF THE SEX AND DRUGS CONNECTION

Phillip is an attractive, 47-year-old, African-American gay man who is HIV-positive. He came to therapy because he had been using crystal methamphetamine and his partying caused him to often miss work, particularly on Monday mornings. His employer had put him on probation for chronic absenteeism, and a social worker at Phillip's EAP (employee assistance plan) told him that he needed to get treatment. For the first few months we worked together, Phillip did not identify his drug use as a "problem," but as the therapy delved into his history, it became clear that in Phillip's life, drug use and sex with men had been linked since age 15. He had come out to himself at a young age, and at 15 he discovered a park near his home where he could meet men for sex, and routinely these sexual experiences also involved marijuana and hallucinogenic drugs. An above-average student who always felt alone, lonely, and different from other children, Phillip treasured his experiences in the park. He told me, "Those moments when men were paying attention to me, either cruising me or while we were having sex, were the only times I ever felt any sort of connection to anyone outside of my family, as fleeting as that connection was."

After college, Phillip moved to Manhattan and began a successful career. He also became active in New York's gay party scene. "My entire social life revolved around the five Ds," he told me, "Drugs, Disco, Dick, Dishing, and Dining, in that order." Increasingly, despite his successes at work and his active social life, he felt unhappy. He had hoped to have a serious relationship with a man yet had never been able to make a relationship last. I assessed him as having symptoms of a lifelong depression, and he was amenable to a psychiatric consultation. He began to take an antidepressant.

As Phillip and I talked about his social life, drug use, and sex life, he revealed that he routinely had unsafe sex with other men. I asked him how he met sexual partners, and he explained that he was quite shy and insecure in gay clubs but had discovered that the Internet was a comfortable way to hook up with partners because on the Internet, "everyone is cruising for sex. So instead of meeting someone at a club when we were both already high and then going home to do more drugs and carry on, I could spend entire weekends with guys doing crystal and having sex. My profile clearly says that I'm HIV-positive and sexually versatile [meaning that he enjoyed both the active and passive roles in anal intercourse]. But that never seemed to matter to any of the guys I played with once we got high." In response to my asking him whether he played safely he explained, "Being HIV-positive I felt badly about not using condoms. But I figured that since they knew that I was Poz, they must also be, since literally never once did any of them raise the issue of playing safe." Phillip also added that if anyone had ever mentioned condoms, he certainly would have used them.

While he was in therapy with me, Phillip was trying to stay clean and sober so he would not be fired. Predictably, this had a significant impact on his social life, which had revolved around partying and using drugs. The first few months, foregoing his usual weekend parties, Phillip felt socially isolated and very lonely. He was used to meeting sex partners online or getting high and going dancing at clubs, but he did not have much of a gay social life outside of those activities. I urged him to find a support group, but he adamantly refused to try 12-step meetings, stating that he had never met a "12-stepper" whom he felt comfortable around. "They all speak as if they were members of the same cult," he told me as I pressed him to explain his discomfort. Eventually, he did join a group for newly sober men, run by a gay community agency. But he did not remain in this group for long because it was an abstinence-based program, and Phillip claimed he did not want to stop using drugs but just reduce the hassles that drug use created in his life.

At first, Phillip was unable to stay drug-free for more than a few weeks. He cited boredom and loneliness as his reasons for calling friends to get high and go dancing or for going online to arrange a hookup. Those nights always ended with unsafe sex. Eventually, it became evident to both of us that the goal of abstinence was mine and not his. As soon as I stepped back from this position and began using a harm reduction approach,[1] Phillip started to respond more positively to therapy. He was willing to explore options for alternative ways to spend his free time doing things he enjoyed without using drugs. He came up with two activities that he felt would help him reduce his intake of drugs. One was to begin training to compete in the Gay Games in figure skating, and the other was to train with a partner to compete in the ice dancing events; the latter idea was to help him not become socially isolated while preparing for the Gay Games. His commitment to train early in the morning and on weekends helped him stay drug-free for longer periods of time. Phillip realized that it was impossible for him to be on the ice and safely lift a partner if he was coming down from crystal.

In response to Phillip's saying that he missed feeling a spiritual connection, I suggested that he try attending Mass at a local Catholic parish known to welcome gay and lesbian people. This suggestion raised feelings of being socially insecure and not knowing how to "homosocialize." I encouraged him to stay after Mass for the coffee hour, and we role-played how to initiate conversations that were not sexual come-ons. This was a slow process. But it eventually led to his being asked to go out for brunch with other gay men after Mass.

As Phillip's life became more balanced, he spent less time on the Internet. He loved to dance and party and did not want to stop completely. Phillip loved attending circuit parties, which are multiday dance parties attended by thousands of gay men where there are high levels of drug use and sexual activity, much of which is high-risk for transmitting HIV (Colfax, Mansergh, Guzman, Vittinghoff, Marks, Rader, & Buchbinder, 2001; Mattison, Ross, Wolfson, & Franklin, 2001; Mansergh et al., 2001). He had not attended any of these events during the first year of therapy and planned to attend an upcoming gay Disney event in Florida. Phillip discussed using drugs but limiting this to small quantities of methamphetamine and Ecstasy. He also planned to bring condoms and have only safer sex.

Upon his return, he was pleased that he had stuck to his plan and taken crystal on only one night. He met someone with whom he partied throughout the weekend. Phillip had told this man that he was HIV-positive before they left the dance floor, and they used condoms for anal sex. In contrast with his previous drug and sex binges, Phillip was not depressed and physically wrung-out for 5 days afterwards. He and the man he met made plans to get together in New York a few weeks later. They spoke on the phone and via e-mail daily since each returned home. Phillip felt excited about learning to date for the first time in his life, even if it was long distance. He relished the conversations and e-mails during which he and his new friend got to know one another in a nonsexual yet romantic way. During the visit by Phillip's friend to New York, they did a small amount of drugs and did not have high-risk sex. That visit was the last time Phillip and this sexual partner got together. Although Phillip was sad and disappointed, or perhaps because he was better able to tolerate feeling these feelings, he did not use chat rooms for about 4 months. When he did go to chat rooms, it was because he was "horny" and wanted to meet someone to have sex with. At this point he always used condoms for anal sex with men who did not also identify as HIV-positive. He was also successful in limiting himself to using a small amount of drugs.

Phillip felt the antidepressants were working, since when home alone with unstructured time, he did not feel desperate. He no longer felt that he was a loser who would never make friends nor have a boyfriend. This change had come about primarily through his affiliation with the church and with his skating partner, who was including him in social activities. Guss (2000) suggests that when doing therapy with gay men who abuse crystal, it is wise to counsel them that sex will almost certainly never be as intense as it was while they were using drugs.

I employed this strategy with Phillip, who shared that my caution that sober sex might never compare to sex while high had been crucial in establishing my credibility in his eyes: "You did not bullshit me about how sober sex could ever be like what sex on crystal was."

Phillip explained that early in our work he had been nervous when very briefly it had seemed as though I wanted him to abstain from drugs or online hookups completely. He knew he was unwilling or unable to do this. Had I continued to push for abstinence, he would not have remained in therapy with me for very long. We discussed his plans to attend three or four circuit parties a year and to continue limiting his use of drugs to small quantities. He had decided to always tell all potential sexual partners about his HIV status prior to arranging a hookup and insist on using condoms with anyone who did not identify as also being HIV-positive. He has stuck with this regimen for over a year. When Phillip used drugs, the use of smaller quantities helped him not get caught up in the heat of a sexual moment and cease to care about having protected sex. After 2 years, Phillip terminated therapy. He had made a few good friends and was learning how to make more, as well as how to date. His drug use was not out of control, and he had completely stopped barebacking except with other men who identified as also being HIV-positive.

CREATING CHANGE: CHAPTER OVERVIEW

Phillip's story of drug use and using the Internet to find sexual partners for barebacking is far from uncommon. In fact, there is now a strong body of research that demonstrates that the Internet and drug use are directly related to barebacking. An in-depth examination of how men meeting men on the Internet facilitates high-risk sexual encounters will be presented in Chapter 5. The current chapter focuses on the connection between drug use and barebacking.

This chapter has three main areas of focus. First, we will examine the research on drug use and high-risk sex among gay men. Is there a link between drug use and barebacking? We will also look at statistics on the frequency of drug use in the gay community and discuss why drug use might create an atmosphere more conducive to barebacking.

We also take an in-depth look at crystal meth. In my practice, crystal use is the number-one predictor of barebacking. Certain properties of that drug, which will be explored in detail, seem to create physiological and psychological changes that make it easier for users to engage in high-risk sex.

After detailing the connections between drug use and barebacking, we will evaluate different treatment models, from abstinence to harm reduction and moderation management. What are realistic behavior-change goals for clients who are drug users? How do the therapists' own reactions with clients get in the way of their work? Therapy is about helping people change, but, as described in the case above, it is easy for helping professionals to fall into the trap of being more invested in the client's changing than he is. I will spend some time discussing the harm reduction model and how it can be specifically applied to men who use crystal meth.

Although this chapter is directed toward mental health professionals, my hope is that all readers will benefit form thinking about the mechanics of change. For each man, barebacking occurs in a unique social, emotional, and psychological convergence. There is no single intervention that will help every barebacker reexamine his choices. If we understand the internal processes and the external stressors and dynamics that may have led men to choose to take risks with their health and the health of others, we may have a chance of being of assistance to them if and when they come in asking for help.

DRUGS AND SEX IN GAY CULTURE

The gay community has a long history of alcohol and drug abuse (Morales & Graves, 1983; Stall & Wiley, 1988; McKirnan & Peterson, 1989; Cabaj, 1992). Stall and Wiley (1988) showed that gay and bisexual men use a wider variety of drugs than heterosexual men do, but the frequency of gay men's drug use is not as high. This suggests that gay men use drugs in specific situations, such as during sex or during visits to specific "homosocial" venues such as bars, clubs, sex parties, or bathhouses. Thus, a unique aspect of gay culture is that drug use is very often specifically connected to seeking or having sex. Purcell, Parsons,

Halkitis, Mizuno, and Woods (2001) note that "The link between gay bars and substance use has a powerful history in the gay community, and many drugs have strong sexual meanings for MSM, meanings that may persist after people know that they are HIV-positive" (p. 186). This is what Phillip meant when he talked about the five "Ds." For men who came of age during the heyday of disco, drugs, dancing (three of the five "Ds"), and sex (or, as Phillip put it, "dick") were a formative part of forging an individual as well as communal gay identity. Peak experiences (often under the influence of drugs) were shared on the dance floors of such legendary clubs as The Sanctuary, Tenth Floor, The Loft, Twelve West, Paradise Garage, and Flamingo in Manhattan; Tracadero in San Francisco; Studio One and Probe in Los Angeles; The A House in Provincetown; The Ice Palace and Sandpiper on Fire Island; Warsaw in Miami; and eventually, what for many was the penultimate gay dance palace, the Saint. These venues, where thousands of gay men created a celebratory (albeit at times self-destructive) tribal rite, live on in today's circuit parties.[2]

BAREBACKING AND SUBSTANCE USE

Studies conducted in the 1990s attempting to correlate the use of alcohol and drugs with unsafe sexual activity had inconsistent results. Some studies reported alcohol use as a factor related to unsafe sex (Boulton, McLean, Fitzpatrick, & Hart, 1995). Others found a statistical relationship between drug or alcohol use during sex and the likelihood of having unprotected sex (McCusker, Stoddard, Zapka, Zorn, & Mayer, 1990; Stall, McKusick, Wiley, Coates, & Ostrow, 1986). In contrast are studies that did not find evidence of this relationship (Bolton, 1992; Weatherburn et al., 1993). Studies of HIV-positive gay men show connections between alcohol use and unprotected sex (Dolezal, Meyer-Bahlburg, Remien, & Petkova, 1997; Kalichman, Kelly, & Rompa, 1997; Purcell et al., 2001; Halkitis & Parsons, 2002; Halkitis, Greene, & Mourges, 2005). Specifically, Purcell and colleagues (2001) describe alcohol and drug use among 456 HIV-positive men, most of whom were men of color.[3] More than 35 percent of these men had unprotected anal intercourse (UAI) while under the influence of alcohol in the preceding 3 months. Halkitis and Parsons (2002) recruited gay and bisexual men for a study to assess the extent of noninjection drug use by gay men. Of the more than half of their sample who reported using more than one drug in the 3 months prior to the study, most reported having UAI while under the influence of alcohol and inhalants.[4]

Yet other studies failed to demonstrate that alcohol use was associated with unsafe sex by gay men (Weatherburn et al., 1993; Crosby, Stall, Paul, Barrett, & Midanik, 1996; Parsons, Halkitis, Wolitski, & Gomez, 2003). In the study conducted by Parsons et al. (2003), though alcohol use was reported by both men who had UAI and those who did not, being under the influence of alcohol was not a correlate for having UAI.[5] It appears that alcohol alone is less likely than other drugs to lead to barebacking, as will be discussed further on in this chapter. These studies surveyed men living in large urban centers, and the results may not reflect the lives and alcohol-use patterns of men who live in rural settings or smaller cites throughout the United States.

CLUB DRUGS AND PARTY DRUGS

As the AIDS epidemic has continued, there is no uncertainty about the role that drugs and alcohol play in UAI and the spread of HIV. Like Phillip, many gay men have online profiles stating they are "chem friendly" or want to "party" or "PNP" (which stands for party and play), all of which mean they seek to have sex while using one of the currently fashionable "party drugs" or "club drugs" such as methamphetamine, GHB, ketamine, or Ecstasy (MDMA). Research documents that high-risk behaviors that spread HIV and other sexually transmitted diseases (STDs) occur more frequently among individuals who have poor impulse control, particularly if their sexual activity takes place under the influence of alcohol or drugs (Stall et al., 1986; Leigh, 1990; Stall, Paul, Barrett, Crosby, & Bein, 1991; Stall & Leigh, 1994; Royce, Sena, Cates, & Cohen, 1997; Chesney, Barrett, & Stall, 1998; Halkitis, Parsons, & Stirratt, 2001; Halkitis & Parsons, 2002; Halkitis, Parsons, & Wilton, 2003).

As Woody et al. (1999) state, "Most studies now show a relationship between alcohol or drug use and increased sexual risk among men who have sex with men (MSM), but it is clear that these relationships are complex and difficult to evaluate" (p. 198). For example, one study of 169 gay and bisexual men using Ecstasy found a strong correlation between use of Ecstasy and high-risk sexual behavior (Klitzman, Pope, & Hudson, 2000). Many of this same study's participants reported unprotected receptive and insertive anal sex with men of different or unknown HIV status the last time that they barebacked. Half of the HIV-positive men and more than half of the HIV-negative men described being drunk on alcohol or high on drugs during their last bareback encounter (Mansergh et al., 2002).

The literature that exists on the connection between substance use and sexual risk-taking points to important correlations. For example, individuals who are regular drug/alcohol users or who use drugs or alcohol with sexual activity are more likely to take sexual risks than are people who are not heavy users of substances or do not use them before or during sex. Several studies (Stall & Wiley, 1988; McKirnan & Peterson, 1989; Martin & Hasin, 1990; Woody, 1990) found that of the majority of gay and bisexual men surveyed who did use various substances, the patterns of drug or alcohol use were recreational and did not display a pattern of usage that would suggest either "chemical dependency" or "addiction." Yet even men who report only using drugs and alcohol "recreationally" have been found to exhibit a direct connection between being high and having UAI.

Are some drugs more likely than others to lead to unsafe sex among users? There is literature that demonstrates that use of specific substances is predictive of high-risk sex. As noted earlier, Klitzman et al. (2000) found that frequent use of Ecstasy was associated with UAI during the preceding year. In a study of young MSM, only the use of cocaine actually predicted a failure to use condoms during anal intercourse, and use of alcohol and nine other drugs before or during sex was correlated with barebacking (McNall & Remafedi, 1999). Purcell et al. (2001) and Halkitis and Parsons (2002) report that use of alcohol and inhalants (amyl nitrate and butyl nitrate, both known on the street as "poppers") almost always predicted unprotected anal and oral intercourse. The study by Purcell et al. (2001) only surveyed HIV-positive men. The researchers found high rates of substance use and a higher proportion of sexually risky behaviors among the men in their study who used alcohol, marijuana, and inhalants before or during sex than those who did not use them. Other studies have corroborated the finding linking poppers, barebacking, and HIV infections (Ostrow, Beltran, Joseph, DiFrancisco, & the MACS/CCD Study Group, 1993; Ekstrand, Stall, Paul, Osmond, & Coates, 1999; Woody et al., 1999). Woody et al. suggest that the increased sexual risk-taking associated with use of poppers may be related to the euphoria, impaired judgment, or impulsive behavior that is experienced as a result of using nitrate inhalant drugs. Thus, drugs that are for the most part not injected, whether used regularly or infrequently, have been strongly linked to sexual risk-taking by users. These data may suggest that gay men who inject drugs are less likely to engage in risky sexual behavior, although we know that when people share intravenous (IV) drug-using paraphernalia they are at high risk for contracting HIV and other blood-borne diseases.

INTRODUCING "TINA" (CRYSTAL METHAMPHETAMINE)

Special attention needs to be given to one drug that has become the premium fuel for unsafe sex, and whose particular properties lead users to abandon caution and regularly take sexual risks. Crystal methamphetamine — referred to as crystal, Tina, meth, crank, or ice — more than poppers (amyl or butyl nitrate), cocaine, and alcohol, lowers inhibitions and heightens sensitivity to sensations, making it a desirable aphrodisiac among a growing number of gay men. A study of gay men and barebacking conducted in New York City revealed that crystal meth use is a serious problem for MSM because of its relationship with high-risk sexual behaviors (Halkitis et al., 2001). As Halkitis, Greene, and Mourgues (2005) note, studies of methamphetamine use during the early 1990s showed that use of this particular drug was largely a regional phenomenon that was confined to the western portion of the United States (Heischober & Miller, 1991; Harris, Thiede, McGough, & Gordon, 1993; Gorman, Morgan, & Lambert, 1995; Gorman, Gunderson, Marlatt, & Donovan, 1996; Eggan, Reback, & Ditman, 1996; Reback, 1997). But later investigations have shown that use of crystal meth has reached high levels in the eastern part of the United States as well

(Guss, 2000; Halkitis et al., 2001; Freese, Miotto, & Rebeack, 2002; Hanson, 2002; Semple, Patterson, & Grant, 2002; Halkitis et al., 2005, in press). Rawson, Gonzales, and Brethen (2002) cite evidence of high levels of crystal use in the western and midwestern parts of the United States. Halkitis et al. (in press, d) state, "Methamphetamine use, when coupled with high-risk sexual behavior, foretells that the growing use of the drug in New York City is certain to exacerbate the HIV/AIDS epidemic" (Halkitis, in press, a). Bull et al. (2001) have shown evidence that the connection between use of crystal and the HIV epidemic grows when the drug is injected.

In one California study conducted at HIV counseling and testing sites, the connection between crystal use during sex and UAI was unambiguous, and this was not just a behavior among HIV-positive men. Almost 12 percent of the gay men and almost 7 percent of the bisexual men whose UAI was linked to crystal use were HIV-positive (Molitor, Truax, Ruiz, & Sun, 1998).[6] Another New York City study by Halkitis's team of researchers confirms the findings from California. Project BUMPS is a study of New York City gay men who use club drugs, such as Ecstasy, methamphetamine, GHB, ketamine, or cocaine. Of 192 men who used crystal and who reported being either HIV-negative or unsure of their HIV status at the onset of the study, upon testing for HIV, 10 men turned out to be HIV-positive and the rest were negative. Either they seroconverted since their last HIV test, or they had been HIV-positive but did not know it.

The researchers analyzed their responses and theorized that these 10 men were more likely to use crystal to avoid physical discomfort, to avoid conflict with others, and to have pleasant times with others (Halkitis, Green, & Carragher, in press, d). The researchers concluded that the meth-using seroconverters are likely using the drug to ease feelings of loneliness or depression. "The implication is that these may be men who are so dependent on this drug to be with other men that when they are with men they lose all inhibitions. That feeling of isolation and depression is absolutely key" (Halkitis, 2004, quoted in Osborne electronic version). The data from this study clearly indicate that unprotected receptive anal intercourse is more likely to occur when an individual is high than when he is not high.

Dr. Thomas Frieden, commissioner of the New York City Department of Health and Mental Hygiene, reports that research has found that one in four MSM who are newly diagnosed with HIV infection in San Francisco had used methamphetamine in the prior 6 months (2003). He also states that MSM methamphetamine users are almost twice as likely to be HIV-positive as those who do not use the drug, and that gay men who use methamphetamine are more than one-third less likely to use condoms during receptive anal intercourse than are non–meth users. Nearly two thirds of gay and bisexual men who present for methamphetamine treatment in Los Angeles are HIV-positive. HIV-positive men are 50 percent more likely to use methamphetamine during sex then are HIV-negative men (Frieden, 2003). However, it is difficult to precisely ascertain what the causal status of crystal meth use might be in relation to HIV status insofar as researchers do not know if these men are infected with HIV prior to using crystal or if they become HIV-positive as a result of high-risk sexual behavior while on crystal. As Halkitis, Green, & Carragher (in press, d) state: "Whether the relationship between use of the drug [crystal] and sexual risk behavior among gay and bisexual men is a direct one is unclear. What is more likely is that men with certain psychological profiles are attracted to methamphetamine, use it in environments and contexts that are sexually charged, and as a result are situated to engage in sexual risk. Whether men use the drug intentionally as a way to facilitate sexual risk-taking behavior or whether sexual risk-taking is a natural byproduct of methamphetamine use are issues that need to be further disentangled."

CRYSTAL AND SEX

What is it about crystal that draws men to take it and precisely what is the connection between crystal and barebacking? A pioneering article by Manhattan psychiatrist Jeffrey Guss (2000) gives the most succinct answer to this question in its title, "Sex Like You Could Never Imagine." Illustrating this, John, a 33-year-old AIDS educator client of mine described an evening he spent at a bathhouse.

"I did a few lines of crystal with the first guy I hooked up with, and then smoked some more with one other man. I don't know how many men I carried on with that night, and I know that I did not use a condom with any of them. Before arriving at the baths I promised myself that I would ask everyone what his HIV-status was, and I lived up to this. Everyone told me that they were positive, and nobody seemed to be bothered by my asking them this question. I had anal sex with every man I was with that night, whether as top or bottom, and never used a condom."

Guss writes: "Stimulant drugs, particularly cocaine and methamphetamine, are particularly appealing to gay men in a highly sexualized subculture that exists within the broader gay community" (pp. 107–108). Guss states that a major attraction of stimulant drugs for gay men lies in the fact that preexisting sexual anxieties are absent, and having sex for 6 to 12 hours becomes "realistic and predictable" (p. 109).

In earlier chapters, I discussed the longing some gay men feel for the pre-AIDS days of sexual adventure and worry-free exploration. What we may be seeing now is that crystal meth use has become a vehicle that allows some users "to reclaim a sense of pre-AIDS sexuality" (Reback & Grella, 1999, p. 156). Reback (1997) suggests that gay men who use crystal meth often create a self-identity that integrates men's sexuality, drug use, and HIV status. She also suggests that crystal use is a means of coping with feelings of isolation and loneliness. Reback's observations suggest that some gay men use sex and drugs as attempts to self-medicate difficult feelings, as was discussed in the previous chapter. Dominic Davies, founder and executive director of Pink Therapy Services in London, sees another possible appeal of the drug for some gay men: "The demonization of crystal within the gay community makes it seem attractive to a group of people who feel they are outsiders from mainstream society and a segment of the gay community who have dedicated their lives to hedonism. The way moral panics operate creates a wave of interest and a rejection of the moral panic by some people. There is also a curiosity to try 'new' drugs whatever they are, and with the immense dopamine high and extra energy one gets from crystal then it's a drug perfectly suited to intense and extended sex sessions" (D. Davies, personal communication, March 31, 2004).

In order to understand crystal's appeal and seductiveness it is necessary to become familiar with its physiological and psychological effects.

Whether an amphetamine is pharmaceutically produced or illicitly man-ufactured like "crystal," primarily this class of drug produces stimulat-ing effects on the central nervous system. Methamphetamine has been described as the "most hyperstimulating of the amphetamine analogues (Drug Enforcement Administration, 1989). As Gawin & Ellingwood (1988) state: "This kind of stimulant creates a neurochemical amplifica-tion of the pleasure experienced in most activities." Crystal accomplish-es this by affecting neurons that release serotonin, norepinephrine, and dopamine, which produces major changes in a person's emotional state (NIDA, 1996). The drug intensifies the senses, elevates mood, increases sex drive, and gives the user energy while suppressing appetite and the need for sleep (Halkitis, Greene, & Mourgues, 2005). Men who use crystal also report an increase in sensitivity in the anus, which leads to an increased likelihood of receptive anal intercourse (Semple et al., 2002). Crystal users report the following psychological effects: hypersexuality, euphoria, lower sexual inhibitions, increased self-esteem, and increased confidence (Reback, 1997; Murray, 1998; Guss, 2000; Halkitis et al., 2001). Crystal meth use also increases a sense of escapism and sexual adventurism that men who frequent dance parties, sex clubs, and sex parties value and desire (McKirnan, Ostorw, & Hope, 1996; Halkitis et al., 2001; Parsons & Halkitis, 2002).

A majority of 48 men surveyed by Halkitis, Greene, & Mourgues (2005) in New York City used methamphetamine for specific sexual encounters and felt that using the drug enabled them to achieve what they sexually desired during those encounters. An example of this was given by one of the men in the study who, when asked why he used methamphetamine, replied, "I want to be penetrated. It enhances that feeling" (Halkitis, Greene, & Mourgues, 2005). Other men reported that they used methamphetamine because it allowed the sexual encoun-ters to last for longer periods of time. One man reported that his sexual encounters while on the drug lasted from 11 to 15 hours. Guss (2000) reports that the men in his practice told him that the intensity of sex while on crystal is far superior to even the most satisfying sex while not on crystal. The men I see in my therapy practice who use methamphet-amine routinely describe the sex as "mind blowing," "phenomenal," and "awesome." One man described it in these words: "I would say that the only way to explain to someone who has not had sex on crystal is that all of the sex I had while not high on Tina is like watching a black-and-white television during the 1950s. In comparison, sex on crystal is like watching one of the new, high-definition color televisions with surround sound." Another man told me that crystal made him feel like a "sexual superman."

PSYCHOLOGICAL EFFECTS OF CRYSTAL

While the physical effects of crystal are attractive to men who take it, it is the psychological effects that may have the most appeal, perhaps unconsciously, for gay users. Crystal meth makes cruising for sex and making contact with other men for sexual liaisons less fraught and simpler, since preexisting sexual anxieties and inhibitions disappear. Guss (2000) notes that many men report that once they are high on crystal, other men are more attracted to them, thus confirming the sense of feeling sexier and more attractive (p. 108). Guss also states that "when sex is added to the stimulant experience, its meaning and value are heightened and transformed" (p. 108). Because crystal meth breaks down inhibitions and enables users to have sex for longer periods of time, the result is that crystal meth users participate more often in group sex as well as other "extreme"[7] sexual behaviors (Gawin, 1978; Gorman, 1998; Guss, 2000; Halkitis et al., 2001).

If people set out to invent the almost "perfect" gay party drug, they would have created crystal meth. Crystal seems to be an ideal drug for many gay men despite certain sexual side effects that will be discussed later on in this chapter. Halkitis et al. (2001) note that the combination of sexual effects in combination with the emotional effects of crystal makes it the "quintessential gay drug." Michael Siever, director of the Stonewall Project, a San Francisco treatment program specifically targeting gay crystal users, agrees, saying, "Crystal is the perfect drug for gay men. What else allows you to party all night long whether you're dancing or having sex? At least, at first, before it becomes a problem" (quoted in Heredia, 2003, electronic version). Once the effects wear off, a crystal user can suffer from severe depression that can last for several days, depending on how many days he was taking the drug. Regular users can become addicted (Yoshida, 1997; Jacobs, 2002; Halkitis, Parsons, & Wilton, 2003b; Heredia, 2003). Long-term use of methamphetamine has been linked to acute psychotic episodes characterized by paranoia, delusions of persecution, social withdrawal, flattening of affect, and auditory, olfactory, visual, and tactile hallucinations (Ellenhorn, Schonwald, Ordog, & Wasserman, 1997). As Howard Grossman, a prominent Manhattan physician specializing in HIV who is also chairman of the Academy of HIV Medicine, has said, "It's frightening. I've seen a huge increase of newly infected gay men that got HIV from unprotected sex during crystal meth binges. Our community is self-destructing with this drug. This drug is destroying our community. It just seems to be getting worse and worse and no one is doing anything about it" (quoted in Jacobs, 2004, pp. B1, B5).

ESTEBAN AND THE CRYSTAL-SEX EQUATION

I gained insight into the equation between crystal and sex when I worked with Esteban, whose use of crystal was a main rationale he stopped practicing safer sex. This 39-year-old, HIV-negative, Cuban-born gay man immigrated to Miami with his mother and her family when he was two. He now works as a banker. He had never tried crystal until 1997, while on a holiday to New York's Fire Island to attend the Pines party, one of the many well-known circuit parties. At the time, he was single and was offered a hit of crystal on the dance floor. Many hours later, he was invited to join a group of men going to someone's house to do more crystal and have sex. At first, he was surprised that no one raised the issue of using condoms or of HIV status. But as he took more drugs and continued to have sex for hours, he just surrendered to the sensuousness of the sexual freedom with a group of very attractive men. Prior to this occasion, he had almost always used condoms for anal sex, only barebacking twice before.

For the next 5 years, until he joined Crystal Meth Anonymous (CMA) to stop his drug use, he never had sex with condoms and he also almost never had sex unless he was high on crystal. Living in Miami, he soon became part of the crystal/sex scene there and threw himself into it with gusto. He felt that sex on crystal was vastly more fun and more intense than sober sex. Sex always was euphoric when he was high, and he lost all his inhibitions. Doing crystal allowed him to live out sexual fantasies, which gave him more sexual self-confidence, resulting in rougher and more extreme sex. "Everything I was doing sexually was right. I knew that I was going to give them the best fuck they ever had," Esteban told me. "When we were done, in fact, they told me that this was true." He got so caught up in the crystal/sex party scene in Miami that he lost his business and moved to New York to live with some family members and go back to school.

Esteban told me that in all the times he had sex while on crystal, not once, ever, did a partner ask him about his HIV status, and he never inquired about the HIV status of any of the men he played with. Similarly, no one ever raised the issue of using a condom. Of all the sex parties he went to while doing crystal both in Miami and in New York, he could recall only one that had condoms available in a bowl, but he does not remember seeing any men using them. He met one man at a club in Miami while both were high on crystal, with whom he started a relationship. After a few dates, this man told Esteban that he was HIV-positive. Even this information did not cause Esteban to start using condoms. He says he was not worried about his own health. He believed that since he never swallowed semen and was never penetrated anally (that act was uncomfortable for him after surgery to remove hemorrhoids), he was protected from contracting HIV. After a few months, Esteban's partner expressed concerns that not using condoms might compromise Esteban's health, but Esteban did not want to think about using condoms and continued to have condomless sex until they broke up.

When I asked him, Esteban was very clear that he never wanted to become HIV-positive. He said the powerfulness of the increased pleasure and ease of not using condoms while high simply took over the better part of his decision-making process. Since he became sober, he has always used condoms for anal sex. As with many men in recovery from crystal use, he feels that sex is not as enjoyable or as intense as when he was high on crystal, and he blames a small amount of that on wearing condoms, which reduces sensation. But when questioned further on this topic, he admitted that even if he were not to use condoms, he was certain that sex would never be as extraordinary as it always was while on crystal. The other change for Esteban is that now that he is sober, he once again asks potential sex partners about their HIV status, and he misses the days of being high on crystal when he never had that uncomfortable conversation. When he does try to avoid the conversation about HIV and condoms, his partners, who are also always sober, raise the issue. When he was using crystal, no amount of sex or of crystal was ever enough. "I wanted more and more sex. I would finish with one person and immediately find someone else to have sex with. While on crystal, I would have sex with one man right after another, often nonstop for hours. I would always seek someone better, bigger, hotter or more interesting. Now, when I finish having sex with someone, even if it is not great, I feel satisfied. I was so totally caught up in it all that, I did not realize how insane it all was."

Esteban told me that while he was on crystal it was all-consuming, both the drug-taking and the sex. "I never cared what anybody's health was. I just wanted to get off. I don't know why, but I am certainly lucky that I am still HIV-negative."

CIRCUIT PARTIES

If there is a recurring theme in interviews with crystal users, it is that the drug is nearly ubiquitous at circuit parties. Circuit parties are no longer solely an American phenomenon. They are now starting to occur regularly in Holland, England, Spain, Greece, Australia, and Canada, with men flying in from all over the world to attend. This represents only the most current aspect of the globalization of contemporary gay culture, initially exported from the United States, which has already resulted in a homogeneousness of many gay clubs, fashions, values, and trends throughout the Western world. Thus it seems possible that it is only a matter of time before the current fashion for crystal meth, so popular in the United States and contributing to incidences of high-risk sex there, also becomes popular among gay men throughout Europe and Australia. Even though there is no current evidence to document that the use of crystal methamphetamine is anywhere near as prevalent among gay men outside of the United States as it is among gay men in the United States, all health care workers in industrialized countries

need to be alert to the possibility of this trend being
countries. Contemporary gay culture and comm
are increasingly international in nature, with a l
ment between countries by gay men with enough dispc
travel. The use of crystal meth by gay men in the United States m
began escalating into a dangerous epidemic on the West Coast. Despite
publicity about the dangers of this drug in national and local gay media
throughout the United States, eventually its popularity has spread across
the American continent, although it took many years to do so.

IS THERE A LINK BETWEEN CRYSTAL AND UAI?

With all the well-documented links between crystal and other drug
use and unsafe sex, we still must ask whether drug use leads to barebacking, or if they simply tend to cooccur? After all, we know there
is evidence that risky health behaviors cluster together into groups
(e.g., smokers also drink). Research by Halkitis and colleagues (2005,
2005c), has found that men who use crystal are exceptionally sexually active. Halkitis, Greene, & Mourgues (2005) — label these men
"hypersexual."[8] What is unclear from their research is whether the men
who used crystal were highly sexual prior to beginning use of the drug
and were attracted to crystal after hearing about how it enhanced the
intensity of sex, or whether they became hypersexual only after beginning to use crystal. What does seem apparent is that many of the men
who are drawn to using methamphetamine seem to exhibit characteristics that would label them as high sensation-seekers. High sensation-
seekers, as has been previously noted, are more likely to bareback than
are men who do not rate high on that scale.

Halkitis, Shrem, & Martin (in press, c) offer a wise and cautious
note, "While the most current knowledge points to a strong relationship between drug use and risky sexual behaviors (Romanelli, Smith,
& Pomeroy, 2003), the emergence of methamphetamine, specifically
its influence on sexual behavior, warrants more scrutinized investigation." Their findings suggest that methamphetamine does not in and
of itself induce gay men to take sexual risks, but that certain hypersexual gay men who are already predisposed to risky sex are attracted to

ing crystal. One of Halkitis' studies was of 48 gay and bisexual men who identified themselves as active methamphetamine users who used the drug for sexual purposes. The aphrodisiac quality of meth was the most common reason given by the participants for why they used the drug (Halkitis, Fishgrund, & Parsons, in press, a). Halkitis notes that while research has shown that the use of methamphetamine can be a predictor of unprotected sex, it therefore has a high correlation with HIV transmission. "In other words, methamphetamine use may lead to unprotected sex, which may cause HIV transmission" (in press, a). Halkitis and his colleagues also have discovered that it is not only middle-income, well-educated white men who are attracted to taking crystal and that in fact use of this drug cuts across all economic and racial groups.

"CRYSTAL DICK" AND VIAGRA

Using crystal meth is a risk factor for contracting HIV, and not just because it induces unmindfulness and euphoria. Gawin (1978) reports that use of methamphetamine in high doses by men may impede their ability to obtain a full or even partial erection. Many male methamphetamine users report impaired sexual functioning manifested by temporary erectile dysfunction or delayed ejaculation. This side effect of crystal use is commonly known as "crystal dick" (Whitfield, 1996). Gay men who experience erectile dysfunction while using crystal are more likely to be the receptive partner in anal sex (Frieden, 2003), thus increasing their risk of contracting HIV. Some crystal users report that the combination of increased anal sensitivity and crystal dick tends to make them "instant bottoms" (Frosch, Shoptaw, Huber, Rawson, & Ling, 1996; Heredia, 2003). Yet, since Viagra first became available by prescription in the United States in 1998, men who use crystal report simultaneously also using one of the drugs used to treat erectile difficulty in order to function as both the insertive and receptive partner during anal sex (Tuller, 2001; Halkitis, Wilton, Parsons, & Hoff, 2004; Halkitis, Shrem, & Martin, in press, c), increasing the possibility of spreading HIV if they engage in UAI. Dr. Jeffrey Klausner, director of STD prevention at the San Francisco Health Department, stated: "Viagra can turn people with chemically induced erectile dysfunction into more effective transmitters of HIV and other STDs" (quoted in Tuller, 2001).

Statistics on rates of new HIV infections seem to bear out a possible correlation between Viagra (and drugs like it) becoming available and an increase in rates of new HIV infections among MSM. New diagnoses of HIV in MSM have increased 17.7 percent since 1999 (approximately a year after Viagra first became commercially available in the United States) after having either declined or remained stable in the population of MSM between 1999 and 2002 (CDC, 2003). "For a subset of gay men, Viagra's definitely found its way into the mix of party drugs," said Dr. Ken Mayer, a professor of medicine at Brown University and a past board member of the Gay and Lesbian Medical Association. Dr. Mayer, who is also medical director of research at the Fenway Community Health Center in Boston, one of the premier medical facilities devoted to providing quality medical care to gay, lesbian, bisexual, and transgender people in the United States, also stated, "And in a bathhouse or other setting where there's an opportunity to have sex with multiple partners, to have a longer-lasting erection can be a prescription for HIV transmission" (quoted in Tuller, 2001, electronic edition).

TREATING DRUG ABUSE TO REDUCE UNPROTECTED ANAL INTERCOURSE

The news is not all bleak about drugs and barebacking. Woody et al. (1999) found that if men who in the past had a problematic pattern of using drugs and/or alcohol stopped using drugs, or in the case of alcohol greatly reduced their level of use, sexual risk-taking decreased. Woody's finding strongly suggests that stopping or reducing problematic drug or alcohol use is directly associated with a reduction in sexual risk. In light of this good news, public health officials, mental health professionals, and those in the HIV/AIDS prevention field would do well to ponder two questions: What needs to happen in order for individuals who abuse drugs and alcohol to admit that they have a problem? And then, what can be done to help them reduce or stop using?

ABSTINENCE

When I first began graduate school and training as a psychotherapist in the mid-1970s, the conventional wisdom was that there was only one way to work with individuals who were abusing or addicted to drugs or alcohol — abstinence from all substance use. The variety of 12-Step programs that began with Alcoholics Anonymous (AA) and expanded into Narcotics Anonymous, Cocaine Anonymous, Marijuana Anonymous, and most recently Crystal Meth Anonymous are all examples of abstinence-based approaches to helping an individual recover from his or her dependence on substances.

Therapists were trained to be very confrontational with substance abusers in an attempt to break through any denial they might have about the problematic aspects of their substance use and to help them stop using. As MacMaster (2004) states; "Implicitly or explicitly, the goal of most substance abuse services is the elimination of nonmedical substance use" (p. 357). While this approach is very useful for scores of individuals, as with any treatment approach, it is not appropriate or helpful for everyone. This is especially true for people who have no desire to stop using drugs but only want to limit the harmful effects on their lives. The major drawback for therapists using an abstinence-based approach is that it has the potential to create a highly adversarial relationship between the therapist and client. The traditional abstinence-based approach is very hierarchical and reinforces shame that the individual may experience about his or her usage. Therapists may find themselves labeling individuals who are not interested in complete abstinence as "resistant" or "unservable" (Miller & Rollnick, 2002) and rather than empowering the individual, they may further exacerbate the sense of personal failure that the client already is feeling.

HARM REDUCTION

Skilled therapists must have more than one way of intervening with clients with any problem. Harm reduction is an extremely useful and welcome addition to my therapeutic tool box. The model was first developed in Merseyside, England, by two professionals concerned with preventing and reducing the spread of HIV among active intravenous (IV) drug users and to better serve those who had already contracted the virus (Newcombe & Parry, 1988; Springer, 1991). In the early days of the AIDS epidemic, most AIDS service organizations would only offer services to people who had contracted the disease through sharing intravenous drug paraphernalia if they were either "clean," meaning drug free, or in a methadone maintenance program. Thus, many of the individuals who were most in need of counseling and education about HIV and AIDS were denied services simply because they were active drug users. This resulted in increased public health risks resulting from these individuals transmitting HIV to more people (Springer, 1991). One concrete and unfortunately still controversial harm reduction approach is needle exchange, where active users are given new needles when they return their used ones (thus preventing them from being sold to other addicts and spreading HIV and hepatitis C). Additionally, needle exchange programs provide counseling and HIV education and increase the likelihood that if someone does wish to address his or her drug use they can be guided to an appropriate drug treatment program.

One study of substance abuse treatment centers in the United States found that 99 percent reported using an abstinence-based model of treatment. Ninety-three percent of all drug and alcohol treatment centers in the United States base their programs on the 12-Step model of treatment (Roman & Blum, 1997). Harm reduction is now expanding into a therapeutic modality employed with individuals engaging in any kind of potentially self-destructive behavior that they are reluctant to stop doing (Denning, 2000; Tatarsky, 2002). In the past decade, harm reduction has gained widespread acceptance as a viable treatment approach to substance abuse around the United States and Europe (Tatarsky, 2002; MacMaster, 2004). Donald McVinney, director of education and training at the Harm Reduction Coalition in Manhattan, informed me that harm reduction is a central part of the official policy for treatment efforts aimed at men who abuse crystal in the cities of San Francisco and Seattle, which will be described later in this chapter (D. McVinney, personal communication via e-mail April 12, 2005). In addition to being an effective treatment strategy for substance-abusing clients, I have found that a harm reduction approach is also an effective way of working with gay men who bareback, as I will describe in detail in Chapter 8.

STAGES OF CHANGE MODEL

Whatever counseling model one uses, it is essential for the therapist to pay attention to where the person is in the change process so that appropriate interventions to *that* stage of change can be offered, neither lagging behind the client nor pushing the client ahead prematurely. Prochaska and DiClemente (1982) developed the Trans-Theoretical Stages of Change Model, which conceptualizes concrete stages that both client and therapist can identify in order to understand exactly where the client is in terms of "recovery readiness." The result is that the therapist and client collaborate, which strengthens their alliance and therefore increases the positive impact of the therapeutic relationship. In traditional therapy with substance abusers, that relationship can become adversarial, confrontative, and shaming of the client. The client often felt beleaguered by "interventions" and having his or her "denial" confronted by the therapist.

MOTIVATIONAL INTERVIEWING

In 1992, Prochaska, DiClemente, and Narcross expanded the Stages of Change model specifically to address substance use. The expanded model posits that people go through the following stages in the process of changing: precontemplation, contemplation, determination/preparation, action, and maintenance (Prochaska, DiClemente, & Narcross, 1992). Motivational interviewing, a therapeutic approach based on the Stages of Change model, was developed by psychologists and substance abuse treatment professionals William Miller and Stephen Rollnick (1991). It is a set of strategies for intervention based on which stage the person is in; fundamental to its successful utilization is that the worker takes a nonjudgmental stance that allows and encourages the client to move through the stages of change at a comfortable pace. Motivational interviewing is an ideal tool for use with men who are barebacking.

What follows is an overview of the stages of change with intervention strategies for each stage.[9] In the following section, when I discuss motivational interviewing, harm reduction, moderation management, and motivational enhancement therapy, it may seem as if at times they blend together. In clinical practice they indeed often do overlap. Similarly, when I give specific examples of interventions that utilize motivational interviewing I am being purposefully ambiguous regarding whether I am talking about using motivational interviewing for barebacking or for drugs because the two are so intimately intertwined.

Precontemplation

The precontemplator is not ready for change and has not expressed a commitment to change. The person may not acknowledge having a problem or may be demoralized by life, personal history, or failures. An example could be a drug-treatment client who has been coerced by the legal system or by intimates to enter treatment, yet the person has no strong internal desire to become drug free. For a barebacker who is in the precontemplation stage, if he even arrives in a therapist's office (and at this stage it would be very unusual for a barebacker to seek counseling), it is because the physician or HIV test counselor has strongly urged the individual to do so after repeated HIV tests following high-risk behavior.

Working with precontemplators in therapy, the main goals are engagement (developing a positive relationship with the client or potential client), assessment (starting to figure out what the person needs), helping with safety issues and survival needs as requested, offering education about important issues or areas of concern, and developing discrepancy. Discrepancy can be defined as the difference between what the client wants and what exists now. For instance, a man who barebacks and acknowledges that he does not want to become infected with HIV but is not sure that he will be able to commit to using condoms for anal sex is exhibiting signs of discrepancy. This can be reflected back to him by the helping professional in order to engage him in the process of change. Until he sees his own discrepancies, change will be almost impossible.

Contemplation

The contemplation stage centers around ambivalence. The person has some awareness of a problem and considers change while at the same time rejecting it. The helping professional works with the client to create a "decisional balance" or a cost/benefit analysis of the particular issue. I always start with the positives: "What is good about your use of crystal?" or "What is good about sex without condoms?" A list is created of the positives, and when the items on it are fully explored, I delve into the negatives. "What is not so good about taking crystal?" "What kinds of difficulties arise from your having anal sex with strangers without condoms?" A list is created for the minus side of the equation. With no rush, the positives and negatives are explored nonjudgmentally. It is important to help the client remove himself from judging the situation and instead try to objectively analyze it, without any particular outcome established as the correct one.

Ambivalence on the part of users about stopping all use of the substance has been greatly underestimated in traditional behavior change work, especially around drug problems. We too often assume that drug use or barebacking is unambiguously negative, and that anyone would want to get off drugs or should always want to use a condom to reduce the risk of contracting HIV. It is possible that a part of the client probably feels that way, but another part enjoys the benefits of drug use or barebacking and wants to continue. These two opposing stances push and pull the client, often leading to a stalemate without any progress being made toward positive change. A barebacker who is in the contemplation stage is highly anxious about possibly having become infected during a recent unsafe sexual encounter, goes to an HIV test center or physician's office requesting an HIV test or PEP (postexposure prophylaxis, which was discussed in Chapter 3), and comes to therapy consumed with anxiety because of having taken sexual risks. At the same time, on some level he knows that most likely he will continue to take the same risks in the future.

Preparation/Determination

During this stage the client makes strong statements about the need to change but has not yet begun to change. The helping professional must help the client set goals, perhaps both long-term and short-term, and make a commitment to the selected goals. Sometimes, when trying to tackle drug abuse issues, a person may decide that cutting down and managing the drug use better are the short-term goals for now, and that someday total abstinence may be the best choice, but not now. Regarding barebacking, a short-term goal might be to try only to have unprotected anal sex with people of the same HIV status, or if the man is HIV-positive, not to ejaculate inside of anyone and not have partners ejaculate inside him.

After goals are established, a plan for change must be constructed. How will these goals be reached? First, therapists can empower the client by reminding him that the plan is up to him, that there are any number of plans that could work, and that only he can be the judge of what will work for him, but that the therapist is available to suggest some things that have worked for others. Depending on the issue, therapists use traditional interventions, alternative or complementary interventions, a range of counseling models, spiritual paths, or whatever appeals to the client and is accessible. For example, for a drug problem, clients can go to traditional drug treatment programs (inpatient or outpatient) or detoxification, or one could join a 12-step self-help group. Alternatively, there are acupuncture, Reiki, nutritional interventions, various models of counseling, or drug-use management groups. The client might also decide to attempt a "geographical cure," literally moving away from the people, places, and things that are temptations influencing him to use drugs or bareback, though this method is almost always doomed to failure. The client might decide to go for psychotherapy to work on underlying problems that drive the drug use (such as past trauma) or combine these various modalities to achieve a plan that is unique for this individual. A plan for barebackers, for instance, might include the men carrying condoms with them, or might entail broaching the topic of "playing safely" with potential sexual partners even if they are not committed to foregoing a potential sexual adventure if the partner refuses to use condoms. When the plan is established and the person is ready, it is time to take action.

Action

Without all the previous stages of preparation, the action stage can fail miserably, and unfortunately all helping professionals are quite familiar with this reality from failures with clients. Simply put, the action plan will not work if the client is not motivated and if the client has not resolved his ambivalence. That being said, it is also true that no one ever *completely* resolves ambivalence, and some ambivalent feelings will generally remain even after change is achieved, but it must be *sufficiently* resolved before attempting to take action, and the person needs to be much more on the change end of the continuum than the stuck-in-ambivalence end. For instance, if a man who has regularly been barebacking with strangers does begin to use condoms, he may never stop missing how much more spontaneous and pleasurable sex was without a condom, even though he now engages in whatever plan or intervention he created to get himself to stop the risky behavior. One example of a plan might be for a man who is either HIV-negative or HIV-positive who is not ready to stop barebacking, but who has decided that he will only bareback with a person of the same HIV status. Thus, a man who decides to ask about HIV status before having sex may discover that while he wants very much to be able to do this, he cannot do it in person. His plan should be revised so that he starts making the inquiry about HIV status in a safer venue, such as during online chats with potential partners, rather than face to face. If he cannot bring himself to use condoms, he might choose only to have sex with individuals who identify as having the same HIV status as his own in their online profiles. While foregoing condoms, he also understands he puts himself at risk, but it may be somewhat less harmful than having sex with a man without asking his HIV status.

I often use a technique in my practice that combines harm reduction and motivational interviewing. I ask clients to determine what quantity of crystal they think is a moderate amount for them and whether they can make a plan to try to limit their use of crystal to that amount. Similarly, I also ask them how often they want to be using crystal. After they make these determinations, I ask if they are ready to make a plan to stick to the limits of how much and how often to use that they have set for themselves. If they are confident of their ability to do that, then I formally call that "the plan." If I hear or sense any ambivalence about their trying to commit to this plan, then I back up and explore what they feel is getting in the way of their sticking to their self-defined limits. Over the course of the following weeks, I ask them to report honestly how successful they were in keeping to the plan. If they are unable to maintain the limit they set, I ask them what they think it means. I always try to remain nonjudgmental when they report not sticking to their own limits. Not infrequently, the client will report eventually that it means that he is unable to limit his intake and has to stop using altogether.

Maintenance

Behavior change, especially when it first commences, is fragile. It is essential to reinforce the change and support the client to maintain the new behaviors. It may be helpful with certain types of behavior change to build lapses into the maintenance stage. For an uninfected individual who is trying to stop barebacking with strangers of unknown HIV status, a lapse might be trusting someone he knows enough who says he is HIV-negative to have bareback sex with him when his goal is to move toward regular condom use except within a committed partnership.

Therapists as well as agencies should consider designing their programs and treatment strategies in such a way that people can come back as needed for reinforcement and support without a lot of red tape and without shame or stigma. The 12-Step structure is very good for the maintenance stage. People can go to meetings and get group support as much or as little as they need, for the rest of their lives, without intakes, fees, or hoops to jump through.

HARM REDUCTION AND CRYSTAL

Crystal meth greatly complicates life for HIV-positive gay and bisexual men in ways that go far beyond barebacking. Many of the problems that an individual experiences as a result of taking crystal occur because, when high on crystal, the person becomes so preoccupied with dancing or having sex that he becomes oblivious to normal bodily sensations like thirst and hunger or medication schedules. For HIV-positive men who are taking the class of antiretroviral drugs known as protease inhibitors and who use crystal, missing medications is not the only concern. Methamphetamine has been shown to interact with this class of antiretroviral medications in such a way that the effect of methamphetamine becomes two to three times greater for men on combination therapy. This is especially true for men taking the protease inhibitor Ritonavir (Out, 1997; Horn, 1998; Urbino & Jones, 2004). The implications are alarming. Men infected with HIV are likely to feel the effects of crystal more profoundly than other users do.

With individuals who use crystal and are not ready to contemplate stopping, I take a harm reduction approach with the goals of reducing the physical damage that they may do to themselves or others as much as possible and educating them about the effects of meth when combined with their medication. For instance, I make the following suggestions to HIV-positive men who are planning to use crystal:

- Purchase a pocket-sized medicine case that can be programmed to beep when it is time for them to take a dose of their antiretroviral medication.
- Disclose their HIV status to prospective sex partners.
- Stay hydrated in order to minimize bodily damage.
- Carry protein bars or other nutritionally complete and portable sources of nutrition that they can easily eat while partying at a club, the baths, a sex party, etc.

It is not uncommon for men who take crystal to begin partying on Friday evening and not stop until Sunday night or Monday, having had little if any food, water, or sleep. As happened to Phillip, when Monday morning comes, they are in no shape to go to work. There are two other suggestions I make to clients when I take a harm reduction approach to their crystal use. If it is the weekend of a big circuit party that a client plans to attend and where crystal use is a sure thing, I urge him to take the following Monday and possibly even Tuesday off as vacation days. For clients who begin to use crystal while partying sexually over the weekend, I urge them to begin on Friday night and end by Sunday morning, which will allow them sufficient time to recuperate before they need to be back at work on Monday. If they are not able to follow these suggestions, I then use this as a way of reflecting to them their discrepancies about their relationship to crystal. It is so common for men who have used crystal throughout a weekend to feel so physically and profoundly depressed on Monday that in Manhattan one CMA (Crystal Meth Anonymous) meeting scheduled for Tuesday nights has been named the "suicide Tuesday" meeting. I also never schedule appointments with clients who use crystal for Mondays, as they often do not show up, or if they do manage to drag themselves to a session they are not in any condition to make productive use of therapy since they are so strung out from the after effects of a crystal binge. My colleague, Dr. Jeffrey Guss, finds that psychotherapy sessions with men in the immediate aftermath of a crystal binge can potentially be powerful (personal communication).

MODERATION MANAGEMENT

A modified version of harm reduction is known as "moderation management." Moderation management (MM) is a behavioral change program and national support group network for people concerned about their drinking and who desire to make positive lifestyle changes. MM empowers individuals to accept personal responsibility for choosing and maintaining their own path, whether moderation or abstinence, and in this it differs from the 12-step abstinence-only model. MM promotes early self-recognition of risky drinking behavior and sees moderate drinking as a more easily achievable goal than no drinking at all. MM offers a supportive, mutual-help environment that encourages people who are concerned about their drinking to take action to cut back or quit drinking before drinking problems become severe (Moderation Management Web site, 2004).

MM was designed to address the problems of early-stage problem drinkers. Though originally conceived as a strategy to help problem drinkers, its tenets can easily be translated to clinical work with any person who is not yet chemically dependent or addicted but who has a problematic relationship with a substance, especially crystal. Identifying the early onset of a problematic pattern of use may help prevent a man from becoming addicted. The MM Web site explains: "Nine out of ten problem drinkers today actively and purposefully avoid traditional treatment approaches. This is because they know that most traditional programs will label them as alcoholic, probably force attendance at 12-step and abstinence-based meetings, and prescribe lifetime abstinence as the only acceptable change in drinking." The Web site also states that approximately one third of people who get help from MM meetings do eventually go to a 12-Step program, further reinforcing the harm reduction concept that as long as the individual feels free to choose which option is best for him or her, some will see the utility of choosing abstinence. Employing a moderation management approach with men who enter treatment with questions about their use of crystal is ideal for enabling them to assess for themselves whether they are able to moderate their use of the drug. Once a person has come to the conclusion for himself that his drug use is either out of control or causing a problem in one or more areas of his life, he is often more ready to address his substance use problem.

Critics may wonder how useful MM can be in the face of a highly addictive substance. From observations made by numerous men engaged in various levels of crystal use, it seems apparent that not everyone who uses crystal becomes addicted to it, though almost all crystal users are at some risk of becoming addicted (Urbino & Jones, 2004). It has been argued that if someone is addicted to crystal meth, then a harm reduction model may not be as practical or helpful as an abstinence model. Petros Levounis, M.D., psychiatrist, and director of the Addiction Institute of New York, does not feel that harm reduction is an appropriate intervention for men who are addicted to crystal (personal communication, August 16, 2004). I agree with Dr. Levounis that for men who are crystal addicts harm reduction may not be an appropriate treatment strategy. Yet, for men who can moderate their use of crystal, harm reduction is an essential component of treating them. I have also found that taking a harm reduction approach with men whose use of crystal is clearly out of control allows us to create a therapeutic alliance and earn the client's trust. For crystal addicts who are unable, unwilling, or simply not ready to stop using, harm reduction is a way to engage them in treatment until such time as they are ready to make changes pertaining to their crystal use. I have found that attempting a moderation management approach for men whose use is clearly out of control is an excellent step in helping them see that they are not able to return to using crystal moderately once they have become addicted to it.

ANDREW, A RATIONAL BAREBACKER

The following case illustrates how moderation management, harm reduction, and eventually abstinence led to significant behavior change in one of my clients. Andrew is a 43-year-old, HIV-positive businessman who had educated himself about the scientific and medical aspects of the illness as well as transmission over the many years he had lived with HIV. He is on combination therapy and in good health and is in a committed partnership of many years that has always been sexually nonexclusive. Prior to first trying crystal in 2000, Andrew would go to one of the local sex clubs or bathhouses to have sex with outside partners while doing a small dose of Ecstasy, a stimulant drug not chemically related to crystal. Eventually, he began to need almost a full week to recuperate after a weekend of taking Ecstasy. When he discussed this with a friend at the gym one day, the friend told him about crystal and (erroneously) said that if he only did a little bit, he would not have any ill effects afterward.

Andrew began using crystal during a period in his relationship when his partner had to relocate out of New York, which meant he had more time on his own. The first time he did it, he inhaled a small amount at home and then went to the baths where he met two other men who offered him more, and the three of them went home to party together for the next 24 hours. He described immediately falling in love with the sex and crystal combination. Prior to starting crystal, he almost always had safer sex but occasionally did lapse into barebacking. In order not to have any moral or ethical qualms about barebacking, he never allowed himself to ejaculate inside anyone unless the person identified himself as already being HIV-positive.

The weekend after his first experience with crystal, he did it again and even smoked it, realizing that he needed twice as much to feel as good on it as he had felt just 1 week earlier. He immediately became part of an entire "Don't ask, don't tell" culture in the world of crystal sex partiers with regard to his HIV status. Since he was using the Internet to find sex partners, he added HIV-positive to his online profile and stated that he preferred that his partners also be HIV-positive so that any men with whom he hooked up would know that he had HIV before they ever met in person. When he went to sex parties while high on crystal, he would only disclose his HIV status about half the time, but if he was playing with more than one man at a time, he almost never raised the topic.

He remembers that at several parties, after hours of people having unprotected sex, someone would admit that he did not know what his own HIV status was. Andrew thought that this was sad and shocking since with the advances in HIV treatment early diagnosis was an important aspect of managing the disease. He also comforted himself with the thoughts that he remained adherent to his medication regime even while high and that his viral levels remained below the level of detectability. He felt that especially since he was never coming inside partners who did not tell him that they were also HIV-positive, he was not placing anyone else at a high risk for becoming infected. He describes an interesting bit of cognitive dissonance in this regard when he explained: "I did not consider myself infectious even though I did think that men who allowed themselves to be fucked at those parties were placing themselves at risk for becoming infected if they were not already. The reason I thought the men who didn't know their status were at extreme risk was because I often spoke with poz guys at these parties who must have had high viral loads since they were not taking any antiretrovirals. Strange as it seems, during cigarette breaks between rounds of sex, I'd have some quick conversations with guys about their HIV status, and their T4 counts and viral load counts, and what treatments they were on. I would always share the information I discovered and told them where they could go online to educate themselves. There were plenty of poz guys who hadn't started treatment yet, with viral loads over 50K. So I always felt the environment was risky for a negative guy; I just didn't think I was the most infectious person in the room. In fact, of the poz guys, since I didn't ejaculate into my partners' mouths or butts, and I was always undetectable, I was probably the least infectious poz guy at most parties."

Within a month of beginning to use crystal, Andrew realized that he had a serious drug problem and began therapy specifically to address his crystal use. But his original goal was to be able to scale back his use to a moderate amount of drug and to do crystal less often so that it would not interfere with his life. I told him that I did not know if this was possible, but perhaps he would be the first one for whom this approach worked.

Andrew began to go to CMA meetings and struggled to control his crystal use but was not successful. He describes himself as a "chronic relapser" during his first year in CMA. When he began to do things that he specifically said he would never do, like take crystal every day while his partner was in New York, use drugs while on his job, and have the kinds of sex at sex clubs that he would never have engaged in had he been sober, he became frightened and checked himself into a residential drug treatment program. After two years of being abstinent, he still barebacks but now will only have condomless anal sex with men who are also HIV-positive. He will let uninfected men top him, but only if they tell him that this is something that they regularly do, that they know his HIV status, and they are not high on drugs or seem to be doing this impulsively.

Andrew's case is interesting to me because he is clearly a very intelligent and well-informed individual who regularly reads the scientific literature about HIV/AIDS as soon as it is published either in journals or on the Internet. He also has taken it upon himself to educate the men he has sex with so that risks of HIV transmission can be greatly reduced. He is also an ethical person who does not want to spread HIV, and he bases his behaviors on information he has gleaned from his readings about what minimizes and maximizes the risk of transmitting the virus. Now that he only has sex when sober, he will not permit himself ever to allow a man who says that he is uninfected to be his bottom. He once told me that he has "as much knowledge about the scientific aspects of HIV and AIDS as practically any infectious disease resident," and from our conversations this is not an idle boast or merely a rationalization that allows him to continue to bareback while not feeling badly about what he is doing.

Andrew is also an example of someone who does not fit many of the typical profiles of someone who barebacks. A highly functioning gay man who has deep friendships with other gay men, Andrew has a strong and positive gay identity. Although he did present with some symptoms of depression, these abated after he became sober. Unlike many barebackers, he practiced some sexual self-control even while high on crystal by not ejaculating inside of sexual partners who had identified themselves as HIV-negative. His motivation for this restraint may have been conscience. Drawing this boundary seemed to make it easier for Andrew not to feel as conflicted about barebacking and possibly spreading HIV to others. Perhaps it allowed him to maintain a self-image of someone who was ethical and caring despite engaging in sexual behaviors that could put others at risk.

DIFFICULTY FOR THE THERAPIST

When I first presented Andrew's case to a peer group of gay male therapists, each of the seven other therapists voiced dismay at his behavior and the likely futility of getting him to stop barebacking even after he became sober. The conversation made me uncomfortable, and I voiced my concerns that there were a lot of negative judgments being expressed that might be a counterproductive influence on my work with Andrew. Several of my colleagues suggested that perhaps I was not being judgmental enough with this client, which gave me pause. Then one of my brave colleagues, who had been the most vociferously judgmental, admitted that he was envious of what Andrew was doing and was in fact turned on by the descriptions of his sexual adventures. An immediate silence descended on the group. We sat there uncomfortably until another therapist and then another admitted that they too had similar feelings. Soon I too shared something I had not been aware of prior to this supervision. I was envious of Andrew. He was in a partnership and was also having sex with men outside the relationship. I was in a monogamous relationship where my partner and I had explicitly agreed not to have sex with other men. I also found myself titillated by

Andrew's descriptions of his exploits. This began a rich conversation of our own therapeutic limits with patients whom we found attractive or sexually provocative, whom we envied or simply liked very much, which was the case with how I felt about Andrew. During this supervision session it became clear to me that I was experiencing a classic case of countertransference that had been interfering with my ability to be as clear and effective as good therapy requires. My liking Andrew so much had resulted in my idealizing him and buying into his defensive presentation about how ethical and noble he was being in the way he barebacked. This supervision session also explored our concerns about vicarious erotic titillation and how to best cope with those issues when they spring up during treatment. One of the most valuable things I took away from this supervision was that I had not been aware of how much I identified with, liked, and respected Andrew, and how my affection had interfered with my ability to correctly assess the dynamics of his behavior.

In the next session with Andrew following this supervision, I suggested to him that all of his rationalizing and explaining about how careful he is not to spread HIV to partners might just indicate that he is not as at peace with barebacking as he would like to be. Hearing this, he bristled. Eventually, he began to admit there "just might be some truth" in what I suggested. I began to ask him to consider what role if any his being HIV-positive might be playing in continuing to bareback. This did seem to strike a chord with him as he grew quiet and seemed to become sad as he thought about this and admitted that this would need to be explored. My goal is not to get Andrew to stop the behavior but only to be as mindful as possible about why he is doing it and of how he evaluates the benefits as compared to the risks of continuing to bareback.

Andrew's experiences on crystal are fairly typical of other users of crystal. Almost all addicts find it easy to rationalize behaviors that they would not engage in if they weren't high. Andrew seems to me to fall into the category of a "rational" barebacker, insofar as he was always aware of the risks both to himself and to other men, as evidenced by his use of serosorting and withdrawal before ejaculating as methods to minimize the risks to other men. It would be easy in Andrew's case to conclude that it was the seductive power of crystal that transformed a rational and previously not self-destructive individual into a regular barebacker. We would have to rethink that theory in the face of the truth that now that Andrew is sober, he continues to bareback. Perhaps the truth is that drugs alone are not the only seducer of gay men in terms of barebacking. According to the now-sober Andrew, even without crystal, he is drawn to having unprotected sex. Sex without condoms can be risky, but it can also be powerfully intoxicating, even for the sober, well-informed gay man.

COMPULSIVITY AND BAREBACKING

Might barebacking itself be a compulsive behavior for some men? Pleasure and excitement seem to have been the major motivations for Andrew's barebacking, first when high on crystal, and later when sober. Men like Andrew seem to more readily be able to admit they have a problem with drugs than to admit they cannot or do not want to stop high-risk sexual behaviors. At first, Andrew was reluctant to admit that barebacking was self-destructive (though he readily identified his crystal use as being so). He obviously compartmentalized much of his knowledge about the risks to his health from other STDs or a multidrug-resistant strain of HIV. Even though he sought therapy knowing that he had a serious drug problem, it took Andrew a long time to accept that his use of drugs had caused his life to spin totally out of control. He still has difficulty acknowledging or admitting ambivalent feelings about barebacking. I sympathize with him as it is hard to view activities that he once did with no negative consequences as possibly being either self-injurious or harmful to others.

CRITIQUE OF THE HARM REDUCTION MODEL

The connection between drug use, particularly the use of crystal meth, and barebacking has been clearly demonstrated. Not everyone will agree, however, on how best to address the problem. I understand that the harm reduction model has its critics. The most common criticism is that it actually enables clients in their drug use and sexual risk-taking. After long consideration, I have come to the conclusion that engaging with my clients where they are, not where I wish they would be, is the most effective intervention I have found. From a practical viewpoint, the therapist cannot and should not make decisions for the client, and should make therapy a safe place for clients. Being patient can be very frustrating and even frightening at times to those of us on the front lines who are watching the AIDS epidemic start to heat up again.

CONCLUSION: INTERNET OUTREACH

Part of psychotherapeutic work with clients is to help them evaluate to what extent they want to reduce or eliminate their risky behaviors. Barebacking and drug use are two community-wide problems, and I believe we need a community-wide movement to address the crystal meth problem, which is fueling the barebacking phenomenon. There are several innovative projects going on right now that use the Internet to educate the gay and bisexual male community about the risks of crystal meth and its connection to barebacking. So far, I have only briefly touched on the role of the Internet and its use as a vehicle for cruising by vast numbers of gay men. The myriad influences of the Internet will be examined in more detail in the next chapter. But in addition to being a venue where gay men meet one another for sexual liaisons, which often take place under the influence of drugs, the Internet provides opportunities to educate gay men about health risks. There are two Web sites that are specifically aimed at gay men who use crystal and that take a harm reduction approach:

In June 1997 the Web site tweaker.org was launched. It states, "We recognize that people use crystal meth. We're not here to condemn it. We're not here to promote it. Instead, we offer information, support, and resources to help gay and bisexual men better understand crystal and how it affects physical, mental, and sexual health" (www.tweaker.org, 2004). This site offers a variety of educational information about how to make crystal use safer and also resources for treatment in the San Francisco Bay area. It has online forums specifically dedicated to men who think that they contracted HIV while doing crystal and true stories of men who did. A similar Web site out of Seattle is crystalneon.org. It also takes an educational and harm reduction approach to crystal use by gay and bisexual men. These Web sites are concrete attempts to meet gay and bisexual crystal users directly where they are in order to provide them with ways to learn about various options that exist to help them.

In response to the rise of both new cases of syphilis and crystal use among gay men in New England who met in Internet chat rooms, Manhunt, one of the largest gay male Web sites in the United States, began to provide space on the Web site where gay men could become educated about issues that were vital to their sexual health as well as educated about substance use and where treatment was available. Initially, Manhunt posted banner advertisements alerting users of the site to the rise of syphilis in New England and where they could go for free screening and if necessary treatment. In March 2004, Manhunt revised its profile so that members' profiles could no longer contain PNP (party and play, which signals directly a desire to have sex while under the influence of drugs), and that any profiles that did not delete this would be removed. Manhunt also collaborated with the Fenway Community Health Center in Boston and developed a series of public information messages about crystal that appear as banner advertisements on the site. A button was also added that reads "Need Help," and when this is clicked a list of local AIDS service organizations and drug treatment facilities appears. Finally, just before one logs off of Manhunt, the following banner ad appears: "If you use crystal, you are digging your own grave." As of this writing, Manhunt works with 15 departments of health and more than 50 community-based organizations that can do partner notification. When a man goes to a clinic and tests positive for an STD, he is now asked if he met his sexual partner online. If the man says yes and states that it was on Manhunt, the group will log on and anonymously let the partner of the infected individual know that he may have contracted an STD (Adelson, 2005). In Chapter 8, I will describe a variety of creative and innovative interventions that have been designed to reach gay men online. In the following chapter, I will explore the connections between barebacking and the Internet in-depth.

CHAPTER FIVE

Cruising the Internet Highway

"Cute Bottom 4 Barebacking Top – 24"

"Looking for White Bareback Jock Tops Under 40"

"Hot, Sweaty, Bareback Sex, Loads of Fun– 36"

"Insatiable Dom Bondage Top Needs Submissive Bondage Bottom – 49"

"Need A Load In Me Today – 32 (Your Place)"

"Positive Men – 32"

"Burly, Butch, and Barebacker"

"Suck Me Off At My Place – 33"

"I Want To Have Some Fun! – 29"

"HIV + Looking For Hot Mouth (Uncut) – 34"

"Asian for Asians"

"Wanna Know. How I Got HIV? – 49"

"Hot, Uncut Latino Into Juice – 37"

"Poz Seeks Same for Raw Sex – 44"

"Athletic and Sexy Seeks Same – 34"

The above headlines came up when I went to the "personals" section of craigslist.org, chose "men seeking men" and specified a search for barebackers. This is only one of many Web sites where men who desire condomless sex find one another on the Internet. The fact that this particular site is not even specifically for barebackers provides a glimpse into how easy and pervasive using the Internet to locate partners to bareback with has become.

MARIO, CYBER CRUISING, AND BAREBACKING

Mario was a 30-year-old professional referred to me by his physician after his third HIV test in as many months had come back negative. Concerned, Mario's doctor asked him why he was getting tested so often. Mario admitted to having frequent unsafe sex with partners he met through the Internet. During my first session with Mario, we talked about his sexual adventures, which included barebacking, and I asked him if he was afraid of contracting HIV. Shrugging, he replied that he didn't want to get infected, but on the other hand it wouldn't be the end of the world if it happened. A friend of his had recently become HIV-positive and was taking combination antiretroviral therapy. The friend had told him that the drugs did not create any adverse side effects. Mario's feeling was that HIV was not a death sentence these days, and if he did become infected he would just get on the drug treatments and that would take care of it.

I was taken aback by his nonchalance and also the misinformation on which he was basing his actions. True, the drug treatments can be effective, but side effects are the norm, and the medications are expensive and a major intrusion on one's life. Also, no one knows how long the drugs will work to keep HIV-positive people from developing AIDS. I became more concerned as I heard Mario describe how this same friend had regaled him with stories about the exciting sex parties he was attending where HIV-positive men were all having unprotected sex with one another. The friend was making HIV infection sound like a great idea. When I reflected this back to Mario, he told me that he did not (at least consciously) want to become infected with HIV, but on the other hand he did not want to give up barebacking, despite some ambivalence.

It took a lot more probing before Mario admitted that he had more than just "some ambivalence" about taking sexual risks, and after 2 months of therapy he admitted that he had a lot of anxiety, which he had to work hard to ignore. But while he was afraid of getting HIV, he was also enormously pleased with his sexual successes. His sex life was the predominant aspect of his social life — in other words, sex is where he received most of his affirmation, affection, camaraderie, and self-esteem. In his mind, the benefits of his sexual adventures outweighed the risks he knew he was taking.

Since I knew that being confrontational or judgmental would not enable Mario and I to form a therapeutic alliance, I employed motivational interviewing (Miller and Rollnick, 2002), which was described in Chapter 4, to explore Mario's complicated motivations about his sexual behavior. I found him to be refreshingly open when we discussed his barebacking. He readily explained that there was a specific rationale to why he barebacked: it made him more sexually popular. "By not even raising the issue of condoms or HIV status with sex partners, I feel that my sexual currency is increased," he told me. "This way, I get to have sex with men who are more attractive than I am. If I were to ask guys their HIV status or bring up safer sex, those guys might not be interested in hooking up since there are plenty of guys who don't bring up safer sex or HIV status with someone they're interested in playing with. I just don't want to take the chance of messing up my opportunities to hook up with such sexy and exciting guys. And besides," he told me, "I never chat online with people whose profiles say they're HIV-positive."

Because his barebacking was linked to his need to feel desirable and popular, I asked questions about his early years. Growing up, Mario never felt he was popular. Although he was a high achiever in academics, he was unathletic and lacked social confidence. In high school he had associated with "the other nerds and brainy types." During college, he met other gay students on campus, made friends, and even dated some of them. He began to work out regularly at the college gym, but although he gained muscle, his self-image remained that of a skinny, unattractive man.

When he first came to New York to begin graduate school, he began to meet people with whom he became friends as well as sexual partners. When one of his sex partners complimented him on his body and offered to photograph him with his digital camera, Mario agreed on a lark. He told me he was not just pleasantly surprised but thrilled with how he looked in the photos. He decided to do something he had never done before: create an online profile. He wrote a short statement about his sexual tastes and the kind of men he was interested in. He began to send his bare-chested photo to men he chatted with when they asked if he had a picture. Soon, he found that men whom he never would have had the confidence to approach in bars or clubs were inviting him to hook up for sexual adventures. It was not long until Mario stopped going to bars or clubs and spent most of his free time cyber cruising and hooking up in person with men he met online. This has been his primary recreational pastime for the last 2 years. Now at age 30, he finally felt he had come into his own, socially. He was sought after by hot gay men he met on the Internet, and he was enjoying newly elevated self-esteem.

Like Andrew in the last chapter, Mario employed serosorting (Suarez & Miller, 2001) as a kind of self-constructed harm reduction approach to barebacking (see Chapter 4). Serosorting is well documented in the social science literature (Hort, 2000; Suarez & Miller, 2001; Mansergh et al., 2002), and is often described by barebackers who are clients of mine. While he came to admit that he was not exactly blasé about contracting HIV, Mario still felt powerfully drawn to seeking out high-risk sexual liaisons; I believe, however, that this was not because he needed the thrill of the risk, but because he needed the boosted self-image that came with partnering with men he considered hot. Interestingly, he never said that the sex was better with these men, but he said honestly that he felt better about himself because his partners were powerfully attractive.

COMPUTERS, SEX, AND HIV: CHAPTER OVERVIEW

I have had a computer since the early 1980s, and by the mid 1980s I was using it regularly for writing and managing my practice, although I did not get e-mail until 1990. I remember being surprised the first time a friend confided to me that he was meeting men online, and the whole point was to have phone sex, masturbate while e-mailing one another sexually specific fantasies, or meet in person for a liaison. Naively, it had never entered my mind before this that the Internet was a tool for getting dates or hooking up. A few years later, it became more common to hear men talk about foregoing the often intimidating bar scene for the relative ease of meeting men online.

An entire online gay culture has blossomed in the last decade, transforming how gay and bisexual men meet one another. It is as dramatic as the change from gay bars being underground hideaways that were periodically raided by the police to becoming hip, chic, clean, and well-lit clubs that exist in most urban centers around the world in developed countries today. The Internet has streamlined the whole pickup and mating ritual. Since online profiles explicitly state sexual desires and preferences, no longer does a man have to engage in idle chatter while trying to figure out what the sexy man with whom he is talking might like to do in bed or worry that this man he has just met might freak out once he learns what you want to do with him. There was a time when men would wear hankies of various colors to signify what sexual behavior they were looking for. Now, the search engine has replaced the hanky, and men are able to more easily find men who share their sexual interests.

In preceding chapters, we read about studies that found that barebackers primarily find other barebackers on the Internet. In this chapter, we will take an up-close look at how barebackers are meeting, what kinds of information they are exchanging (about HIV status and sexual tastes) before they hook up, and what level of consciousness of risk-taking exists on the Web sites.

The most disturbing side of barebacking for anyone who is concerned about the spread of HIV and AIDS is those who are intentionally spreading HIV or who seek to become infected. We discussed this very briefly in Chapter 1 when I mentioned "bug chasers" and "gift givers." In this chapter, we will take a look at what percentage of barebackers fall into these categories and review research that investigates the psychological motivation of bug chasers.

Finally, we will look at how the gay culture is changing. Sex parties for HIV-positive men and "conversion" parties are now part of our community. What does this mean for the future of gay men in the age of AIDS?

HOOKING UP ONLINE

There are a lot of reasons why gay men have embraced online chat rooms as a way of hooking up. It cuts through the uncomfortable small talk men traditionally had to endure in face-to-face encounters. It alleviates social anxieties, and for bisexual men or men who are struggling to come out, affords more privacy to figure out one's feelings about one's queer attractions while talking about them in the safety of virtual reality. For the majority of men, these benefits seem to outweigh the immediacy of cruising bars. Drawbacks to using the Internet to meet include the lack of real-time erotic flirtation that precedes an actual first encounter and often, the absence of romance. It may be convenient, but seeking sex on the Internet can contribute to a person's remaining isolated and not developing requisite social skills that come with face-to-face conversation and real, face-to-face interactions.

A whole generation has grown up and come out in the world of online Internet chat rooms. Internet chat rooms have been hailed as "the new gay bar" (Fries, 1998, p. 24), and the Internet has made it simple and straightforward to find sexual partners. Because people can anonymously and confidentially advertise for partners to act out their sexual desires and interests, it makes men like Mario — who were put off by feeling easily intimidated in real-life settings such as bars — more bold about pursuing their sexual fantasies and approaching men whom they would have thought beyond their reach in a bar or club. Men like Mario, who felt overwhelmed by the potential of face-to-face rejection in bars and clubs, have experienced a kind of liberation on the Internet.

Men meet in gay chat rooms across the Internet. The sites are easy to find, and there are a wide variety of types of chat rooms based on sexual preferences. Just as men who are into sado/masochism (S/M), muscle boys, or bears would have frequented a local bar that catered to men with the same specific sexual interest, men can now visit Internet chat rooms that are filled with others who share the same interests and turn-ons. Gay chat rooms have replaced gay bars and clubs as places to meet, mingle, and flirt. Different kinds of sexual activity take place in cyberspace. Cyber sex[1] can be a session of virtual sex while exchanging instant messages (IMs), or men exchanging telephone numbers, engaging in telephone sex, or arranging to meet in person for real-world sexual liaisons. Another popular sexual sport online occurs on numerous Web sites that offer either pornographic photographs, videos, or live Web cams, which an individual can watch while possibly masturbating.

WIDESPREAD USE OF THE INTERNET TO MEET MEN

The Internet has quickly become one of the most popular venues for gay men to find sex partners (Simao, 2003). Over the course of the past 15 years, there has been a massive proliferation of online profiles. The practice of gay men meeting sexual partners online has become so popular that it is referred to by some men as "gay takeout" (Tuller, 2004). Research in the United Kingdom found that use of the Internet by gay men doubled between 1999 and 2001, and that in 2001, the Internet was the second most popular venue where men had met a new partner in the previous year (Weatherburn, Hickson, & Reid, 2003). As John Bancroft, former director of the Kinsey Institute in Bloomington, Indiana, noted: "The Internet presents us with the latest and, in many respects most powerful form of new technology to impact on sexuality" (2002, p. x). My sense of what Bancroft was referring to is that the explosion of the Internet as a way of meeting sexual partners has been the single biggest development of the sexual revolution since the birth control pill freed women from unwanted pregnancy.

Michael Ross, a professor of public health at the University of Texas, Houston, who has been conducting research on the prevalence of using the Internet for sexual purposes, has estimated that in the United States the Internet is used far and away most often for sexual purposes (Ross, 2002). He provides the following statistics regarding Internet use by people who visit sites specifically targeting gay men: "On any given weekday afternoon, there are approximately 10,000 people signed into sexual chat rooms on gay.com. The number participating during the evening hours and weekends is much higher" (Ross, 2002, p. 4). Ross was only citing numbers from one popular gay cyber cruising site. When all the other gay-specific Web sites that gay men visit are considered (such as gaydar.com; manhunt.net; and so forth), the number of visitors to gay sites rises dramatically. As of February 2005, manhunt.net had close to 300,000 active members in the United States alone (Adelson, 2005). All of the major Internet service providers (AOL, MSN, and so on) have gay-specific chat rooms where men seek social, romantic, and sexual relationships.

Accessibility, affordability, and anonymity — the "triple-A engine," according to Cooper and Griffin-Shelley (1997) — are the three most prevalent factors driving sexual contact on the Internet. For gay men, there are two additional factors, according to Tikkanen and Ross (2000): acceptability and approximation. Acceptability refers to the Internet being an acceptable way gay men meet one another and either hook up or date, and approximation refers to a dynamic important to men who have sex with men (MSM) who are unsure of their sexual identity or who may not yet have come out even to themselves. The Internet allows them a safe way to experiment with their sexual identity by approximating being gay either through fictitious selves or by having virtual sex on the Internet.

Texas psychologist Michael Ross feels that the Internet's creating the dynamic of "approximation" is like a one-way window into a gay bar; men who struggled with their same-sex sexual orientation prior to the development of the Internet did not have access to such a window. Many of those men took years to find and then go into a gay bar, a struggle that the safe space of virtual reality provided by the Internet now ameliorates (M. Ross, personal communication, 2004). These five factors combine to "turbocharge, that is, accelerate and intensify, the experience of using the Internet to seek sexual gratification" (Cooper & Griffin-Shelley, 2002, p. 5). As Ross and Kauth (2002) note: "these Quin-A engines [meaning five factors beginning with an "A"] are likely to make MSM use of the Internet more common and serve important psychological functions as well" (p. 53).

Psychologically, it may feel vastly safer for a man who is in a stage of pregay identity formation to test the waters by chatting online with men either to homosocialize or to arrange a sexual liaison, rather than having to actually brave going into a gay bar, club, or community center or having real-life sexual or social encounters, which were the only available options in the days prior to the Internet. Benotsch, Kalichman, and Cage (2002) describe how MSM individuals in general have relatively few places to meet without fear of negative social consequences. Therefore, especially for bisexual men or those who are either experimenting with or questioning their sexual orientation, the Internet can be an "important gateway for men who may not immediately feel comfortable in an overtly gay environment, but are seeking social support from individuals with similar preferences" (MacMaster, Aquino, & Vail, 2003). Perhaps not surprisingly then, one San Francisco study found that gay men were more likely than heterosexual men or women to use the Internet to meet sexual partners (Kim, Kent, & McFarland, 2001).

A Swedish study compared the differences among Swedish men who never, occasionally, and frequently visit Internet chat rooms. The findings indicated that men who used the chat rooms were younger, more likely to live at home or with a woman partner, more likely to be bisexual, less open about their homosexuality, less likely to be members of gay organizations, and more likely to engage in unprotected anal intercourse (UAI) with casual partners. The authors conclude that with these findings in mind, the Internet may be a useful place to reach younger gay and bisexual men, and those who use the chat rooms to meet sexual partners, with HIV and sexually transmitted diseases (STDs) prevention messages, often before they have publicly come out (Tikkanen & Ross, 2003).

In the United States, many men who use the Internet to meet sexual partners have well-developed gay identities and participate in the gay community. Yet, studies conducted in England show that some of the men who seek sexual partners on the Internet are not integrated into the gay community and may be using the Internet as a way to meet social and emotional as well as sexual needs. British gay men who were out to relatively few people were more likely to meet sexual partners on the Internet than were men who were out to more people in their lives. Men diagnosed with HIV were among the most likely to meet sexual partners of different or unknown HIV status on the Internet (Weatherburn et al., 2003).

BAREBACKERS ON THE INTERNET

Research on barebackers has shown that the vast majority find partners on the Internet. The rationales they gave to researchers Halkitis and Parsons (2003) include that it is easy to find sex partners who want to bareback on the Internet and that the Internet is anonymous. These men also stated that they were more likely to seek bareback sexual partners on the Internet than in bars or clubs, since online profiles often state HIV status and thus remove the awkwardness of needing to disclose or ask about HIV status. This finding seems to support the previously discussed concept that many barebackers are using "serosorting" as a way of attempting to limit the risks they take having bareback sex with other men.

Serosorting creates an interesting dilemma in how we categorize behavior as barebacking. As mentioned in Chapter 1 and Chapter 3, many social scientists differentiate between barebacking and sex without condoms or unprotected sex, where barebacking specifically refers to sex that is intentionally unsafe and carries the potential for risk of HIV being transmitted. Is it barebacking if an HIV-positive gay man has UAI with another HIV-positive gay man? There may be a risk of reinfection, but is that the same thing as becoming infected for the first time? And do HIV-negative men having UAI with each other risk transmitting HIV? Serosorting points to the fact that there are men who seek UAI but do not seek the risk of HIV infection, although the risk may be present.

Barebackers have made use of the Internet to hook up with others who are interested in UAI. As of late 2000, there were 80 different bareback electronic mailing lists (Goodroad, Kirksey, & Butensky, 2000). The Internet has become a place that offers people with a desire to engage in barebacking, whether with someone of the same or different HIV status, opportunities to meet other like-minded people and to develop both a virtual as well as real community for mutual support around it. But beyond providing opportunities to meet, Web sites that existed as early as 1998 were popularizing (and some would say glamorizing) sex without condoms. Men who wanted to bareback openly advertised this sexual preference. Visitors to any of these sites could watch bareback videos and look at bareback photographs. There are now numerous Web sites that are frank and open havens for men who want to know about, seek, and find bareback sex.

Several studies conducted both in the United States and Europe have shown that people who use the Internet to meet sexual partners are more likely to practice high-risk behaviors (Halkitis & Parsons, 2003; McFarlane, Bull, & Rietmeijer, 2000; Elford, Bolding, & Sherr, 2001; Kim et al., 2001). Factors such as loneliness and depression contribute to "cyber cruising" (using the Internet to find sexual partners) and also seem to contribute to high-risk sex. Some men, like Mario, lack the sexual self-confidence to tolerate the host of anxieties that face-to-face cruising brings up, and the Internet provides a margin of safety and comfort for them. They may use their willingness to take sexual risks as a way of becoming more attractive to other men and feeling more sexually desirable. Some depressed clients have described not having the energy or self-confidence to go out and search for sexual partners. From the comfort of their own homes they can seek out sexual partners using the Internet. Both the search for sex and the actual experience also frequently serve as ways of self-medicating against depression and isolation. Chatting with men online provides the illusion of connecting and being socially engaged. Both Weatherburn (2003) and Elford (2002) found that the HIV-negative men in London who were seeking sex on the Internet reported being twice as likely as other men to have UAI with a person of unknown or different HIV status, increasing the risk of possibly transmitting HIV. These findings were replicated in the San Francisco study (Kim et al., 2001). Elford, Bolding, and Sherr (2002) do note that neither the London nor the U.S. studies actually established whether the high-risk behaviors for HIV and STDs occurred with sexual partners whom the men actually met online or in other venues; they just established that men who used the Internet for meeting sexual partners took more sexual risks than did men who did not use the Internet in this way.

There is conflicting research about the Internet as a contributing factor to the rise in unsafe sex by gay men. One study of 150 men from 14 states conducted over a month at a gay sex resort found that 57 percent reported using the Internet to seek sex. There were no statistical differences found in this sample between the men who did and did not use the Internet to find sexual partners and whether they had unprotected anal sex or in the number of sexual partners they had. The one big difference between men who used the Internet to find sexual partners and those who did not was that the men who used the Internet to find sex used more drugs and engaged in higher levels of what these researchers call "extreme" sexual behaviors such as fisting and group sex (Mettey, Crosby, DiClemente, & Holtgrave, 2003). A study conducted at a Denver public HIV testing clinic found increased levels of high-risk sex among people who seek sex on the Internet.[2] This same study discovered that the people who did seek sex on the Internet were more likely to be male and gay and to report having engaged in UAI (McFarlane et al., 2000).

The San Francisco Department of Public Health documented an outbreak of syphilis among men who visited a specific M4M (man for man) chat room. Two gay men, each with a new case of early syphilis, met most of their sexual partners in a chat room called SFM4M and only knew their partners' screen names. In an effort to reach other men who might be infected and spreading the disease, the Department of Health sent e-mails to participants in this chat room informing them that they may have come in contact with men who could have given them syphilis and encouraged them to seek medical evaluation if they had had unprotected sex with men they met through this chat room. The number of men evaluated at the particular clinic in San Francisco where the original two cases of syphilis were diagnosed rose 18 percent for the month following the e-mail alert, and an additional five cases were identified among SFM4M participants (Klausner, Wolfe, Fischer-Ponce, Zolt, & Katz, 2000). This is viewed as conclusive evidence that at least some men who meet sexual partners on the Internet engage in risky sexual activities. One report, from Rhode Island, documented two cases of acute HIV infection after these individuals met their sexual partners in Internet chat rooms (Tashima, Alt, Harwell, Fiebich-Perez, & Flanigan, 2003). Another study explored the link between Internet cruising and high-risk sex among 4507 young adults ages 18 to 24. The results found that those who sought sex on the Internet were at significantly greater risk for STDs than their peers who did not use the Internet to find sex partners (McFarlane, Bull, & Reitmeijer, 2002).

THE BAREBACKING LABEL AND CYBER CRUISING

When one examines the profiles gay men post on bareback Web sites, it is clear that the limited definition of barebacking used by social scientists is not shared by many men who place ads in search of partners for unprotected sex. There are numerous ads from HIV-negative men who only seek unprotected sex with other uninfected men but nevertheless describe themselves as barebackers. Gauthier and Forsythe (1999) argue that barebacking is a sociological as well as sexual phenomenon insofar as social structures are in place to recruit and train participants; to gather people together to engage in sexual acts; to provide social support systems for participants; and to provide opportunities to exploit new technologies. The Internet is the newest of the technologies that contribute to the ease and frequency with which men who are attracted to this kind of sex can find one another. As Gauthier and Forsyth (1999) state: "Web sites, chatrooms, mailing lists and personal ads devoted to the subject of barebacking have become part of the Internet landscape in the past few years" (p. 88).

For instance, one bareback Web site bills itself as "A place where you can come inside with pride," while another states, "It's all about fucking raw." One of the Web sites describes itself as designed for the adult gay bareback community, and advises that "If you are uncomfortable with this, please do not continue using this Web site" (ultimate bareback.com). Tewksbury (2003) found that one of the Web sites states; "It's up to you . . . to decide how you want to run your life, who you want to fuck, whom you infect, and what you even believe. Also since you are an adult, you decide to live this lifestyle or not, and accept the consequences for doing so. We are here for those who want to live this lifestyle, and don't feel that they fit into the safe-sex world" (p. 468). Bareback Web sites offer members the chance to review profiles either for a specific geographical location or of all members. These Web sites allow members to IM or e-mail each other to arrange sexual hookups, provide opportunities to watch bareback videos and look at bareback photographs, and list the locations of bareback sex parties. Some Web sites accept advertisements for "escort" services.

AIDS EDUCATION ON BAREBACK WEB SITES

It may run counter to one's assumptions, but bareback Web sites can be very direct about the risks of HIV transmission. The three bareback Web sites I visited were all based in the United States, and each offered educational material about the risks of HIV infection. The site that lists itself as "A place where you can come inside with pride" has a section devoted to bareback health and information that states "You know, this isn't just a sleazy-ass sex site" (barebackjack.com 2004c), and then urges men to read the sections on sexual health, drug taking, and safer bare-backing so that each person can enjoy barebacking while keeping the risks at a level that he is comfortable with. This same site states: "While health information may not be your first reason for visiting this site, it is the underlying motivation of Bareback jack.com. We believe that men can enjoy hot, unprotected sex best if they are informed about the risks involved and what they can do to minimize those risks to them-selves and others" (barebackjack.com, 2004a). The site then posts the following information. "Bareback sex brings with it the risk of contract-ing many STDs including HIV. If you are HIV-negative, you are at a higher risk of becoming exposed to HIV while barebacking than if you engage in sexual intercourse with condoms. If you are HIV-positive, you can reinfect yourself or combine strains of the virus. You should assume any such risk as *your responsibility* when meeting advertisers and having sexual encounters" (barebackjack.com, 2004b). The webmaster goes on to explicitly discuss viral load, stating (barebackjack.com, 2004b):

> The term "Viral Load" refers to the amount of HIV virus active in the body. "Undetectable Viral Load" does not mean "HIV-negative." According to the CDC [Centers for Disease Control and Prevention], a person with an undetectable viral load still has the HIV virus and is still considered contagious even though the amount of HIV virus in their bloodstream may fall below the level detectable by modern methods. While drug therapies may help bring a person's viral load down to the level of being unde-tectable, you should not assume that anyone claiming to have an undetectable viral load has been cured of HIV, or that you cannot

become infected by them. Current opinion is that HIV infection is a permanent condition and is not curable at this time, and even undetectable levels can still be transmitted from person to person.

The Web site then posts the following disclaimer (barebackjack.com, 2004b): "We do not endorse the intentional and unlawful infection of HIV-negative persons, without foreknowledge, by HIV-positive men. Ads referring to 'conversion,' 'infection,' 'bug chasing,' and 'gift giving' regardless of ad category are assumed to be the responsibility and consensual desire of the advertiser."

BAREBACKING PROFILES — HOW IT WORKS

I was curious about how it worked. How did barebackers hook up online? What kind of information did they request of each other? In order to explore their Web sites or to communicate with men who post profiles, one needs to develop a profile that is available for other members to see. For research purposes, I created a profile that identified me as a researcher, author, and therapist writing a book on gay men and barebacking, without responding to any of the questions pertaining to my sexual tastes and HIV status. Among the questions I was asked to create my profile were descriptions of my age, race, height, weight, and geographical location (city and state within the United States). Additionally, one is asked whether one is a "bug chaser" or "bug giver,"[3] one's HIV status, the desired HIV status of potential partners, one's sexual role (top, bottom, or versatile), whether one is single or partnered, and whether one is seeking a long-term relationship, one-on-one sexual encounters, ménage à trois (three-way sexual encounters), sex parties, or social activities. Questions are also posed about whether one is willing to give or receive semen orally or anally, and whether one is into PNP (party and play, which means the use of drugs during sex). On bareback Web sites, some men who identify as either a bug chaser or gift giver use an innocuous-looking graphic symbol on their profile to indicate this preference. The symbol for a bug chaser is shown in Figure 5.1. The symbol for a gift giver is shown in Figure 5.2. Additionally, some HIV-positive men use the

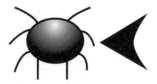

FIGURE 5.1   Bug Chaser

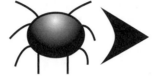

FIGURE 5.2   Gift Giver

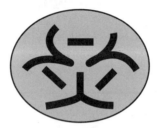

FIGURE 5.3   Online Symbol for HIV+

international biohazard symbol in their profile to visually represent the fact that they are infected, as shown in Figure 5.3.

I reacted with intense shock to the Web site's casual questions about bug chasing, gift giving, and giving and receiving semen. I could not fathom how many thousands of men had responded to those questions. How many of them were surprised, shocked, or possibly relieved to see these phenomena openly queried? Frankly, I am not easily shocked by almost anything to do with sex or sexuality. I have been working on the topic of barebacking intensively for more than a year while researching and writing this book, in addition to listening to clients discuss this issue in therapy for years. When I read the questions about whether I was a bug chaser or gift giver, it was not the first time I had encountered these terms. I think it is safe to assume that my reaction probably is similar to that of many others when they first encounter these terms or hear about or encounter the phenomenon of gay men barebacking. I have come across shock, strong negative judgments, and disbelief among both sophisticated gay men and other therapists. I was not shocked by the openness with which men sought out sex without condoms. What shocked me was first encountering seemingly casual questions about bug chasing and gift giving. While I had read about these terms and men who supposedly were behaving in ways that would result in their fitting one of the labels, I had never before in either my clinical work or social life met any individual who admitted to being either a bug chaser or gift giver. Prior to reading those questions on the Web site, I had just assumed that the reports of bug chasers and gift givers were, if not a myth, then at least hyperbole.

BUG CHASERS AND GIFT GIVERS

Few articles in the professional literature have analyzed characteristics of men who post profiles on bareback Web sites. Tewksbury (2003) analyzed all 880 new profiles posted on a specific Web site within a one-week period in January 2003 in an effort to identify any correlation between a desire for bareback sex and the desire to spread HIV. Tewksbury found that only a very small number of individuals in his sample were actually looking to spread HIV (self-identified gift givers).[4] These results strongly suggest that the vast majority of men who seek to find partners to bareback with online are not looking to knowingly put themselves in high-risk sexual situations. This raises an interesting question about how to reconcile these findings with the research cited earlier that showed that men who met sexual partners on the Internet are more likely to engage in high-risk behaviors. My interpretation of this is that though the vast majority of men who meet other men for sex online are willing to take sexual risks, it is only an infinitesimally small percentage who *actively* seek to become infected or infect another person. This is a subtle but important distinction.

Tewksbury found that although only a small portion of men were directly seeking a partner of discordant status, a fairly high percentage (72 percent of HIV-positive men, 17.4 percent of HIV-negative men, and 78.9 percent of men who either did not know their HIV status or refused to disclose it) had no preference with regard to the HIV status of men they were willing to bareback with. This suggests that many men may be willing to risk either becoming infected with or spreading HIV while not overtly vocalizing any active desire to spread the virus. So once again, while they may not be looking to put themselves at risk, at the same time they also are not making efforts to avoid putting themselves or others at risk.

It is very important to differentiate between men who are willing to expose either themselves or another to the possibility of becoming infected and those individuals who are actively seeking to infect someone or become infected. Grov (2004) visited one of the bareback Web sites specifically to examine only those individuals who participated in an online discussion about intentionally spreading HIV. When Grov visited the site in May 2003, the site claimed to host more than 55,000 active profiles, most of which did not mention spreading HIV. He used the site's keyword search feature in an attempt to identify individuals specifically interested in intentionally spreading HIV. He searched all profiles on the Web site between January and February 2003, and again in June 2003, using keywords "bug," "spread," "breed," "seed," and "gift." To further refine his search, he also analyzed entries in the members' guest books (where individuals are able to respond to members' profiles) who expressed a desire to spread HIV. He was only able to identify 55 original profiles that overtly displayed some form of desire to either infect or be infected with HIV. An additional 26 men were identified by analyzing the guest books of the 55 men whose profiles explicitly stated a desire to spread HIV. These 26 men each overtly implied a desire to spread HIV when responding to a profile that had been explicit about the desire to spread HIV but had not stated this same desire in their own profiles. Grov's findings[5] confirmed Tewksbury's that although a fairly large percentage of men are willing to knowingly place themselves at risk for becoming infected, the actual numbers of men who are actively seeking to spread HIV as either a "bug giver" or "bug catcher" are infinitesimally small.

In September 2004, I visited one of the bareback Web sites to see how many profiles explicitly included references to exchanging HIV. I also wanted to ascertain from a selected number of profiles (n = 57) who indicated a willingness to engage in high-risk behaviors whether they were deliberately trying to either become infected or infect someone who expressed a desire to become HIV-positive. When I selected "show me all profiles" (regardless of geographical location), fewer than 24,000 profiles were available. I searched all of them using the search words "bug chaser," "gift," gift giver," "seed," "conversion," and "breed." I came up with no responses on this Web site for a search of profiles using "bug chaser," "gift," or "gift giver." There were 5 profiles that contained "conversion," 27 that contained "seed" (not all of which referred to seeking to become infected with HIV), and 20 that contained "breed." This was a small percentage of the thousands of member profiles. My results confirmed what both Tewksbury and Grov discovered — that while the bareback Web sites are filled with thousands of men seeking unprotected sex, only a very small minority are actually consciously seeking to either get or spread HIV or state this online. The five profiles that specifically mentioned conversion did seem to belong to either uninfected men or men who did not know or did not state their HIV status who were seeking positive or men of unspecified HIV status to bareback with.

As Grov (2003) states: "the term breed can take on multiple meanings. Breeding has been used by some in context with spreading HIV — breeding the virus in a new host. However breeding could also simply mean sex, like how animals breed" (pp. 338–339). Most of the profiles I examined used "breed" to indicate taking semen in the anus without any indication of a desire to become infected with HIV. One example is a man whose profile stated he was seeking "tops to keep my newly POZ breeding hole sloppy." Since he was already HIV-positive, he was clearly not seeking HIV. Another man who stated he was into keeping his "breeding hole juiced" listed himself as HIV-negative and indicated that he was only interested in other uninfected men, thus indicating that the term "breed" has erotic uses that are not related to spreading HIV. Several other profiles were not specific about their preference regarding the HIV status of sexual partners whm they were willing to be "bred or seeded by," and thus the implicit content of these profiles could be a desire to spread HIV.

INTENTIONALLY SPREADING HIV

I was curious to try to ascertain exactly how many of the ads on the bareback Web sites that talked about wanting to intentionally spread HIV indicated that the men were seeking to either become infected or infect other men. My hypothesis was that many of the ads simply reflected transgressive fantasies, and the individuals who placed the ads might only go so far as to have cyber sex that chatted about spreading the virus. On the same Web site as the one where I used the search feature described above, I examined 57 profiles of men who identified themselves as barebackers in order to see how many were willing to have sex that could place themselves or others at risk for HIV. Out of these profiles, 49 were from various parts of the United States including Alaska and Hawaii, and eight were from foreign countries (Australia, Belgium, Canada, England, France, Germany, New Zealand, and Saudi Arabia). Of the HIV-negative men, two did not specify a preference for the HIV status of their sexual partners, and three said that the HIV status of their partners did not matter. Two of the negative men specified that they were seeking partners who were HIV-positive. The majority of the 15 men who identified as HIV-negative only sought or preferred partners who were also uninfected. I had to conclude that these results suggest that a majority of the men were not interested in becoming infected.

It is uncertain how many men advertising for barebacking partners online are bug chasers or gift givers. Simply analyzing their profiles for preference of HIV status in partners does not provide that information. In other words, just because a positive man seeks to bareback with a negative man, or vice versa, it is not safe to assume that he is actively seeking to become infected or infect. But some assumptions can be made based on men's stated preferences, in their profiles, about their willingness to give or receive semen anally. Since the Web site on which I created an online profile had asked members to indicate their willingness to give or receive semen anally, it was possible to examine profiles of others on the site in order to explore whether their intention was to spread HIV by looking at the HIV status of those with whom they were willing to engage in UAI.[6] Most of the men were not willing

TABLE 5.1

Profiles from One Bareback Web Site

HIV Status	Status of Sex Partners Being Sought	# of Profiles	Give Semen Anally			Receive Semen Anally		
			Yes	No	NS	Yes	No	NS
I Don't Know	Not Specified	3	2	1	0	2	1	0
I Don't Know	Doesn't Matter	2	2	0	0	2	0	0
I Don't Know	Negative Only	3	2	1	0	1	2	0
Not Specified	Not Specified	16	0	0	16	0	0	16
HIV Positive	Doesn't Matter/ Unspecified	5	3	2	0	5	0	0
HIV Positive	HIV-Positive Only/ Preferred	6	5	0	1	6	0	0
HIV Negative	HIV-Negative Only/ Preferred	15	12	0	3	14	1	0
HIV Negative	Doesn't Matter	3	2	1	0	3	0	0
HIV Negative	HIV-Positive Only	2	0	0	2	0	0	2
HIV Negative	Not Specified	2	1	0	1	0	1	1
Total		57	29	5	23	33	5	19

to receive semen from someone who was HIV-positive. A murky area regarding who might be willing to become infected or infect was men who did not state their own HIV status or a preference for the HIV status of a man they would like to have sex with, but who did express a willingness to give and receive semen. (See Table 5.1 for a breakdown of this information.) My conclusion is that there are men who are willing to risk becoming infected, and who are willing to risk infecting others, but this does not mean they are actively seeking to do either. Therefore, I would not count them in the category of bug chaser or gift giver.

I wished to further explore the issue of intentionally seeking to spread HIV, so I e-mailed seven men whose profiles stated that they were HIV-negative and who stated that they were willing to give or receive semen anally with men whose profiles did not state they were also uninfected. I also e-mailed five men whose profiles did not indicate either their own or a partner's HIV status, three men who did not know their HIV status, and the five men whose profiles stated that they were HIV-positive but were willing to have partners who were not also positive. I asked all of them specifically whether they were actually seeking to intentionally spread HIV or were they just seeking to have either phone sex or cyber sex. I received back seven responses. None of the men reported that they were only seeking either cyber or phone sex, thus possibly discrediting my hypothesis that a lot of the online bareback activity was just sex talk and fantasy. One man who publicly identified himself as HIV-positive told me that he did not worry about different strains of the virus. He told me that he finds many guys think that getting HIV is like being admitted to an exclusive club, which he does not understand. But since he openly acknowledges his HIV status, he is willing to convert anyone who asks. Another man who publicly identified as HIV-positive told me that he does not consciously bareback with negative guys, and if someone tells him that he is HIV-negative then "BB is not an option for me." When I asked him whether an uninfected man just wants to do cyber sex or phone sex with him around the topic of becoming infected he replied: "I'm not into cyber or phone sex so it hasn't happened yet. As far as an uninfected man trying to hook up because I'm Poz or looking to be converted, it has only happened twice that I can recall, and both times I've refused."

Another respondent who had not specified his HIV status or that of the men he sought to bareback with admitted that in reality he was HIV-positive but identified himself in his profile as not being infected so that he could enact fantasies that included becoming infected. When I questioned him further about this, he admitted it was a way that he tried retrospectively to empower himself by fantasizing that he was actually in control of when and how he became infected, though in reality that had not been the case. His response reminded me of a quote from the owner of another bareback Web site who was interviewed by a reporter for *Time* magazine. The reporter asked him if he had actually spoken with many men who barebacked and if so what were some of the rationales they gave for the behavior.

It should be pointed out that a number of the "conversionists" who advertise may be men who are already aware they are infected.

Since the underlying commonality among the above seekers of infection is the desire to exercise control over how and when they become infected, it stands to reason that a good number of these men may be creating a fantasy in which they would have "control" over an event that quite probably occurred without foreknowledge. This fantasy extends two ways: the "convertee" (who already knows he's infected) gets the power of control during the act, and the "converter" feels a sense of power in infecting a man who "wants" his disease. Although I believe the bulk of conversion scenes are strictly fantasy, I have no way of knowing for certain. (Barebackjack.com, 2004)

In my own small sample, another man who had never been tested for HIV and sought out sex partners who were either HIV-positive or negative admitted when I queried him that he assumed he was probably HIV-positive. I wondered if he, too, might be retroactively acting out something that he suspects has already happened. One man whose profile stated he was willing to take semen anally did not give his HIV status in his profile but admitted to me that he has been HIV-positive for 14 years and is very serious about hooking up for real and is not into cyber sex at all.

One user whose screen name translated meant that he was primarily a sexual bottom but could be sexually versatile and who barebacks listed his HIV status as negative and wrote that the HIV status of partners did not matter to him. When I asked him whether he was seeking to become infected, his reply was "It doesn't matter to me," and he asked me why I wanted to know. I asked him to briefly try to explain his thoughts or feelings about becoming infected. His response was "Just the thrill of becoming Poz and being able not to worry about it, I guess, and you can have skin-to-skin sex." A few days later he sent me a follow-up e-mail, asking, "May I ask what you think I should do and what you are looking for?" This indicated to me that he may have felt some ambivalence about what he was doing and sought guidance. I introduced the concept of trying to only bareback with men who are negative and said that he might want to consider discussing all of his feelings about this with a therapist who could help him sort through what was going on for him.

He never responded to my last e-mail. The results of my nonscientific survey are elaborated upon in Table 5.1.

BUG CHASERS

I have come to believe that a small percentage of men do want to become infected with HIV. On the spectrum of barebacking, they are the most worrisome to me because this choice seems blatantly self-destructive. But in fact their motivations for bug chasing are a complicated tangle of both conscious and unconscious motivations. Guathier and Forsyth (1999) suggest that four overlapping lines of explanation emerge when one reviews both the literature on active bug chasers and the bareback Internet sites. They feel that the following explanations apply to both barebackers and bug chasers. They postulate that fear and relief motivate some bug chasers to seek out becoming infected. They describe that some men's previous fear of infection so inhibited their behavior that their perceived quality of life had greatly diminished to unacceptably low levels. These individuals seem to validate a point discussed in the last chapter, originally voiced by Odets (1994) and echoed by some of the men who responded to my inquiries, which is that they seem to wish for the relief of finally getting it over with, the relief of knowing that they are infected. Since, to these individuals, becoming infected with HIV is inevitable, they wish to hasten this inevitability and move on with their lives, no longer consumed with the worry. Because many of these men believe HIV is now a medically manageable condition, "inducing a manageable infection is perceived to be the best route to an increased quality of life" (Gauthier & Forsyth, 1999, p. 93).

The following quote from a man who actively sought to become HIV-positive illustrates this point:

> In a way it's a relief. I don't have to wonder anymore. That awful waiting game is gone. So now, if I do find someone, the relationship can be 100 percent real with nothing in the way. That's what I want: 100 percent natural, wholesome and real. Maybe now that I'm HIV-positive, I can finally have my life. (Green, 1996, p. 38)

In the same interview in *Time* quoted above, the owner of Barebackjack.com discussed his impressions about why men are willing to take the risks associated with barebacking.

> The first is one of resignation. Most of the men I have talked to have indicated they wanted the fear of being infected over and done with. This attitude is consistent in men who bareback as well as men who practice safe sex. The barebackers are tired of worrying after every encounter if this was the fuck that might convert them. The routine condom users are tired of fearing the likelihood of a torn or punctured condom. Fear has been a very powerful motivator throughout the AIDS crisis, and it has also been capitalized upon. Some people are simply tired of living their lives in fear when they so desperately want to enjoy sex without fear. These men don't see any other way of releasing the fear of HIV other than by resigning to the virus. And since there have been a few stories available on the Internet that romanticize "gift-giving," they see conversion as something possibly wonderful and meaningful.

A second theory for why some men are "bug chasers" offered by Gauthier and Forsyth is that risk-taking is erotic for some people. They state, "for many individuals, regardless of sexual orientation, the most captivating quality of the sex act is its irrationality" (p. 93). It is important to add that for many people one of the most exciting aspects of good sex is how it taps into darker places in their psyche that bring them close to a place of danger. The late Stephen Gendin (1997) wrote that for him and for many other barebackers, safer sex completely negates the possibility of surrendering to the bliss of being able to be irrational or mindless during sex. Toby, the young architect discussed at the opening of Chapter 3, is another example of an individual who discusses the connection between sexual risk-taking and a more intense release found in sexual play. Journalist Michelangelo Signorile (1997), in describing his own foray into barebacking, put it this way. "The thrill of going bareback makes the sex hotter" (p. 147).

"These individuals perceive heightened sexual satisfaction derived from high-risk sexual encounters wherein they flirt with death" (Gauthier & Forsyth, 1999, p. 94).

"Barebackjack" speaks to this point as well:

Some men look at conversion as a way to have more sex without
barriers. Worry-free and guilt-free fucking, like in the days before
HIV. In urban areas where there are high concentrations of
HIV+ men (like Los Angeles, San Francisco, and New York City),
they feel they will have the sexual candy store open to them if they
share that common affliction. It seems a number of these men
appear to be regular users of drugs like crystal meth, heroin, and
ecstasy, and their overall judgement may be impaired. Then there
are those who find conversion the ultimate kink — to be given the
death fuck is their idea of the pinnacle of sadomasochism. Some of
these men look at this as some kind of masculine ritual that should
be carried out by a "brotherhood" of men. Of course, pricking one's
finger and doing the old Boy Scout "Blood Brothers" ritual might
be as effective, but to these men, the lure is to be inseminated by a
group of infected men.

The entire phenomenon of "bug chasers" brings to mind Susan
Sontag's comment, paraphrased from *AIDS and Its Metaphors* (1988), that
there is nothing so negative as to give a disease a meaning. This seems to
be particularly poignant within the context of a discussion of men who
deliberately seek to become infected. Gauthier and Forsyth also find that
loneliness and group solidarity contribute to why some men become bug
chasers. They report that "many HIV-negative gay men feel that they
have been left behind as lovers and friends have moved on to a status they
do not share" (p. 94). These authors suggest that for some uninfected gay
men, the loss of solidarity and community that they experienced as part
of the gay community prior to the onset of AIDS is imperiled as they
remain HIV-negative. This may have been true in the earlier days of the
epidemic, but I have not heard any man articulate these feelings, or feelings of survivor guilt, in more than a decade.

Gauthier and Forsyth note that HIV has caused a split within
the gay community along HIV status, and to overcome this sense
of exclusion from the gay community it seems that some are willing
to become infected in order to regain a sense of being a member of
the group. The point that these authors are referring to has also been

called "sexual apartheid," by HIV-positive men who were upset that some uninfected men refused to sleep with or date them once they disclosed being HIV-positive. An article that appeared in *Newsweek* put it this way. "A lot of gay men regardless of HIV status feel out of place, put down, worthless. If you're HIV-positive, everybody is generous and there is a sense of community" (Peyser, 1997, p. 77).

I have been living with HIV for almost 30 years now[7] and feel very uncomfortable whenever I hear anyone express sentiments about the benefits of having HIV. Canadian author Ian Young, in his article *The AIDS Cult and Its Seroconverts*, writes, "Many HIV-negative men think HIV positives live richer, more complex, more authentic lives, get more attention, are better able to take risks including, significantly, the risk of intimacy and with such risk-taking, life can be meaningful and full" (1996–1997, online). As an HIV-positive man, I think that this is ridiculous. There are any number of other ways for men to discover authenticity, meaning in their lives, or intimacy that do not have to include voluntarily becoming infected with a life-threatening illness. If an individual was shallow, self-involved, and incapable of intimacy prior to contracting HIV, there are no indications that becoming HIV-positive would suddenly transform that individual into a spiritually rich person with deep introspective qualities who can easily develop a rich friendship network.

The last explanation of why some men are bug chasers, offered by Gauthier and Forsyth, is that some do it as an act of political action. They reason that some bug chasers see the act of becoming infected as politically charged in response to the larger homophobic culture with which gay men have to contend. They cite a study by Ames, Atchinson, and Rose (1995), which states, "A few gay men believed that unprotected anal sex was a required part of truly gay sex and an essential part of coming out. For some of these men, continuing to engage in it was a political act" (p. 64). The following profile I found posted on one of the bareback Web sites seems to support this hypothesis.

> I am a bi-wm who views barebacking as a rite of passage into the gay community, if you are that man that would like to change my world, please reply to this add. Once I get that conversion, I will

no longer consider myself BI, and consider myself gay, its like crossing a barrier for me.

While what Ames et al. describe is undoubtably true, it does not speak directly to the issue of why men become bug chasers. It only describes men who are willing to place themselves at risk and are willing to take the chance that by doing so they may become HIV-positive, but nothing in this one quote or in the rest of the article by these researchers seems to suggest that any of these people are intentionally seeking to become infected with HIV, though the individual quoted above may be equating his seroconversion with an essential rite of passage into becoming a full-fledged gay man.

Grov (2004) makes an interesting point that may be the most helpful lens through which to try to understand bug chasers. "One could argue that men seeking seroconversion have most likely adapted an ideological stance towards the disease. These men appear to believe the disease will benefit them in some way because they discuss it as both valuable and desired" (p. 340). I think that the ideological position discussed by Grov may in fact be what Gauthier and Forsyth were trying to elaborate when they spoke of the desire to seroconvert as a potentially political action. One rationale that may contribute to why some men actively seek to become infected has to do with class or economic privilege. If an individual is poor or socioeconomically disadvantaged, there in fact might be advantages to becoming infected with HIV. These advantages may include entitlements such as access to free or very low-cost health insurance, medical care, and medications to treat HIV, food stamps, housing subsidies, and even welfare payments.

At a 2004 conference sponsored by the CDC, one presentation was on gift giving; it analyzed 281 messages from 17 Web-based gift giver/bug chaser newsgroups that contained postings from September 1998 through February 2003. Rationales for gift giving and bug chasing reinforced the themes found in the general bareback literature, which included:

- Condomless sex is more natural, real, and intimate.
- Risk takers are essentially masculine and hyper-masculine.
- Spreading or contracting HIV is an individual choice.

- Spreading HIV was an act of rebellion and resistance.
- Gift givers/bug chasers were exhausted by safer sex and felt it was inevitable that they would become infected.
- Current treatments made HIV seem like a manageable illness.
- HIV, AIDS, STDS, decay, and illness were all eroticized.
- Ejaculate was fetishized.
- Sex roles were gendered and to be penetrated equaled feminization.

Some men conceived of "The Gift" as facilitating joining the brotherhood of POZ men, even saying they were now "POZ brothers" and had a new life after seroconverting, and that conversion provided the opportunity for the man to become a giver himself as well as denigrating the unawares and the "clean" ones who chose not to take the risk of becoming infected. The key findings included that when HIV is conceived of as a "gift," the meaning of HIV can be manipulated to fulfill the particular social and emotional goals of an individual.

Since many bug chasers view becoming HIV-positive as inevitable, they have shifted the paradigm to make it desirable, and thus the gift of HIV is transformative. Exchanging HIV provides a sense of control, and since gift giving is a form of extreme sex, it provides a sense of sexual transgression that safer sex precludes. One 20-year-old who had sought to become infected, writing in *POZ*, explained part of his rationales for wanting to become infected this way. "Maybe it's because growing up in the Midwest, I was taught through fear: have safe sex or die! Barebacking seemed the ultimate rebellion" (Hitzel, 2002, electronic version). Later on in the same article Hitzel reports, "In some ways I knew I was on a suicide mission — it was my hope to, at some point, wear my body out and die ... because for five months at 19, I had decided I would invite a disease into my life. All because I wanted to fuck any person that walked in that door. Never thinking that one day I wouldn't want just any person, I would want that one person." In the film *The Gift*, Hitzel (2002) gives other details of his wanting to get HIV.

> I always wanted to fit in and to have gay male friends. I tried
> to cruise the M4F chat rooms but wasn't very successful. Once
> I decided to begin having sex with men who are HIV-positive
> I felt like I had struck a pot of gold. There were vastly more people

I could hook up. I would get calls from guys who said there are four people here and I was telling them about you and they want you to come over and play. Hey, people were suddenly talking about me.

Contained within Hitzel's story are also the realities that his seroconversion only resulted in his becoming even more depressed than he had been while seeking to become infected. He described feeling let down that becoming HIV-positive did not positively transform his life. In fact the added burdens of medical tests, treatments, and symptoms did not translate into having been worth the risk he took to get himself infected.

THE GIFT

In 2002, a film entitled *The Gift* was released. The filmmaker hoped to create dialogue within the community and raise awareness of the issues of isolation and division in the gay community around HIV status, thereby leading to a renewed prevention effort. The film documented the phenomenon of barebackers, including bug chasers who host conversion parties where men actively seek "the gift" of HIV infection. The film shows one young man named Ken who answered an ad to come to Los Angeles to live in a house called LASEXHOUSE, which hosted regular sex parties. He discusses throwing a conversion party to get "the gift" so he will not have to worry about HIV any longer. As part of his rationale, he said that he hated condoms. Prior to seeing this film, though I had read articles about the phenomenon, I had never met anyone who admitted to participating in a conversion party. An article in the Los Angeles gay news magazine *Frontiers* reported that one of its reporters, when visiting a bareback Web site, found a posting for a conversion party that read:

> 30-year old neg bottom looking for tops to seed and convert me . . . . I will have a room rented and will be naked and ready to take your charged loads. The more the merrier. (Caldwell, 2003)

Bareback parties, which began in the 1990s, are now entrenched in gay culture, according to Perry Halkitis (quoted in Martinez-Bevin, 2004). In 1999, the HIV/AIDS Web site TheBody.com posted an article written by Rick Sowadsky (1999), which described conversion parties as group sex parties where bug chasers allow themselves to get infected by gift givers, and Russian roulette parties as barebacking parties attended by both positive and negative men. Knowing that there may be HIV-positive men at these parties, negative men take their chances that they will be infected when having sex with the positive men there. Depending on the circumstances, the participants may or may not know ahead of time who is positive and who is negative. It is important to differentiate between bareback sex parties and supposed conversion or Russian roulette parties. Bareback sex parties usually are advertised in one of three ways: as only for men who all identify as HIV-negative; as POZ parties for men who already know that they are infected; or as barebacking parties where people are encouraged not to ask or discuss HIV status and just assume that everyone else is HIV-positive.

This category of sex party was also elaborately described in the film *The Gift*. Speaking about bug chasers and conversion parties, Mario Weinstein, president of the AIDS Healthcare Foundation, stated: "I think that the average, open-minded individual realizes we do self-destructive things. They also realize gay men endure a lot of hatred and that leads to self-destructive behavior. It's not as if we have a monopoly on bad behavior. Throughout the world, in every community, there's antisocial behavior" (quoted in Cadwell, 2003). Weinstein also acknowledged that the bug chaser subset of gay men is probably very small, but that they do definitely exist, and he feels that they are symptomatic of a dangerous mentality developing among some gay men.

Gauthier and Forsyth suggest: "It is possible, even probable, that bug chasers have existed since the beginning of the AIDS epidemic, but that their numbers were extremely small. As the epidemic progressed, claiming more victims, it is likely that bug chasing increased in frequency owing to a variety of reasons. More importantly, however, than the speculated increase in frequency of participation in this activity is the certain increase in frequency of public discourse about participation in this activity" (p. 92). One indication of the extent of the nonprofessional interest in bug chasers is that in September 2004, when I conducted a Google search for bug chasers, 64,400 results came up.

BUG CHASING IN THE MEDIA

One significant contributing factor to the public controversy about bug chasers was a controversial article in *Rolling Stone* (January 23, 2003). Author Gregory Freeman misquoted openly gay San Francisco psychiatrist Robert Cabaj as saying that a mind-boggling 25 percent of new gay male HIV infections were due to bug chasing, and Boston's Dr. Marshal Forstein as saying "bug chasers are seen regularly in the Fenway health system." In this article, Freeman describes a vast and vibrant underground, mostly conducted on the Internet, where bug chasers had a mission to get infected with HIV. It created an immediate uproar with both gay conservatives and liberals pointing out the numerous factual errors in the story. Shortly after the *Rolling Stone* article appeared, Cabaj wrote that the 25 percent estimate was wrong. In an interview with *Newsweek,* Cabaj said he told a *Rolling Stone* fact checker that the 25 percent figure was incorrect (Mnookin, 2003). The day after the *Rolling Stone* story appeared, Forstein told a reporter for the *Washington Post* that he, too, was misquoted and what he was purported to have said was in fact "a total fabrication." He also told the reporter "I have seen two such cases in the last 3 years, and I can count on one hand how many patients like that I have seen in years. I said specifically that this was a small phenomenon" (Sorokin, 2003).

Despite the swiftness with which the experts supposedly quoted had denied what was attributed to them, conservative Web sites such as the Drudge Report quickly began to spread the false allegations in an effort to make it seem like a large percentage of gay men were intentionally trying to become HIV-positive. Even though the figures conservatives were using were disputed, this did not stop some right-wing groups from continuing to cite the original story. The Traditional Values Coalition used the article to urge the Centers for Disease Control and Prevention to curtail its AIDS funding (Mnookin, 2003). In response to the *Rolling Stone* article Lee Klosinski, then-director of programs for AIDS Project Los Angeles, said: "If we're talking about some highly organized effort among a group of men, then that's not been our experience at APLA. My hunch is that the whole bug chaser phenomenon is an Internet-related phenomenon and basically some type of erotic urban myth" (quoted in Caldwell, 2003).

SEX PARTIES FOR HIV-POSITIVE MEN

In June 2003, the New York Lesbian, Gay, Bisexual, and Transgender Community Center cohosted a forum entitled "Sex in the City '70s, '80s, '90s, and Now. Evolution and Revolution: How Drugs, Disease and Prevention Changed the Way We Have Sex." The event was moderated by Robin Byrd, a well-known cable television host of adult programs who always reminds her audience to use condoms. One of the panelists was a man named Brandon who founded and hosts a regular sex party for HIV-positive men. The party is advertised both on the Internet and in New York's weekly gay giveaway magazines. It is listed under the headline "Brandon's Poz Party" and is described as "HIV prevention through Poz playing with Poz only" (*HX*, 2004, p. 64). Like some bareback Web sites, it is an interesting mixture of advocacy, education, social networking, and sex. When Byrd heard that barebacking was tolerated at the party, she attacked Brandon by asking what happened if HIV-negative men came in. He explained that this was advertised specifically as a place where HIV-positive men could come to have whatever kind of sex they wanted with one another.

Brandon was adamant and nonapologetic that he was providing a service for infected men where they could experience stigma reduction. Several men I interviewed who are regulars at these parties confirmed that their experience mirrored what Brandon was saying. One described the parties as an "empowerment zone where it doesn't feel like I am being stigmatized for having HIV." Another spoke of the camaraderie that goes on at these parties, and that though most people do not use condoms, he leaves feeling so good about himself and has increased self-confidence that when he is in bars or clubs and someone asks him his HIV status he no longer hesitates to respond in a truthful way. Even when an uninfected man chooses not to go home with him, he only feels disappointed and not crushed, since he knows he can always go to Brandon's parties and talk about these experiences with other understanding men and always find sexual playmates and even men to date there. Writing about the power of barebacking with other infected men, Stephen Gendin (1997) explained:

It's like being thrown into jail for life and then, while serving your time, having the warden threaten to extend your sentence. The threat has no power because nothing can make a life sentence any worse. You can laugh at the threat, even spit in the warden's face. That time I got fucked by another positive guy, I felt I didn't have to fear HIV any longer. I could taunt it, challenge it by taking it into my body without being further hurt. (Online)

Of course, Gendin was writing without any acknowledgment of the risk of possibly acquiring a multidrug-resistant strain of HIV.

BUG CHASING AS TAKING CONTROL

The relationship of seeking a sense of control to bug chasing has been described by Scarce (1999a), when he describes young gay men who seek to become infected with HIV. He reports that some of these young men describe selecting a "father" who will give them the virus. Scarce reports that seeking out the virus results in the youth feeling empowered since they had control over when, how, and by whom they became infected. Both Scarce and Suarez and Miller (2001) strongly suggest that the intense and rampant homophobia that affects young gay men contributes to their believing that their future will be nothing but dismal, especially when they are just coming out of the closet and are particularly vulnerable. This perspective and information should provide powerful motivation for gay health care, social service, and education professionals to increase the urgency with which programs for gay youth are developed to provide sexual minority youth with access to safe and nurturing environments that offer psychosocial community supports that can hopefully help ameliorate some of the societal and internalized homophobia that contributes to this generation's intentionally seeking to become HIV-positive.

Lee Klosinski, director of programs for AIDS Project Los Angeles said: "If somebody is deliberately looking to become infected, that is pathology. Let's call a spade a spade. This is beyond a targeted HIV-prevention method. It's a behavior that is self-destructive. The response is one that needs to be rooted in mental health services. In the world of diminishing resources, it's hard to say that bug chasers are worth targeting, because it's hard to know if it's even a group" (quoted in Caldwell, 2003, online version). While I agree with parts of Klosinski's statement insofar as any behavior that is self-destructive needs to have a component of mental health to treat it, taking this approach to bug chasers without an additional component of targeted community mental health and community building just pathologizes the individual and does not take into account the dysfunctional and unhealthy system in which he is living that contributes to feelings of worthlessness. We must look at how individuals who cannot see any other options for feeling valued, connected, or cared for may be susceptible to putting themselves at risk of becoming infected. I would add that a community-wide approach that actively attempts to increase community attachment and a sense of being cared about by the gay community, long before one becomes infected with HIV, is what is required to reach people who are knowingly trying to get infected.

THERAPY WITH BUG CHASERS

I have never had a patient tell me that he was either actively a bug catcher or gift giver in all the years I have been doing therapy. Tewksbury (2003) suggests that: "social stigmas or fears of public health policing efforts may lead men to hide their bug chasing intentions" (p. 468). Wanting to find out if my experience was replicated by other professionals, I sent out an e-mail to more than 100 therapists I personally know who work with gay men in the United States, England, and Canada. I also sent the e-mail to Dr. Jack Drescher, editor of the *Journal of Gay and Lesbian Psychotherapy* and asked him to please forward my e-mail on. Dr. Drescher forwarded it to his e-mail list of more than 800 professionals as well as to the listserv of Division 44 of the American Psychological Association (The Society for the Psychological Study of Lesbian, Gay, and Bisexual Issues, which has more than 1500 members in all 50 states and eleven other countries) and to the listserv of the 180-member gay section of the British Psychological Association. Of the more than 100 responses I received, only three colleagues had ever worked with an individual who discussed actively wanting to contract the virus. Two of these cases were men in long-term, committed relationships with a partner who was HIV-positive. Both of these men felt that becoming infected would increase the specialness of the union with their partner. I do not think of these men can be thought of in the same way as men who are single and seeking to become infected. The third was a man in his early twenties who expressed feelings of envy toward the community of HIV-positive men because he felt that they had some kind of privileged status and that he felt excluded from their community. The psychologist who reported this case to me told me that it was as if this young man felt it was chic to be HIV-positive. I was not surprised that there were almost no colleagues who had worked with bug-chaser or gift-giver clients. Part of my speculation about the reasons for this is that in addition to it being a very rare phenomenon, men who engage in the behavior probably have a high enough degree of shame about it that they either are not in therapy or if they are, are not discussing this with their therapists.

The Internet may have increased opportunities for barebackers to hook up, but it also offers unparalleled opportunities to reach its users with AIDS prevention, education, and other health promotion messages as well as the possibility for live, real-time virtual interventions. As Elford (2002) states, "The Internet undoubtedly offers enormous potential for sexual health promotion and HIV prevention" (p. 3). Some efforts to use the Internet to reach men who bareback with educational information and referrals have already been described a bit in this chapter. A more detailed discussion of how the Internet is being used to reach men who engage in risky behaviors will be presented in Chapter 8.

Part Two

TAKING OFF THE CONDOMS:
RAW SEX IN RELATIONSHIPS

CHAPTER SIX

Love in the Time of Plague: Male Couples, Sex, and HIV

A COUPLE IN CONFLICT OVER CONDOMS

Donald and Ted, a white couple in their forties, had been in an on-again, off-again relationship for more than 2 years when they called for a consultation. Both men were HIV-positive. Donald was in excellent health. Ted's health was more precarious. Their presenting problem was that Ted was reluctant to define their relationship as "permanent." He said it was not because he was half-hearted about Donald, but he interpreted Donald's unwillingness to commit to sexual exclusivity as Donald having one foot out the door. As might be expected, Donald did not agree with this assessment of their relationship, citing Ted's lack of commitment to a long-term relationship as his rationale for having sex with other men. The men were entrenched in this no-win cycle of blame.

I was curious about Donald's contention that he would not be interested in sex with other men if Ted would commit to him. As we explored his pursuit of other men for sex, I discovered that Donald used the Internet to locate parties for HIV-positive men who wanted to forego safer sex. "In those venues, I feel a freedom that I don't feel anywhere else, since I don't have to discuss my HIV status," Donald explained. "I also feel a spiritual connection with other Poz guys as we drink each other and come inside each others' butts. I don't even experience this with Ted, since when we fuck we use condoms. During these parties, and for a few hours afterward, I really feel part of one segment of the queer men's community."

It was clear to me that there was more going on for Donald than commitment issues. As the men sat in my office for session after session discussing how frustrated and misunderstood they each felt, a disturbing lack of trust and empathy emerged. Much of it centered around the different meanings they assigned to the act of having unprotected sex. In their sexual relationship, Donald wanted to dispense with using condoms, and he pushed Ted hard to see things his way. But Ted's health was more fragile than Donald's, and the idea of not using condoms made him extremely uncomfortable for two reasons. He didn't want to risk the possibility of becoming infected with an additional strain of HIV from Donald, and he knew Donald was having unprotected sex with other men and was afraid Donald might pass a sexually transmitted disease (STD) to him. Donald brushed away Ted's concerns, insisting that his doctor had told him that it was perfectly safe for an HIV-positive man to stop using condoms with other HIV-positive men. Ted countered that his doctor had told him there could be serious risks to Ted if he participated in unprotected sex.

Donald turned a deaf ear to Ted's concerns and accused Ted of worrying too much. I was surprised by this lack of empathy and shared my reaction with them. Ted appreciated what I said, but Donald became defensive and accused me of siding with Ted. Trying to find a compromise, Ted told Donald that he would be willing to have unprotected anal intercourse (UAI) if Donald stopped having sex with other men, but he added the condition that Donald must not ejaculate inside of him. Donald pouted and complained about this last condition, accusing Ted of not trusting him. Ted remained adamant.

When they arrived the next week, Ted was furious at Donald. That morning, they had been having UAI and Donald broke their agreement and ejaculated inside Ted. It was not the first time, and Ted was hurt, angry, and bewildered by Donald's disregard of his expressed wishes. In therapy, Ted said he felt doubtful about the viability of their relationship. The men came for a few more sessions to discuss whether or not they might find a compromise, and during our final session they mutually agreed to separate.

ALL UAI IS NOT BAREBACKING: CHAPTER OVERVIEW

While this book has so far focused on barebacking outside the context of committed relationships, studies have shown that UAI occurs most often among gay men in ongoing relationships (Doll et al., 1991; Schmidt et al., 1992; Hunt et al., 1992; McLean et al., 1994; Hospers & Kok, 1995; Hickson et al., 1996; Buchanan, Poppen, & Reisen, 1996; Hoff et al., 1997; Hays, Kegeles, & Coates, 1997; Elford, Bolding, Maguire, & Sherr, 1999; Davidovich, de Wit, & Stroebe, 2000; Halkitis, Wilton, Parsons, & Hoff, 2004).

When I titled this book *Sex Without Condoms: Unprotected Sex, Gay Men, and Barebacking*, I was trying to address the reality that the same sexual behavior has different connotations, ramifications, and even labels among gay and bisexual men. Even though, as Morin et al. (2003) have reported, the term "barebacking" has assumed a general usage within the gay men's community to mean any instances of anal sex without condoms, couples who have UAI rarely describe their condomless sexual encounters with each other as barebacking. Men who are coupled frequently have anal sex without condoms, although many may not refer to this as "barebacking." In relationships where both men are HIV-negative and monogamous, UAI carries no risk of HIV infection, since there is no virus to transmit, although other preexisting STDs like herpes or diseases contracted through sex with outside partners may still be transmitted. Because of this lack of risk, those partners often do not label their sexual behavior as "barebacking," which leads me to conclude that many gay men equate the term "barebacking" with sexual behavior that introduces some risk of HIV infection or reinfection, and that many men who are having UAI do not consider themselves barebackers. After all my research and thought on this topic, I too, do not consider all UAI to be "barebacking." I respect the complexity of the issue of condomless sex and the ambiguities and twists and turns of logic and practice associated with both the behavior and the term "barebacking."

This chapter explores some of the themes, beliefs, and behaviors of male couples who engage in UAI. What motivates them to take off the condoms? What kinds of conversations — if any — are they having before they engage in high-risk sex? Central to our discussion is an examination of love, lust, and power. How do romantic notions of love and commitment affect gay couples' decision making? How does lust factor in, and how should we think about nonmonogamy? And how are covert power issues between men part of the equation?

For many readers, gay nonmonogamy is a controversial topic. Although it is a well-accepted and often ubiquitous part of the gay subculture, it is often misunderstood by mainstream society — and some gay people — as a problematic aspect of gay relationships. What is relevant about this topic with regard to our discussion of UAI in couples is how gay men negotiate nonmonogamy, and what constitutes "infidelity" in that context.

Part Two of this book focuses on UAI in couple relationships because it is the most common configuration where sex without condoms occurs. But this is a very tangled and complicated topic, so I have divided it into three sections. This chapter looks more broadly at the prevalence of couples engaging in UAI, and some of the research on why they do it, as well as excavating some of the underlying tensions that come up in relationships when condoms are being discussed. The kinds of negotiations and arrangements used to mitigate the risks of UAI are explored. Chapter 7 investigates two smaller pieces of the picture. The first part looks at seroconcordant couples — partners who both have the same HIV status — and the second part looks at serodiscordant couples — partners who have different a HIV status from each other.

RESEARCH ON COUPLES AND CONDOMLESS SEX

Gay men having a steady partner was one of the most consistent predictors of condomless sex (Doll et al., 1991). Hays et al. (1997) found that in their sample of young gay men — ages 18 to 27 — living in three medium-sized cities on the West Coast of the United States, 51 percent of the men with boyfriends had engaged in UAI in the past 2 months with their boyfriends. Slightly more than one-third of

Swiss gay men in relationships reported engaging in UAI with their partners (Moreau-Gruet, Dubois-Arber, & Spencer, 2001). There is now a substantial body of research focused on sexual risk-taking by men in steady relationships.[1] A variety of factors have been found to contribute to the likelihood of men not using condoms with a regular partner. These include:

- Knowledge of the partner's sexual history (McLean et al., 1994; Boulton, McLean, Fitzpatrick, & Hart, 1995; Misovich, Fischer, & Coates, 1997).
- Familiarity with the partner in general (Boulton et al., 1995; McNeal, 1997).
- Monogamy (Misovich et al., 1997; Hays et al., 1997).
- Trust (Remien, Carballo-Dieguez, & Wagner, 1995, Boulton et al., 1995; Misovich et al., 1997).
- Love (McLean et al., 1994; Boulton et al., 1995; Carballo-Dieguez & Dolezal, 1996).
- Intimacy (Remien et al., 1995; Boulton et al., 1995; McNeal, 1997).
- HIV status (Kippax, Crawford, Davis, Rodden, and Dowset, 1993; Hays et al., 1997; Hoff et al., 1997; Crawford, Rodden, Kippax, & Van de Ven, 2001; Halkitis, Wilton, Parsons, & Hoff, 2004).

Ten percent of Swiss gay men chose to have UAI with a boyfriend of unknown HIV status based on personal assessment of past risks or their being in a monogamous relationship (Moreau-Gruet et al., 2001). In Germany, the corresponding research found 23 percent (Bochow, 2000); in California and Oregon 21 percent (Hays et al., 1997); and in London and Sydney, 12 percent (Elford et al., 1999; Kippax et al., 1997).

What is clear from the research is that various types of male couples have anal sex without condoms, including men in HIV-concordant couples (men who have the same HIV status) as well as men in HIV-discordant couples (men who have different HIV status) (Remien et al., 1995; Hoff et al., 1997; Hays et al., 1997; Halkitis et al., 2004). Within primary relationships where both men have the same HIV status, seroconcordance is commonly reported as the main rationale for having UAI (Stall et al., 1990; Kippax et al., 1993; Halkitis et al., 2004). In other words, the men do not fear infecting the other or becoming infected themselves. Some findings indicate that in long-term serodiscordant couples unsafe sex is prevalent (Remien et al., 1995). However, this is not universally supported, as Kalichman et al. (1997) failed to find any correlation between relationship status (that is, short-term vs. long-term couples) and sexual risk-taking in men who were HIV-positive.

HIGH-RISK SEX WITHIN RELATIONSHIPS

A substantial proportion of new HIV infections occur within steady partnerships (Davidovich et al., 2001). Unfortunately, several studies have shown that steady partners who have UAI with each other often do not know either their own or the other's HIV status, making sex without condoms a risky behavior (Elford et al., 1999[2]; Davidovich et al., 2000). Data from a 17-year study in Amsterdam of young gay men found that nearly 30 percent of those who were in a relationship reported engaging in high-risk sexual behavior with a steady partner whose HIV status was either unknown or serodiscordant from their own (Davidovich et al., 2000).

While little research on this topic has been done in the United States, European researchers have found that there seem to be common considerations gay men make when they decide to have UAI with steady partners. Elford, Bolding, Maquire, and Sherr (2001) suggest that "one, but not the only, factor is the extent to which couples are aware of their own and their partner's HIV status" (p. 1054). In a study of more than 1000 men in central London, Elford and colleagues (1999) found that more than half the men who reported only having UAI with their main partner did not know their own HIV status or that of their partner. Moreau-Gruet et al. (2001) report that in Switzerland, slightly more than half of the couples said they knew their partner's HIV status. Davidovich et al. (2000) found that in Amsterdam, the number of men who knew their partner's HIV status was considerably lower than half, and Van de Ven, French, Crawford, and Kippax (1999) found that in Australia, a considerably higher percentage of gay men in partnerships who were having UAI with their partners knew each other's HIV status. Elford, Bolding, Maquire, and Sherr (2001) suggest that these numbers may reflect differences between countries in both the availability of HIV testing and incentives to take the HIV test — such as how easily available highly active antiretroviral therapy is in each country. Davidovich and colleagues (2004) correctly state that "the customary prevention strategy to promote condom use for all incidents of anal intercourse failed to generalize to the context of steady relationships" (p. 305).

WHY COUPLES TAKE RISKS

Appleby, Miller, and Rothspan (1999) discovered three factors that led partners to choose to have UAI. They looked at 46 long-term male couples in the United States. According to the subjects, the three most prevalent rationales for why they did not use condoms with their steady partners were love, trust, and commitment. Men who scored higher for emotional and social dependence on their relationship and who desired a stable and lasting relationship were more likely to practice UAI. Also, the study revealed that requesting safer sex had negative connotations (such as suspicion of nonconsensual nonmonogamy among partners). In interviews with 20 working-class men in a small town in England, Flowers, and colleagues (1997) found similar results. Many of the men in that study reported that within the context of romantic relationships they often demonstrated their commitment, trust, and love by foregoing the use of condoms, and they made this a priority over their own health.

FRANK AND JESUS: RECOGNIZING POWER ISSUES

A critical factor in discussing UAI within the context of a relationship has to do with power. My review of the research literature indicates that the issue of power and how it relates to condom use by gay men within relationships has not been investigated. But from my own clinical experience, power is frequently a key factor in men's decisions to stop using condoms. People may not love equally, and people rarely have equal power in a relationship. Some men may attempt to prove their love or try to make someone love them more by not using condoms. These imbalances, which are often not overtly acknowledged, often emerge in sexual negotiations — or the lack of such negotiations.

Frank and Jesus, both HIV-negative, sought therapy because of tensions that had arisen about using condoms for anal sex. Frank was a 35-year-old WASP, well-educated and employed as a teacher at a private school. Jesus was a 23-year-old Puerto Rican immigrant who was employed as a dishwasher at a diner. They met while Frank was on holiday in Puerto Rico and fell in love. Jesus relocated to New York so they could be together. Before meeting Jesus, Frank had never had UAI. Now together in a monogamous relationship, they had gone together to be retested for HIV infection and both tested negative. The problem they were experiencing was around how much risk they each felt willing to take, sexually, in their relationship. Jesus repeatedly asked Frank not to use a condom, and despite not being completely comfortable about it, Frank complied. But Frank insisted that Jesus wear a condom when topping him. At times, when Frank decided he wanted to use a condom when topping Jesus, Jesus became upset. Jesus told me, "Since neither of us is supposedly having sex with anyone else, when he wears a condom I wonder who else he has been messing around with. I think that he must not want to give me a disease that he got from another guy."

Frank explained his way of thinking about monogamy, Jesus, and condoms: "It's because I love him so much that I want to use a condom." He addressed Jesus, "I hate it that every time I decide to use a condom, you freak out thinking that I'm cheating on you. Even though I trust you, it's so early in our relationship that it's hard for me to accept that you trust me enough for me not to put on a rubber." Frank said he needed Jesus to wear a condom even though he believed that Jesus had been "faithful."

Two themes emerged that were intimately related to condom use: defining the relationship, and power. Jesus and Frank had different understandings of where the relationship was, developmentally. Having given up his life in Puerto Rico to move to New York to be with Frank, Jesus felt ready to have a commitment ceremony and thought of them as already married. When Frank heard this, he responded: "But honey, we've only been living together for three months! We're still getting to know each other. I feel that it's way too soon to consider us married. We are definitely moving in that direction. Once we're both as sure about the relationship as we can be, I'll probably be ready for both of us to stop using condoms. But up until then, please try to relax about this."

In response, Jesus told Frank that being told he had to wear a condom even though Frank had made love to him without a condom played up all the power inequalities in their relationship. Frank was white; Jesus was a man of color. Frank was older, better educated, and financially secure from both his job and family money. Jesus had not been to college, came from a poor family, and earned considerably less money than Frank did. In addition, Frank was a native of New York, and a native English speaker, while Jesus was an immigrant, and English was his second language. Jesus had only one other friend in New York and felt dependent on Frank socially, financially, and emotionally, which made him feel extremely vulnerable. They lived in an apartment that Frank owned. Most of the things in their home were Frank's.

I admired Jesus for his courage in raising these issues and shared this with them. I have seen gay couples stew in silence about power differences for years and years, to the detriment of the relationship. I congratulated Jesus on his ability to see their condom disagreement in this larger context. Frank was also visibly relieved to have these matters on the table for discussion. Each admitted to having spent time thinking about all of these things independently. Hearing and exploring each other's feelings about power and intimacy and trust took weeks of therapy, and they both felt it strengthened the emotional foundation of their relationship. Instead of putting all in terms of sexual trust, they could start to talk about emotional trust.

Despite his progressive politics, Frank was surprised at how oblivious he was about how aspects of his own unexamined privilege impacted his relationship and the man he loved. During one session, Frank suddenly understood how their different perspectives on condoms looked to Jesus, who had taken so many risks — in every aspect of his life — to be with him, including the ultimate risk of trusting Frank to have unprotected sex with him. Frank burst into tears, deeply saddened by how out of touch he had been to how the issue of using condoms affected his beloved. This conversation was the real beginning of their learning how to negotiate a host of complicated issues, only one of which was their use of condoms.

Although Jesus was hurt that Frank did not think of them as married, he said he believed Frank did share the goal of being in a long-term, committed, monogamous relationship with him. Believing they shared the same relationship goal and values around love, intimacy, and trust allowed them to begin discussions about ways that the power and control inequalities could be addressed. They explored how to restructure decision making about household chores, spending money, socializing, and even what language to speak, since both were bilingual. These conversations led to Jesus saying he would try not to make an issue of Frank's condom use. At their last session, Jesus told me: "I guess that when Frank stops using a condom, it will be all right for me to stop using them also, and that will mean that our relationship has really moved to the next level."

FACTORING IN LOVE AND LUST

In order to understand how couples make the decision about whether to have condomless anal sex, it is important to consider the broader context of sexuality and male couplehood, and how HIV plays a role in couples' sex lives whether or not they have the infection. Love is one of the most complicated of human experiences to describe and to quantify, and it is often a totally idiosyncratic reality that varies from person to person and relationship to relationship. While subjects who were asked to say why they did it cited "love" as the rationale for why they engaged in UAI with a steady partner, it is not at all clear how these men are defining "love," since other men may use condoms with beloveds and give the rationale for doing so as "love."

Research conducted with Norwegian gay men (Prieur, 1990) discusses the symbolic meanings unprotected anal sex has within couples: it is a demonstration of affection, intimacy, and trust, and it creates a feeling of oneness. That research sample consisted of men in their twenties, and therefore it is not clear whether the same factors affect older partnered gay men who do not use condoms, but in my experience older couples (those in their thirties, forties, and fifties) have the same underlying expectations of unprotected sex as a way of building or confirming emotional intimacy. Also, Prieur's research was conducted during the height of the epidemic and it is unclear whether a similar study conducted today, more than a decade later, would confirm these findings, but I believe it would.

Negotiations about condom use have the potential to be highly fraught. After all, men are talking about whether or not, how often, under what circumstances, and when they would be willing to trust their partner with their health and ultimately their life. The problems that Donald and Ted experienced at least in part were created by their inability or unwillingness to really look at the issues of power, combined with lack of empathy and a sense of entitlement. The result was their decision to end their relationship. All of my efforts to try to get them to examine these issues only resulted in greater anger, hurt, and digging in of their heels so that neither felt heard or understood by the other. Inherent in the mix for Donald and Ted was confusion about love, with both wrestling with what it meant to love and be loved and asking themselves questions like, "If I love him, do I have to prove my love, or does he have to prove his love? And will I be loved back the same way?" Part of Ted's dilemma before they split up was his rationalization that Donald loved him and therefore could not possibly mean to "fuck me over this way, because he says he loves me and I know that I love him."

We cannot talk about sexuality without talking about one of the biggest engines that drives it: lust. This powerful human desire is another extremely difficult and complicated experience that is impossible to quantify. Often, people who experience love or lust confuse the two sensations and experiences and are unsure of how to tease them apart. Lust can make people do seemingly irrational things. But when it comes to irrational behavior (and I am by no means saying that when two men in a loving relationship decide not to use condoms that it is irrational), love and/or the desire to experience love combined with lust can make people behave in ways they would not normally choose. This seems to be consistent with the research that confirms that men are more likely to forego using condoms with men they either feel in love with or a desire to be in love with than with casual partners.

LOVE AND SELF-SACRIFICE

As a therapist, I have been privileged to witness how powerful and healthy love can be for those who are lucky enough to find it, surrender to it, and nurture it. I have also been discouraged, pained, and sorrowful at how some clients confuse love with an unhealthy loss of their autonomous sense of self. Many people, across the spectrum of mental and emotional health, find that romantic love is the organizing principle of their personality and self-concept. For these people, sex and this kind of love become inextricably linked, and rather than risk losing love they may have unprotected sex, like the men interviewed by Appleby (1999). People outside any particular relationship may ponder whether it was "really" love between the two men if one man fears that his boyfriend will stop loving him if a condom is not used. But the reality is often not as simple or direct as that. Yes, in some extreme cases one partner might bully or threaten a partner with the end of a relationship or retaliate by going out to have sex with someone else who will not insist on using a condom. But these cases are, in my experience, rare, and are an example of partner abuse. More often the pressure comes from inside the partner who would prefer to use a condom, but for whatever reason (for example, lack of self-confidence, a sense of powerlessness, financial inequality, loving someone more than they are loved in return) is unable or unwilling to raise the issue or insist that condoms are used. Thus, in these kinds of situations, the man who wants to use a condom but is going along with UAI is often doing so to hold onto his own feelings of — or illusions of — love and being in love.

Sometimes, these decisions take place on a conscious level, but more often it happens on an unconscious level as the man feels fearful and anxious that he might be rejected by his beloved. He may be telling himself he is agreeing to UAI out of love, but it may have little to do with love or desire and more to do with his fragile self-esteem.

For people unable to differentiate between lust and love, unprotected sex is often an effort to hold on to the illusion of love or the potential for love. "Is love, in fact, self-sacrifice," asked the deceased actor Charles Ludlam (quoted in Kaufman, 2002, p. 138) "or is there another way of expressing love?" Though he was not speaking about sexual risk-taking, this question is one that all people concerned about gay men who have sex without condoms, especially within a committed relationship, would do well to ponder. Obviously, love within a healthy relationship is not just about self-sacrifice but also about sharing and compromise. So while self-sacrifice may indeed occur, it is probably best not to have that be the foundation upon which a relationship is built.

FOUR AGREEMENTS ON CONDOM USE

In the worst-case scenario, couples never directly talk about what they are going to do sexually. Sometimes these couples will use condoms and sometimes they will not. The problem is not whether or not they use condoms but their inability to discuss with each other what each is comfortable with and willing to do in regard to protecting themselves and each other from possible risk. Crawford et al. (2001) suggest that agreements regarding anal sex within and outside a relationship can be classified as such:

- None — where men have no agreement with their partner about how anal sex will be conducted either between them or with outside partners.
- No unprotected anal intercourse — where the men have agreed always to use condoms with each other or outside partners or to abstain from anal sex entirely with each other and outside partners.
- Negotiated safety — which will be described in detail further on in this chapter.
- Unsafe — where the men agree not to use condoms either sometimes or all the time within the relationship and where (a) one of the men is HIV-positive and the other is uninfected or the HIV status of one or both partners is unknown or (b) both men have the same HIV status but there is no agreement about not engaging in anal sex without condoms outside the relationship.

UNDERSTANDING GAY NONMONOGAMY

Ever since HIV was discovered to be transmitted sexually, AIDS prevention experts, public health workers, and mental health professionals have generally advised gay men, even those in committed relationships, always to use a condom. They made no exceptions for men in committed and explicitly monogamous relationships. In addition to being unrealistic, there was a level of unexamined homophobia and negative attitudes about gay relationships reflected in this advice. For one thing, it reflects negative stereotypes of gay men and a double standard: the same message was not given to committed opposite-sex couples. Gay men continue to be stereotyped as sexual animals who are unable to commit to sexual exclusivity or to honestly discuss with a partner their outside sexual activity and HIV status.

Research has shown that heterosexual married couples who identify as monogamous actually report a high degree of covert sexual non-exclusivity at some point during their marriage — in other words, straight married people routinely and frequently have sexual liaisons outside of their marriages (Hunt, 1974; Hyde, 1982; Blumstein & Schwartz, 1983; Glass & Wright, 1985, 1992). Blumstein and Schwartz[3] found that a sizable minority of heterosexual married and cohabiting couples they studied had sex outside the relationship even though their spouse or partner believed the relationship was sexually exclusive.

In the face of this evidence that monogamy is not the norm for approximately one quarter of opposite-sex couples, the stereotype is still that heterosexual couples are faithful and monogamous for life. Gay men, on the other hand, are so routinely viewed as incapable of or disinterested in monogamy that even professionals who are activists, gay-affirmative, and sympathetic to gay cultural norms accept it without question. Those gay and gay-friendly professionals who create AIDS prevention campaigns have assumed that male couples would not be able to maintain their sexual exclusivity. The reality is that, for decades, couples have been figuring out for themselves how to address the question of whether or not to be monogamous and whether or not to use condoms, whether they do or do not have the same HIV status. Being able to choose to do what they wish, even if it is to share infection, is often difficult for outsiders to accept without having strong negative judgments.

Though some couples of whatever sexual orientation do remain sexually exclusive, many others do not. I agree with Manhattan social worker Donald McVinney (1998) who writes: "Gay male couples are highly diverse. Various social and historical conditions combine with constructs of eroticism, gender, and intimate relationships to create the rich constellations of gay male couples" (p. 209). Still today, in the third decade of the epidemic, HIV prevention campaigns continue to advise even long-term monogamous male couples to wear condoms no matter what their HIV status. Without retracting what I said above about the homophobia inherent in the message to all male couples that they should never take off the condom, it is also true that, like all couples, male couples might break monogamy agreements, either openly or in secret. But the fact remains that this is not exclusively a gay male phenomenon, and pathologizing those who choose negotiated nonmonogamy reflects heterosexual cultural biases and not gay cultural norms.

PATHOLOGIZING GAY MEN'S SEXUAL CULTURES

Even after homosexuality was removed from the American Psychiatric Association's list of diagnosed mental disorders, some mental health professionals, such as notoriously homophobic psychoanalyst Charles Socarides (1978), have portrayed gay men as deeply disturbed people and have unethically tried to use psychotherapy to change people's sexual orientation from homosexual to heterosexual. One of the most often-cited examples of homosexual men not being as developed or mature as "normal" heterosexual men was the supposed inability of gay men to form long-term, stable, and committed relationships. Socarides and other homophobic therapists cited the high incidence of nonmonogamy to support their belief that gay men's loving relationships are inherently unstable and used such pejorative terms as "narcissism" and "preoedipal relatedness" to describe a different cultural norm than that of the majority of opposite-sex couples. The gay men's community evolved an easier acceptance of nonmonogamy than the mainstream world. That does not mean gay men suffer from psychopathology, arrested development, or immoral values but only that some male couples are more realistic about the limitations of sexual exclusivity when combined with a committed love relationship.

Johnson and Keren (1996) describe that even supposedly liberal branches of the mental health field, such as family therapy, often used judgmental terms like "triangulation," "difficulty with intimacy," and "male objectification" to try to come to terms with nonmonogamy. Not specifically addressing the sexual orientation of the people involved,

Murray Bowen, a pioneering family systems theorist, wrote that when tensions arise between two people in a couple, there is a tendency to engage outsiders, resulting in an emotional triangle that deflects tension and stabilizes the original couple (Kerr & Bowen, 1968). For years, family therapists tried to reconcile this theory with the primarily happy nonmonogamous male couples they were seeing (Kurdek & Schmitt, 1985/86; Green, Bettinger, & Zacks, 1996; Greenan & Tunnell, 2003; Cheuvront, 2004). It is also true that power issues come up in negotiating nonmonogamy, much as they do when negotiating UAI (Shernoff, 1995; Morin, 1999; Shernoff & Morin, 1999; Greenan & Shernoff, 2003). But the point is that in itself, nonmonogamy is not inherently unhealthy or a sign of dysfunction when it is openly discussed and mutually agreed upon by all parties involved.

MALE COUPLES' SEXUAL DIVERSITY

One of the biggest differences between male couples and heterosexual couples is this cultural difference regarding sexual exclusivity. As family therapists Johnson and Keren (1996) note: "Monogamy seems to be hardwired into spoken and culturally sanctioned norms for heterosexual relationships. The gay community's normative acceptance of casual sex, anonymous sex, and nonmonogamy in couple relationships represents a dramatic departure from heterocentric norms and values" (pp. 238–239). This acceptance of sex outside a primary partnership has direct and urgent implications for gay men's emotional and physical well-being, especially when the realities of possibly contracting and spreading HIV are factored in. This is why I will spend the bulk of the rest of this chapter looking at how the issue of sexual exclusivity or nonexclusivity may be played out by male couples.

Research conducted prior to the onset of AIDS showed that many gay men were in couples in which both members agreed to be sexually nonexclusive (Blumstein & Schwartz, 1983; McWhirter & Mattison, 1984; Kurdek & Schmitt, 1985/86.) Studies conducted both in Australia[4] and the United States[5] just as the epidemic started to spread confirmed that a large percentage of male couples were not monogamous. Other studies confirmed these findings (Hickson et al.,

1992; Bryant & Demian, 1994; Bringle, 1995, Crawford et al., 2001, Davidovich et al., 2001). More recently, Coleman and Rosser (1996) discuss that though a majority of male couples are not sexually exclusive, they are in fact emotionally monogamous. Within the gay men's community, so many male couples are not monogamous that there is often an assumption that nonmonogamy is the norm for most male couples, which research seems to confirm, and that nonmonogamy in and of itself does not create a problem.

As a therapist working with male couples, I routinely explore how each member of the couple feels about monogamy and whether the couple has explicitly discussed the issue. If they have reached an understanding about how sex outside the partnership will be handled, asking about this can elicit important information about the couple's decision-making process and values as well as clarifying any possible confusion or miscommunication that may have occurred. It is not uncommon for couples to come to therapy in crisis because one member of the couple has either had sex or an affair outside of a supposedly monogamous relationship or one man wants to open the relationship up to outside sexual partners and the other does not and fears that this may mean a diminishing emotional attachment.

One form that nonmonogamy takes is called polyamory. Polyamory literally means many loves. Anapol (1997) suggests that polyamory can be understood as responsible nonmonogamy. I think that this is simplistic as negotiated nonmonogamy is very definitely responsible, even when it pertains to relationships that are primarily sexual. Bettinger (2005) states that "some gay men in committed relationships have other sexual relationships which involve a degree of emotional intimacy, commitment and/or longevity" (p. 98). My clinical experience is that some male couples are polyamorous and may form a variety of relationships that are often overlapping and sometimes become their primary families of choice. Speaking to this reality, Bettinger (2005) reports that "the sexual and romantic mating patterns of gay men are more complex than domestic partnership connotates. The lack of monogamy results in some gay men having primary and secondary partners. There may be more than one primary or secondary partner" (p. 98).

NONMONOGAMY MAY NOT BE INFIDELITY

Nonmonogamy challenges many basic assumptions about love and commitment. Some heterosexual therapists (for example, Charny, 1992) referring only to heterosexual couples, suggest that sex outside a primary relationship is *always* a sign that the primary relationship is troubled. Indeed, there is some research suggesting that sex outside a male couple's relationship may be related to dissatisfaction about the partnership (Sagir & Robins, 1973; Bell & Weinberg, 1978; Kurdek & Schmitt, 1985/86). Yet, subsequent studies have found no significant differences in relationship quality or satisfaction between samples of sexually exclusive and nonexclusive male couples (Blasband & Peplau, 1985; Kurdek, 1988; Wagner, Remien, & Carballo-Dieguez, 2000). For therapists who work with male couples, inquiring about whether or not the couple is monogamous and how they negotiated this issue is a perfect segue into conversations with the couple about whether or not they use condoms and the comfort level each has pertaining to this decision.

Research has shown that a minority of male couples are monogamous. Even so, this does not justify the public policy message to male couples that they should never take off a condom with their partner if both know their own and the other's HIV status. Male couples who are monogamous may be sexually exclusive either for certain periods of their relationships or for the duration of their relationships (Blumstein & Schwartz, 1983; Kurdek & Schmitt, 1985/86; Stulberg & Smith, 1988; Kippax et al., 1993; Bryant & Demian, 1994; Shernoff, 1995; Crawford, 2001). A variety of social scientists have documented that the majority of male couples they surveyed did not believe that sexual nonexclusivity threatened their relationship and differentiated between negotiated sexual nonexclusivity and infidelity (Mendola, 1980; Silverstein, 1981; Blumstein & Schwartz, 1983; McWhirter & Mattison, 1984). Yet the research I just cited all took place prior to AIDS, which changed the potential impact that sexual infidelity could have upon a relationship. As far as I am aware, no research has specifically examined whether one partner breaking the agreement to be monogamous after the onset of the age of AIDS has a different impact upon a male couple than it did prior to the epidemic.

In the past several years, among the couples I have seen who were in a crisis due to one of them having sex outside of their supposedly monogamous relationship, the realities of STDs and especially HIV certainly contributed to the intensity of the crisis. Again, terms and definitions are slippery areas. For example, "fidelity" may be used by male couples differently than by heterosexual couples. Generally, heterosexual couples use the term "fidelity" synonymously with "monogamy." If the male couple has explicitly agreed to be sexually exclusive, then fidelity has the identical meaning for them. Yet, for other male couples, "fidelity" means "honesty." Thus, for male couples who are not sexually exclusive, "fidelity" often means the emotional primacy of the relationship. For example, two men may live together and jointly own property, share a rich social and emotional life, celebrate holidays together, and be integrated into each other's families. This couple may or may not still be sexually active with each other. Perhaps together they go to sex parties or the baths and either play together with a third person or participate in group sex or have sex separately there. Or they may have an understanding that one night of the week they are each permitted to have a night off from the relationship. These are only some of the possible ways that male couples may set up how there will be sexual nonexclusivity while remaining committed to each other.

Well-known gay writer Edmund White wrote about these kinds of situations in a 1983 — pre-AIDS — article on sexual culture in *Vanity Fair* (White, 1983, p. 164):

> If all goes well, two gay men will meet, most probably through sex, become lovers, weather the storms of jealousy and the diminution of lust, develop shared interests, and end up with a long-term, probably sexless camaraderie that is not as disinterested as friendship or as seismic as passion or as charged with contradiction as fraternity. Needless to say, such couples can wreak havoc on the newcomer who fails to grasp that Bob and Fred are not just roommates. They may have separate bedrooms and regular extracurricular sex partners or even beaux, but Bob monitors Fred's infatuations with an eye attuned to nuance, and at a certain point will intervene to banish a potential rival.

While the kind of relationship described by White certainly does exist, and I have known such couples socially and worked with them as clients, I also know and have worked with many long-term male couples who do remain sexually active with each other, whether they are sexually exclusive or not, for years and decades.

NEGOTIATING OPEN RELATIONSHIPS

One important aspect to keeping a nonmonogamous relationship healthy is explicit and clear communication between the partners in order to establish a set of rules or guidelines for both to follow that set the parameters about how sex outside the relationship is to be conducted. In the context of couples who have condomless sex, either only with their partners or also with men outside the couple relationship, it is essential that these agreements be predetermined and explicit. Infidelity within this context means breaking the rules that the couple has agreed upon for how sex outside the primary relationship is conducted (Shernoff, 1995).

Examples of the kinds of rules that some couples set up regarding nonmonogamy may include:

- Always use a condom for anal sex outside the relationship.
- No anal sex with outside partners.
- No affairs.
- Don't ask, don't tell.
- Full disclosure.
- No sex with friends.
- No sex in the couple's home.
- Sex is allowed in their home but not in their bed.
- Mutual participation in the outside sexual relationships (three-way or group sex).

For example, if the couple has decided that sex outside the relationship is permitted when either partner is traveling, and one man steps outside the relationship when both men are in their home city, this would constitute a sexual infidelity. Some nonmonogamous couples in which partners have confirmed that they are HIV-negative have an explicit agreement that if either does have sex outside the relationship either anal sex is not permitted or if it is, then condoms must be used for anal sex. This arrangement is part of what has been labeled "negotiated safety" (Kippax, Crawford, Davis, Rodden, & Dowset, 1993). Negotiated safety will be discussed at length near the end of this chapter. Engaging in unprotected anal sex with an outsider would then be considered an infidelity.

STAGE OF RELATIONSHIP AND SEXUAL RISK-TAKING

Male couples living in the age of AIDS need to balance different desires, sexual tastes, and levels of comfort regarding what sexual risk-taking, if any, is acceptable and how the couple decides whether or not to be sexually exclusive. Thus, monogamy in the age of HIV and AIDS is an even more important issue to be discussed openly than it was historically for male couples. How these issues are raised, discussed, and negotiated are indications of the emotional climate created in the couple's daily interactions and shared emotional life. Hendrick and Hendrick (1983) and Brehm (1985) both suggest that relationship dynamics vary depending on the developmental stage of the relationship. As Hays et al. (1997) note, "It is reasonable to expect that the factors contributing to high-risk sex at early stages of relationships may differ from those associated with high-risk sex in relationships of longer duration" (p. 322). Research on unprotected sex by gay men in boyfriend relationships found that gay men's sexual behaviors become increasingly risky as they progress (Hays et al., 1997).

NEGOTIATED SAFETY

Why would relationship longevity increase partners' willingness to take sexual risks? The answer lies primarily in the fact that the longer male couples stay together, the more likely they are to develop trust and better communication, and the more likely they then are to attempt the delicate negotiations around sexual nonexclusivity and sexual safety.

As mentioned earlier, "negotiated safety" (Kippax et al., 1993, 1997; Crawford et al., 2001) is an agreement between two HIV-negative gay men in a relationship. It is a process of discussion, inner contemplation, and further discussion which leads them to decide whether or not to stop using condoms when they have anal sex. The discussions are premised on the mutual knowledge of their own and their partner's HIV status. As originally defined by Kippax et al. (1993) in its simplest form, negotiated safety was safer sex with a partner until mutual testing at least several months after either partner's most recent high-risk encounter showed that both men were uninfected. Once this had been established, then nothing unsafe was permitted with outside partners. While there may be varieties of negotiated safety agreements, the most commonly accepted one is as follows. The only time the men do not use condoms is when they have sex with each other, making this an acceptable safer sex option. They agree not to have unprotected sex outside the relationship; if either partner does so, then he must immediately inform his partner prior to their having sex again. They then agree to resume using condoms until subsequent HIV tests prove that the partner who had unprotected sex is still negative (freedoms.org.uk, 2002).

For couples I work with who are considering adopting a negotiated safety agreement, I always provide them with the Web site of freedom. org, a British organization that has developed a sample negotiated safety agreement, so they can download a copy. This agreement is reproduced with permission in Appendix 1. I urge them to go through it together when they are not in a session with me, and then come back to therapy so we can talk about what the experience of completing the questions on the agreement was like for each of them. We can then also discuss any additional concerns they might have, as well as any feelings that may have arisen in reading and talking through the sample agreement. If they agree not to use condoms, then only their agreement protects them from contracting a life-threatening virus. In other words, the trust they have for each other has to be strong. Sometimes one or both become very frightened and wish to revisit the entire issue of opening up their relationship sexually. Some couples decide that they are not ready or able to trust each other to that degree and decide to remain sexually exclusive and continue to have UAI with each other.

HOW SAFE IS A NEGOTIATED SAFETY AGREEMENT?

Does negotiated safety actually protect HIV-negative men in sero-concordant relationships from becoming infected? Limited social science research has studied precisely this question, and none of the studies published to date on negotiated safety have examined male couples in the United States. Michael Ross, the U.S. editor of the prestigious journal *AIDS Care,* told me that in his opinion part of the reason for the absence of any U.S. studies on negotiated safety was a healthy skepticism about negotiated safety among researchers and AIDS prevention professionals in the United States. He described negotiated safety as "something that sounds sensible in practice but is normatively dangerous. If properly applied, it would work (safer sex until mutual testing), but in practice it provides a scientific-sounding justification for asking 'Are you HIV-negative?' and then acting on that" (personal communication, November 22, 2004). I do not disagree with Dr. Ross, but I believe that there are additional reasons why information on negotiated safety is not provided in the United States and why it is not researched here.

My sense is that negotiated safety makes AIDS prevention professionals in the United States nervous. This nervousness is reflected in an unwillingness on the part of U.S. AIDS service organizations to address honestly the issue that increasing numbers of gay men are not using condoms for anal sex, and if both men are uninfected and only having sex with each other this is not a high-risk behavior. U.S. AIDS service organizations and prevention messages reflect a timidity in avoiding the kind of honest harm reduction information about barebacking that appears in England and Australia out of fear that if they were to do so it would be construed as an endorsement of barebacking, just as conservative politicians accuse needle exchange programs of being an endorsement of intravenous drug use. Under the Bush administration, AIDS researchers and sex researchers have found their funding threatened, withdrawn, or not available. "Social scientists say that for all its diverse tastes and freedoms, the nation that invented Viagra and *Sex and the City* is still queasy about exploring sexual desire and arousal, even when this knowledge is central to protecting public health" (Carey, 2004). Carey (2004) states that in July 2003, the U.S. Congress threatened to shut down several highly regarded sex studies and refused to finance a widely anticipated proposal backed by three large universities to support and train students interested in studying sexuality.[6]

Luckily, researchers in other countries are not working under constraints similar to those in the United States. There is now research that demonstrates that negotiated safety agreements are fairly widespread in England and Australia and once entered into, are in the vast majority of cases kept (Kippax et al., 1993, 1997; Davidovich et al., 2000). One study in Sydney surveyed the sexual practices of 1037 gay and bisexual men and found that a significant number of men used negotiated safety as an HIV prevention strategy.[7] Kippax's team also found that 11 percent of their respondents did not keep their agreements never to have anal sex without a condom with a casual partner. These authors found that the integrity of the negotiated agreement was related to the nature of the safety agreement reached between the men and on the acceptability of using condoms with outside partners. Agreements between HIV-negative, seroconcordant regular partners prohibiting anal intercourse, even with a condom, with casual partners or any form of sex with a casual partner were typically complied with, and the men who had such negotiated agreements were at low risk of HIV infection (Kippax et al., 1997). In Amsterdam,[8] of the men who met all the criteria for inclusion in a study on negotiated safety agreements, only two had engaged in UAI with a casual partner in violation of the agreement they had made with their primary partner. Other studies from Amsterdam (Davidovich et al., 2001; Xiridou, Geskus, de Wit, Coutinho, & Kretzschmar, 2003) and Australia (Kippax et al., 1997; Crawford et al., 2001) reveal that approximately 90 percent of men in HIV-seroconcordant relationships have negotiated safety agreements. These same studies report that the rates of noncompliance with negotiated safety agreements are consistently around 10 percent.

Despite the impressive statistic that roughly 90 percent of gay men who negotiated safety agreements honor them by not having risky sex outside their relationships, it must be added that Davidovich et al. (2000) included an important caveat in their conclusions when they stated that they assumed that the reported rates of noncompliance with negotiated safety agreements are an underestimation of the actual noncompliance rates. There are two reasons to strongly suspect a higher level of noncompliance with negotiated safety agreements. The first is that in trying to ascertain levels of compliance, the researchers have to rely upon self-reports from their study subjects. Davidovich et al. (2000) suspect that there may be a social desirability bias that interferes with some subjects' willingness to be honest about their engagement in UAI with casual partners, especially since it means noncompliance with a negotiated safety agreement they made with their primary partner. The second reason is that typically only one member of the relationship is a participant in any of the cited studies, leaving the possibility open that the man who is not a study subject may be noncompliant with the negotiated safety agreement.

Even though the estimated 10 percent of men who are noncompliant with negotiated safety agreements is a relatively low percentage, it still raises important public health issues as a potential vector of new infections, as demonstrated by the two Amsterdam studies. To clearly illustrate how much of a public health risk this is, I want to discuss a third study out of Amsterdam. Davidovich et al. (2001) questioned 144 men who had recently seroconverted. Men under 30 who seroconverted between 1994 and 2000 had greater odds of having been infected by their steady partner than did those who seroconverted between 1984 and 1987, when men were more likely to have been infected by a casual partner. By 2000, the proportion of HIV infections that can be attributed to steady partners reached 67 percent of the young men who had recently seroconverted. In trying to explain why younger gay men became infected from their partners, Davidovich and colleagues offer a few possibilities. They suggest that a previous study they conducted (Davidovich et al., 2000) found that younger gay men engage in more high-risk behaviors with steady partners than with casual partners. They also suggest that young gay men may practice less negotiated safety and/or lack the ability to remain compliant to these agreements when they do make them with their primary partner, which exposes them to more risk. "It could also be that young gay men have more romantic or infatuated attitudes towards relationships, which facilitate risk-taking behaviors" (Davidovich et al., 2001, p. 1307). Younger gay men also do not know, because they have not observed it firsthand, the kind of real and lasting damage that HIV and AIDS can cause.[1]

Davidovich et al. (2000) provide an appropriate cautionary note about negotiated safety when they write that negotiated safety "can provide the necessary protection from HIV infection, but incidents of noncompliance do occur and can involve risk" (p. 704). Both Kippax et al. (1997) and Davidovich et al. (2000) remind all who either practice or advocate negotiated safety that the rates of noncompliance must be taken into consideration. Davidovich et al. feel strongly that negotiated safety agreements should not leave out the condition of reporting noncompliance to a partner, as the freedom.org Web site's agreement model suggests. The researchers write: "It must be made clear that the disclosure of incidences of risky noncompliance is an inseparable part of the negotiated safety agreement. Furthermore, it should be emphasized that after an incident of risky noncompliance the negotiated safety process must start anew if the steady partners wish to continue to engage in UAI with each other" (p. 704).

How men in relationships conceive of what is sexually risky varies greatly. In discussing negotiated safety, Michael Ross told me that he suspects for many men there appears to have been a shift in what people now mean when they think about what has become known as negotiated safety. The original premise of negotiated safety was safer sex until mutual testing proves that it was safe for the men to stop using condoms and then nothing unsafe took place outside the relationship. For some couples negotiated safety has evolved into "let's agree not to have unsafe sex outside the relationship." Ross suggests that this has shifted the paradigm of negotiated safety from something that was safe to "something that relies on trust and a belief that one is negative [due to an outdated test result]. This is in fact a move from 'negotiated safety' to 'negotiated trust,' which is not the same thing" (Ross, personal communication, November 24, 2004). The studies conducted in Amsterdam show that a majority of men who become infected with HIV were infected by a steady partner. Some of these men were infected because they did not know either their own or their partner's HIV status and were having UAI. Some were infected because one of the men was not compliant with a negotiated safety agreement. Thus, what Ross refers to as "negotiated trust" is clearly not an effective way of stopping the spread of HIV.

For all gay men who seek a committed relationship or who are already in one, love, the desire to love and be loved, sex, and the specter of HIV infection are inextricably bound together and most likely will be for the foreseeable future. Psychologist and researcher Leo Wilton (2001) has stated that how two men behave within the context of their coupled relationship is a complex equation and that decisions about sexual practices within the couple may be influenced by numerous biomedical, psychological, and sociological factors. With what Wilton points out in mind, Halkitis et al. (2004) suggest that at times some decisions to practice UAI may in certain situations be without risk, as when the men have the same strain of HIV-1 and are monogamous. "In other instances, however, misperceptions about health risks (that is, beliefs that superinfection cannot occur) and dyadic miscommunications (that is, misunderstandings about how monogamy is defined in the relationship) may lead some members of the couple to make faulty decisions that place them at high risk for adverse health consequences" (Halkitis et al., 2004, p. 100).

CONCLUSION

The simple advice to "just say no" to UAI is not realistic, practical, or followed by large numbers of gay men in relationships. Partnered gay men are caught in multiple and often conflicting vortexes, some of which are unique to same-sex couples and some of which are common to all couples. The internalization by male couples of the predominant (heterosexual) norms of romance and coupledom are often in conflict with gay cultural norms. Male couples are constantly bombarded by gay cultural pressures to have lots of hot sex, with and without their partners. Simultaneously, most have grown up or become sexually active with messages about the importance of using a condom every time and not to trust others to be honest about HIV status. On top of all of this, each individual has his own expectations and assumptions about his partner, who experiences all of these forces as well.

Male couples also have to contend with each man possibly being in a different phase of gay identity formation, and how out each is about being gay. All couples have to find ways to cope with differences in life stage and the relationship's various developmental stages, to negotiate relationships with their families and friends, and to balance autonomy and togetherness. Differences about communication, problem solving, and negotiation of power, as well as cultural differences, also need to be factored in. In the best of all possible worlds, male couples would learn how to enter into skillful verbal negotiations about sex, intimacy, and emotional trust, while becoming mindful of their own and their partner's internal psychodynamics. The following two chapters will discuss how all of these issues play out around condomless sex in three different types of male couples: those where both men are HIV-positive, those where both men are HIV-negative, and those where the men have different HIV status.

CHAPTER SEVEN

Love, Sex, and Trust

SECTION I: SEROCONCORDANT MALE COUPLES

JAKE AND MARK: POSITIVE NEGOTIATIONS

In the two years that Jake and Mark had been together, they always practiced safer sex. They were healthy, HIV-positive white men who came to see me for therapy to talk about their plans to move in together. They were both in their fifties and financially successful, and each had lost a long-term partner to AIDS. From the first session, I was impressed by how loving and tender they were with each other. They had a maturity that I do not always see in clients; they were able to listen deeply and absorb what the other was saying before responding.

One of the main concerns that came up around their plans to move in together was whether they would continue to have protected sex or whether they would now start having oral and anal sex without condoms. While neither had a detectable level of HIV, they practiced safer sex with each other in a sexually exclusive partnership. They both described their partnership as rich, interesting, and sensual, but Mark said he felt some frustration that they were still using condoms. One of his hopes for moving the relationship to a deeper level — cohabitating — was that their new level of commitment would open the door to new sexual intimacy, namely that they could start loosening the strict rules they had about safer sex. I asked Mark what his best-case scenario would be for this next phase of their relationship. "I really want to drink him," Mark answered right away. "Since we have undetectable HIV, there's no way we can test to see if we have the same strain of the virus. That's why we've practiced safer sex for two years — we don't want to risk reinfecting each other." When I asked him to explain why semen exchange was so important to him, he said it would be a kind of "spiritual communion" with Jake. "Being able to do these things would make me feel even closer to him than I already do," said Mark. He also shared that historically, prior to AIDS it had been his absolute favorite sexual thing to do and he really missed doing it.

I noticed that Jake looked uncomfortable as Mark spoke, so I asked him what he was feeling. Jake said that he had grown up in a conservative Southern home, and hearing Mark speak in such a sexually explicit way to me, a virtual stranger, made him uncomfortable — even though he knew that this was one of the areas they had come to therapy to talk about. Mark looked sheepish and said, "Sorry, honey," and Jake smiled at him and said, "No, no, it's me, not you. You should say whatever you want to say. I'll have to get over it."

When I asked Jake what his feelings were about relaxing their rules around safer sex, Jake shook his head and said he wished he could give Mark what he wanted, but he was not willing to have sex without a condom. The first reason was that he did not want to take even the smallest chance that he could reinfect his beloved. "To me, it wouldn't be worth the pleasure of the moment to do something that could hurt Mark," he said. The second reason was more pragmatic — he could not imagine relaxing enough to enjoy the unprotected sex. "I'd be thinking the whole time about the possibility of AIDS, and it wouldn't be fun." I nodded, remembering the many times I had heard other couples speak over the years about how unsafe sex brought thoughts of death into their sexual play.

Mark listened carefully to Jake, although clearly he had heard his lover's arguments before. I asked him what he had to say about

Jake's position, and Mark turned to Jake and said, "Honey, we are now middle-aged queens, something I never expected to become when I first found out that I was HIV-positive in the 1980s. Even if we did get reinfected with another strain of the virus, it could take 15 or 20 years to have a negative impact on either of our health. How long do you want me to live?"

Jake smiled a little as Mark said this. I privately thought that Mark had been very strategic to remind Jake that even reinfection would not necessarily mean death — having HIV today is not like it was a decade or two ago. Jake had obviously heard this argument from Mark previously, but still he did not dismiss it. He was quiet for a moment and then said that while intellectually he also wanted to dispense with condoms for anal sex, he was deeply conflicted about it. On the one hand, he missed the kind of completely uninhibited sexuality he had experienced prior to AIDS. But on the other hand, he said again that he worried that if he did not use condoms he would not be able to let himself go and enjoy sex with Mark. He spoke about his deep loss — of the many loved ones now gone from AIDS, as well of the carefree part of his own sexuality that he had cherished but could not express now because of AIDS. He told Mark, "Considering how many people have died, it's going to be hard not to think of either my own or your semen as anything other than a drink of death." Mark was visibly touched hearing this and reached over to hold Jake. After a few minutes Mark said that if Jake wanted him to continue to use a condom, he could live with that.

My assessment of Mark was that he was not depressed, impulsive, or self-destructive. He understood that there was some possibility of becoming reinfected by Jake with another strain of HIV. He was conversant with the medical debates on the issue of reinfection, which in the current medical terminology is labeled HIV superinfection.[1] My assessment of Jake was that he was emotionally autonomous enough for it to be unlikely that he would feel pressured or forced to engage in behavior with which he was uncomfortable.

While it seemed that Mark had given in to Jake's needs, I had a sense that the discussion was not over. I could tell they had expressed their positions to each other several times before coming to therapy. "I'm guessing that, since you're sitting here today, one of the important points of contention is that you aren't completely resolved about the status quo regarding continuing to use condoms," I said. The men looked a little uncomfortable. I realized that it is normal for men at this phase of a relationship to want to avoid or minimize conflicts that arise from their having different needs and feelings. I reflected this back to them and shared that I believed that if we talked more about this issue, and the impact their decision would have on their lives and sexual intimacy, they might come to a place where they both felt positive about the outcome. They smiled nervously at each other and at me. Knowing that part of my job as a couples therapist was to try to give voice to fears that may not have yet been spoken, I said, "Mark, I think it's noble that you're willing to give up your need out of respect for Jake's feelings, but I wonder if you might not resent it after a while?" I turned to Jake. "Jake, I wonder if you are worrying that your not giving Mark what he craves from you in this very intimate area might push him to look for it elsewhere?"

They both looked a little stunned that I had voiced their secret fears, but there was also relief that it was now out in the open. I urge clients to tell me if my guesses are wrong, and these two men did not contradict me. Mark reassured Jake that as much as condomless oral and anal sex were his absolute favorite things to do, he would never want Jake to fear that he might seek this from other men. He was committed to monogamy with Jake no matter what. Hearing this, Jake let out an intense exhale and admitted that he had feared just that, and in fact until the moment when Mark relieved this anxiety, he had felt an internal pressure to do something he was not comfortable with in order to keep his boyfriend from straying. It was a pivotal moment — the underlying tension had relaxed and now they could start to look for a win–win solution.

Mark once again said that as much as he was not thrilled with their sexual status quo, he could live with it. Hearing this, Jake looked hurt and pained. I asked Mark if he saw the look on Jake's face, and Mark nodded, looking worried. I asked him to ask Jake to explain what the facial expressions represented. He did, and then Jake explained that he had thought that they were having great sex and was hurt and surprised to hear that Mark had complaints about their sex life. I thanked Jake for being so vulnerable and honest with Mark and asked Mark to respond. Mark began by saying that he did not really have complaints. Before he could continue, Jake interrupted him by saying: "It certainly sounds as if you have complaints!"

At first Mark was dumbfounded. But he broke the tense silence by reaching over, hugging Jake and telling him that he loved their sex, and thought it was all great, but that he was greedy and wanted more. "I want all of you, especially your juice, which I've never had. It's much more important for me to get your juice than to give you mine, though of course I'd love to do that as well," Mark said in a sexy and boyish way that caused Jake to crack up and melt. Mark reiterated that he could live very happily with Jake without adding in this one thing that he longed for. I noted first to myself and then to Mark that during these interactions Mark had been both holding onto his need and trying to let go of it. I did not know how to interpret this and asked Mark about it. "When the goddess created cocksuckers, I was the prototype," he said. "I certainly have had my share of it during my long and rich sex life, only never with this man, whom I plan on spending the rest of my life with. I can't deny that having him give me that is a very deep need of mine, but I get so much out of our relationship that without denying my need, I can choose to forego it. I know by now that one never gets everything one wants, nor should one expect to." I was impressed by his wise perspective and told him so.

Hearing this, Jake broke into tears. "Honey, I never realized how profoundly you missed not getting this one thing that you love so. As you can see, I'm literally moved to tears that you love me so much that you would be willing to live without this. How about if, for right now, I promise to be open to possibly doing this and let's see what happens?" With what appeared to be a possible breakthrough moment at hand, I asked Jake if he was willing to speak more about one of the two concerns he stated earlier — that he wouldn't be capable of enjoying sex without condoms because of worry about HIV reinfection. I asked him if he thought he might have sexual performance problems. Jake said yes, he did wonder if he might lose his erection. I asked Mark to respond to Jake's concern. Mark very sweetly told him that there were a whole lot of things they could do if indeed Jake went limp and then said,

"Whoever said that a soft penis didn't have feelings and need attention also?" We all laughed at that.

With all of this good feeling to draw on, I wanted to clarify what I was hearing was their new agreement. "So, tell me if I am saying this right. You are agreeing that the possibility is now open for you both to cum in each other's mouths, and in the future the possibility of unprotected anal sex will also be considered. Is that it?" Mark corrected me, "We're agreeing that I can drink Jake, but he doesn't have to reciprocate." Two things surprised me. I asked Jake how he was handling the fear of possibly reinfecting Mark, as well as any fears he had about possibly becoming reinfected himself as a result of having Mark's semen inside him. He responded he wasn't that worried about himself because his health was excellent and he did not really believe that if Mark stopped using condoms it would have any negative impact on his health. On the other hand, Mark's health was not as robust as his, he explained, and this was a major contributing factor to his not wanting to give Mark his semen.

Hearing this, Mark said, "I'm a big boy and have taken plenty of risks in my life. If this is one I am willing to take, while I appreciate your protectiveness, I would rather have a fuller and richer sex life with you even if it meant a shorter life, which I am not convinced it will!"

"I really hear and understand what you're saying. I just don't want to lose you prematurely," Jake told Mark.

"I know, honey, but just think about how much more of you you'll be giving me if you do decide to stop using a condom," Mark replied.

"I like that idea a lot," Jake told him. "But it still does not seem to balance the equation."

"Perhaps there is no balancing of this equation at all, but only living as fully and as courageously as we can with whatever time we may have left to enjoy each other," Mark said in a manner that was both flirtatious and earnest.

I asked Jake how this made him feel. He said that Mark's insistence that a shorter life would be preferable if it was more satisfying was beginning to thaw his resolve. I asked him whether he felt he was being worn down by Mark's arguments. He responded, "Only a little. But I really want to do these things also but am just very nervous about it." I was never able to get Jake to say whether he had somehow managed to set aside his own misgivings or whether he had just given in to Mark.

After a few more sessions, the men left therapy with a new agreement that they would begin trying oral sex that might culminate in ejaculations inside of each other's mouths. Over time, as Jake became more comfortable with this idea, they tried unprotected anal intercourse (UAI) with both ejaculating inside of the other. For a short time after dispensing with condoms, Jake did occasionally lose his erection. Because he had talked about this possibility in therapy, neither man became overly concerned about it, seeing it as a normal part of the transition. This resulted in it very quickly ceasing to occur. Both came in for the last session reporting that relaxing of safer-sex practices greatly enhanced their sex life and made them feel closer than ever. They both reported that dispensing with condoms made them feel like they were each reclaiming a part of their youth and pre-AIDS sexuality, while obviously understanding that what they were now doing was not risk-free.

At our last session, Jake told me, "I feel that I am being so bad by not using condoms any longer, and I really love that it is Mark who's helping me indulge in my private secret naughtiness. I have allowed AIDS for so long to be a central part of my life. Taking meds on a precise schedule, being sexually cautious, I still have my fears, but I'm having so much fun I think Mark is right — more of this pleasure may be worth a few years less of life. If I get too uncomfortable with our not using condoms, Mark has agreed that we can always revisit beginning to use them again. I don't feel locked into what we are now doing sexually for the rest of my life, unless we both are comfortable with this arrangement."

COUPLES AND CONDOMS: CHAPTER OVERVIEW

Jake and Mark were hardly the first couple I have worked with who were both HIV-positive and wanted to change the rules of their sex life to dispense with condoms. What strikes me about their case is their thoughtfulness combined with empathy, and how the respect they showed for each other's positions allowed them to negotiate effectively. Mark and Jake's process was vastly different from that of

Ted and Donald — the HIV-positive couple described in the previous chapter.

The kinds of conversations Jake and Mark had about changing the rules about condom use are happening in and out of therapists' offices. These kinds of conversations seem to me normal and appropriate for all male couples to have at some point in their relationship, no matter what they decide regarding whether to use condoms. The presence of HIV or the specter of HIV cannot be underestimated and needs to play a huge part in these discussions, as do assumptions and insecurities and questions about monogamy, desirability, and all the factors discussed in Chapter 6, such as love, trust, intimacy, and power. How well informed are couples when they begin these conversations about either's desire to change the rules? What beliefs are influencing their decisions — from the possibility of reinfection to the risk or safety of unprotected oral sex?

This chapter explores the intimate dialogues about condoms, risk, and health among couples where both men are HIV-positive, where both are HIV-negative, and where one is positive and one is negative. How do the different configurations change the nature of the conversation? What are some of the most successful ways men negotiate their needs and desires and some of the most destructive ways? Individuals' own intrapsychic issues always play into partners' decision making, and in this chapter we will look at several examples of clinical work with men who came to understand how their past experiences influenced their decision whether to take sexual risks. We will also examine some common relationship issues and how they create pressure on some men to change the rules about condoms when they do not feel ready or willing. I will also describe what I believe to be the most useful tool for couples talking about their sexual lives, called negotiated safety agreements.

In Section II of this chapter, we will look at specific issues for serodiscordant couples, including disclosure of HIV status, how combination therapies change partners' thinking about the risks of HIV, and — returning to one of the thorniest questions of the book — how some men are turned on by high-risk sex. We will also hear from men for whom barebacking resulted in seroconversion. I see over and over again that loving, committed gay partners want unsafe sex to be a step in the deepening intimacy between them.

The literature on HIV and AIDS lacks research and discussion about the rationales why HIV-negative seroconcordant couples choose to have condomless sex. There has been much more emphasis placed on rates of frequency of UAI than on the internal decision-making process of men who make that choice, although that information would be very helpful to mental health, public health, and AIDS prevention professionals. It is interesting to conjecture on the reasons for this lack of research. One reason may be that in the United States, research most often does not focus on "healthy" individuals, and since neither man in a HIV-negative seroconcordant couple has an illness, there is no funding to study them. This is part of the general medicalization and pathologization of research that results in the underfunding of research on the reasons people make choices that enhance their health and wellness. Another factor might be that to fund studies of uninfected gay men in relationships would mean legitimizing those relationships by studying them. With political and religious conservatives having unprecedented access to the legislative branch of the federal government, it is highly doubtful that large-scale studies of uninfected male couples are considered a priority.

ROMANTIC RATIONALITY

Flowers, Smith, Sheeran, and Beail (1997) discuss a phenomenon they call "romantic rationality," which is a collection of motivations that influence sexual decision making by men in relationships. Once most people are in love, their definition of normal shifts, so that they think differently about issues than they did when they were single. Romantic rationality also speaks to the fact that when individuals are in love, they can rationalize almost anything they or their beloveds do. People in love also often put up with situations they would never endure if they were single, based on the benefits they derive from being loved or loving.

Flowers et al. also discuss that traditional understanding of sexual behavior comes from the field of health psychology. Health psychology studies individuals' reactions to becoming ill or what influences them to make decisions that will increase the likelihood of staying healthy and how health care professionals can be better attuned to the emotional and psychological aspects of staying healthy and being ill. Traditional conceptual frameworks such as the health belief model (Rosenstock, 1974), the theory of planned behavior (Ajzen, 1991), and the theory of reasoned action (Fishbein & Ajzen, 1975) all have as their foundation the assumption that most people are in pursuit of health and the avoidance of illness. Applied to the discussion of barebacking and UAI in relationships, we can see that changing a behavior (in this case using a condom for anal sex) will result in a single benefit to the individual of maximizing his likelihood of maintaining health. In sexual health research this is thought of as an individual's disease prevention beliefs (condom use). This is weighed against the person's beliefs in sexual pleasure (loss of sensation and spontaneity from use of a condom).

Health psychology has previously only utilized a health rationality approach, which uses a health promotion approach to encourage condom use. Health rationality takes as a given that most people would rather make rational decisions about things they can do to remain healthy or prevent illness, like not overeat, exercise more, or not smoke. Health promotion refers to attempts to motivate people to make choices that will increase their ability to remain healthy. But as is now clear, this approach has only had limited success, with even less success when targeting male couples. Flowers and colleagues strongly suggest that gay men in relationships may prioritize romantic rationality and make informed decisions regarding HIV risk-taking not to use condoms. This choice would demonstrate commitment, love, and trust but nevertheless place some men in relationships at risk for becoming infected.

MONOGAMY AND MALE COUPLES

Every relationship is unique, but I think it is safe to say that when couples come to therapy at least in part to discuss whether or not to stop using condoms, one person is less comfortable than the other with the idea. Usually, as in the case of Mark and Jake, one partner is pressuring the other to give up condoms. As in the case of Ted and Donald in the previous chapter, this pressure may create considerable stress within the relationship. There have been many couples with whom I have worked who after talking decide to continue to use condoms because one or both partners' discomfort with the idea of having unprotected sex is so high — no matter how sexy and appealing it seems.

Similarly, several couples have consulted with me where one was pushing for a sexually open relationship, and his partner was feeling pressured into going along so that he would not end up losing his spouse. When therapy has been able to get both men to look at issues that range from power imbalances between them to emotional vulnerability, the couple is more likely to find a satisfying way to keep their erotic fires lit and their trust and communication strong. At the very least, once these conversations are begun about power and how it is played out in the sexual realm, couples can approach the issue of whether to be monogamous with increased clarity about why they are at this place in their relationship at this time. With almost all couples who arrive in my office with issues about diminished sexual satisfaction in their relationship, I normalize the reality that for many couples the sexual intensity does indeed diminish over the years. But then, I also use a concept first articulated by San Francisco psychologist Jack Morin (1999) by asking them: "What is wrong with a steady supply of good warm sex when hot sex is not happening?" This often opens up frank conversations about each of their expectations about sex with each other and the numerous options for addressing sexual dissatisfaction. Many male couples like Jake and Mark have subtle and covert expectations that increasing emotional intimacy should or will or might also lead to increased sexual intimacy, including unprotected sex. Manhattan couples therapist Esther Perel has been speaking (2003a; 2004) and writing (2003b; in press) about a dynamic that is central to these issues. She discusses that most people become part of a couple for a complex variety of reasons that almost always include a search for safety and comfort. Yet she strongly suggests that comfort and safety also are paradoxically antierotic, and too much closeness and safety can smother and kill a couple's erotic life. How this dynamic might be played out regarding condom use is a very useful area for therapists to introduce with couples wrestling with the issue.

"IS IT SAFE IF WE'RE BOTH HIV-NEGATIVE?"

Another memorable couple who grappled with the question of whether to stop having safer sex was Willis and Larry. They were both HIV-negative African-American attorneys in their mid-thirties and had been a couple for 3 years. They had just bought an apartment together prior to our first consultation and came to therapy to talk about how living together was affecting their relationship. Among the issues they raised was the possibility of stopping their use of condoms with each other, since they had been monogamous for the past 2 years and since each had recently retested negative for HIV.

As usually happens, one member of the couple was more ready than the other to make the transition to unprotected sex. In this case, Willis admitted that he began pressuring Larry to be sexually exclusive after they had been dating for 6 months. This coincided with their first saying that they loved each other. I asked Larry what it had been like to hear that Willis loved him and wanted them to be monogamous. Larry said, "While I knew I had fallen in love with Willis, wanted to spend my life with him, and had told him this, when he first raised the monogamy issue it just felt wrong. It was too soon. Even though I was not having sex with other men, I didn't want to make a promise that I didn't feel ready to keep. It felt like too much pressure. At the time, I wasn't ready to make that kind of commitment. Now it's different." He further explained that he had not felt ready to commit to monogamy until they decided to begin to look for an apartment to buy together, but nonetheless he had chosen not to have sex with anyone besides Willis.

Willis said that one of the reasons he wanted a monogamous relationship with another HIV-negative man was so that they could forget about safer sex. Willis described how neither he nor Larry had ever had anal sex without a condom, nor experienced anyone ejaculating in their mouths, and the prospect of both was exciting. Larry agreed that being in a sexually exclusive relationship with a man he loved provided him the perfect opportunity to expand his sexual boundaries while not having to worry about HIV (or other sexually transmitted diseases [STDs]). "Having that latex barrier between us seems like such a metaphor for our love and relationship not being able to grow any stronger or closer,"

Larry said. When I asked them why the issue of condoms had come up now, Larry explained that until he was ready to commit to not having sex with anyone else, which had only happened in the past few months, he did not even want to open up the condom conversation, though they had come very close to not using one on several occasions. It was after the last time that they had physically flirted with not using one that he finally began to talk with Willis about this issue. Their initial conversation about wanting to have unprotected sex had prompted them to go together and get retested. When I asked Larry what he meant by having physically flirted with not using one, he told me that they had "gone inside for a few good pumps but pulled out way before the point of no return." I told them that this was known as "dipping," and many men used it as a method of keeping anal sex without condoms safer than "going all the way." They both grinned and nodded.

I could see that, like most couples, Larry and Willis were moving at slightly different paces with their commitment, and that Larry needed more time to feel safe and confident about his decision to commit to Willis. I often see that gay men equate jointly investing in real estate with getting married. It is a big step, but it doesn't have to mean more than the men want it to mean. In this case, Willis wanted it to mean "married," and Larry wanted it to mean "engaged." There was no right or wrong here. I helped them understand that their different viewpoints did not signify a betrayal or lack of commitment, and that practicing patience with each other would go a long way toward helping them build an even more loving and compassionate foundation for their relationship.

The men liked this assessment and Larry, in particular, seemed more lighthearted after I "let him off the hook." In fact, once Willis had reassured him that he did not have to see moving in together as married for life, Larry became more willing to think about changing their agreement about anal sex and condoms. "But how will we figure out how to do this so we both feel totally safe?" he asked. It was a good question.

I asked them how far each was willing to trust the other, since the potential risks were so high. They gave almost identical responses. They had purchased their condominium and merged their finances, which involved an extremely high level of trust in each other and in the relationship. They also had a realistic understanding of the potential limits of monogamy, meaning that they were confident that if either did have sex outside the relationship, it would be a serious issue but would not necessarily bring the partnership to an end. When I asked each of them in an individual session about whether they had been sexually exclusive, both responded that since they met, neither had had sex with anyone else.

Having worked with numerous couples who have elastic definitions of monogamy, I knew that there was the possibility that, like many male couples, Larry and Willis might be practicing what San Francisco psychologist Jack Morin has labeled "modified monogamy." Morin defines modified monogamy as when a couple values monogamy and strives to be monogamous. At the same time, the men recognize that the goal of monogamy may not be realistic or achievable, so the couple devises certain accommodations that reflect the tension between their desire to be sexually exclusive and practical realities (Morin, 1999). One example of "modified monogamy" is when a couple who define themselves as sexually exclusive together have sex with a third person or a group of other people. With Morin's work in mind, I asked if their definition of monogamy encompassed having sex together with another person or with other people. At this point, they became noticeably uncomfortable. I commented on their squirming, and asked what it was a response to. In an uncharacteristically sheepish manner, Willis asked, "Are we monogamous if we occasionally have played together with another guy?" I asked if they had done that, and when both nodded affirmatively, I responded, "The rules and definitions of your sexual relationship are up to you to decide. But this raises an important issue about safer sex that we need to talk about."

I proceeded to explain the concept of "negotiated safety" (Kippax, Crawford, Davis, Rodden, & Dowset, 1993), and provided them with the URL of a British organization's Web site that has prepared a sample negotiated safety agreement (Freedoms.org, 2003). I suggested that they download the agreement and spend time talking about all the issues raised in the questionnaire. They did this prior to our next session, and the next few visits were spent discussing all of their feelings about the issues that the questionnaire raised for each of them. During the session, when I introduced the concept of negotiated safety,

I explained that if they decided to incorporate this kind of protocol into their relationship, they would not just be agreeing to have anal sex with each other without condoms, they would also be agreeing to make a serious effort to make anal sex without condoms as safe as possible for both of them. I stressed that such an understanding would be premised on their knowing each other well enough to deal with difficult situations together — for example, if one of them should have unprotected sex outside the relationship — and that it would work only if they had the willingness to trust in each other. I told them that previously during anal sex, it was the condom that had provided protection from HIV; now it would only be their partner's honor and integrity that would protect them. In other words, the agreement would have to be strong, and the commitment to following it exactly as agreed upon would have to be just as strong.

I did not want to scare my clients but very much felt it was crucial for them to take very seriously the potential for doing harm and being harmed. Frankly, no couple in the blush of love wants to believe that he or his partner could ever do something willfully or otherwise to harm him. For this reason, most couples do not bother engaging in simple conversations about their relationship that include the equivalent of prenuptial agreements that talk about how they will divide up their possessions or real estate if they split up. There is a general denial and avoidance of thinking the worst when lovers are happy, but with the reservoirs of good will full to overflowing, it is an ideal time to encourage couples to begin to think about these difficult issues and plan for their possibility. I find that therapists may have slightly more leverage getting partners like Willis and Larry to negotiate their sexual agreements because of the fears of contracting HIV. I try to be very real with the men that this is a very big step they are taking so they do not go into it with a casual attitude.

Willis said, "While we're talking about condoms, what about Dan?" Dan was a semiregular third partner, also HIV-negative, whom they occasionally invited into their bed. Willis wanted to know if there was a point at which they could stop using condoms with Dan.

Hearing this, Larry became angry. "Are you nuts? If he's screwing around with us, we can only assume there are other men he's sexual with as well. Even if he tells us he's uninfected, I, for one, am not willing to trust either my health or yours to some other guy. I don't even want us to go there."

At first, Willis was taken aback by the intensity of Larry's response. "I was just thinking out loud," he told Larry.

"I know how your brain works," Larry told him. "The only way I will agree to take the condoms off with you is if you promise me that you will never again raise the issue of going bareback with anyone other than me, even if it's someone we both know well and play with."

When I asked Willis how Larry's position made him feel, he thought for a few moments and eventually smiled. "I feel like you are my main man and are really looking out for me and us. I love it! You've got yourself a deal." He said this in a flirtatious way.

The couple spent four additional sessions talking through all of their feelings about a negotiated safety agreement, and they ultimately decided to forego using condoms with each other. During a follow-up session 18 months later, they reported having completely unprotected sex with each other, as well as occasional "play sessions" with other men, during which they used condoms. They had retested HIV-negative and were thrilled with the arrangement. "It's great that we have all these special sexual treats that we only indulge in with each other. Yet we also enjoy a bit of safer sexual variety," Willis explained the last time I saw them.

THE RISKS OF REINFECTION

Hoff et al. (1997) found that in relationships where both men had the same HIV status (whether HIV-positive or HIV-negative), there were higher rates of UAI, both with and without ejaculation, as compared with men in serodiscordant relationships. They suggest that two HIV-positive men in a primary relationship who do not use condoms for anal sex with each other often believe that the degree of harm from reinfection is negligible or inconclusive among HIV-positive men. Halkitis and colleagues' research (2005b) confirmed Hoff's findings. This brings us directly to the question: how high are the risks of reinfection?

In a study conducted in New York City and San Francisco from 1997 to 1998 (Halkitis, Wilton, Parsons, & Hoff, 2004),[2] the sexual practices of HIV-positive men who were in a primary partner relationship with another man who was also HIV-positive were investigated, and a majority were found to have had unprotected sex with their partners because they did not believe that there was a significant risk of reinfection with a drug-resistant strain of HIV. Halkitis et al. (2004) offered a cautionary note to men in HIV-positive seroconcordant relationships who do not use condoms: "The ultimate health outcomes for HIV-positive men in primary partnerships who practice unprotected sexual behaviors are still an area of biomedical research that require further study" (p. 100).

While the caution sounded by Halkitis and colleagues (2004) is appropriate, there is now some evidence to suggest that superinfection is not that common. In a small study of HIV-positive couples,[3] most participants were infected with a strain of HIV that was genetically different from his or her partner's. Among those who engaged in frequent unprotected vaginal or anal sex with each other, no evidence of superinfection was found.[4] Until the rates of reinfection with an additional strain of HIV are well researched, it would be premature for therapists, doctors, or HIV prevention experts to assure men like Mark and Jake or Donald and Ted that not using condoms for anal intercourse does not pose any risk of reinfection. When patients ask about the risks of reinfection, I can only convey to them that there are very few reported cases in the medical literature and that they have to weigh the potential risks for themselves.

The overarching question for seroconcordant HIV-positive couples who have unprotected sex is "How safe is safe?" and what are the real risks of reinfection? At this moment the research appears to be mixed on this crucial question. An additional question for men in HIV-negative seroconcordant relations who do not use condoms is: "How do we trust that when an HIV antibody test is negative that this means it is safe to take off the condoms?"

It is understandable that men like Willis and Larry, who both have consistently tested negative for HIV, would believe that relaxing their safer-sex standards with each other would not put them at risk for HIV infection, but Appleby, Miller, and Rothspan (1999) offer the cautionary reminder that a man may believe that he is uninfected when he is actually HIV positive, even if he tests negative for the virus. This is because there is a period of time when, despite being infected, the body has not yet produced enough antibodies to HIV to be detected by blood tests. Also, a man might have a change in his HIV status — in other words, he might have tested negative but afterwards engaged in high-risk sexual behaviors and been retested. In Australia, Kippax et al. (2003) found that partnered men in their study were most likely to contract HIV during the early months of a regular relationship.

CONDOMS, INTIMACY, AND TRUST

Appleby et al. (1999) suggest that especially regarding HIV, trust, risk, and commitment are often interwoven themes in today's intimate relationships. For many years, the message "Use a condom every time" implied that by doing so you demonstrated caring and love for your partner by protecting both of you from possibly transmitting HIV. The other part of this message was that caring and love are associated with not taking chances by "playing it safe." Yet, in order for any relationship to grow and deepen, both parties need to develop trust by taking increased risks based on the trust earned by both members of the couple. At times that means financial risk — like buying property together or financially supporting each other. At times it may be emotional risk — showing a beloved your fears and feelings of shame or self-doubt. In the world of AIDS, the risk may be sexual in nature. Appleby et al. discuss that though traditionally, unprotected and possibly risky sex was never one of the risks that two men would engage in to build trust and subsequent closeness in their relationship, condomless sex may very well have come to symbolize evidence of love, trust, and commitment between two men.

In fact one study conducted in various cities in England found that the main feature of those who had UAI with a regular partner was the depth of their emotional involvement with their partners. Three quarters of the men reported being in love with the man with whom they had not used condoms and two thirds were committed to the relationship continuing indefinitely (McLean et al., 1994). These findings led the researchers to suggest that "greater emotional involvement between the men is the most important factor in accounting for higher rates of unprotected intercourse in regular relationships" (McLean et al., p. 339). They also concluded that intercourse without a condom is often seen as more intimate, bringing partners closer together and creating a feeling of oneness with a partner. Prieur (1990) has written about how, in an act of love that wishes to convey warmth, closeness, giving, sharing, and trust, using a condom can convey the opposite. Protected sex can be experienced by one partner as evidence that he is not to be trusted, that he is thought to be diseased; the refusal to accept semen can be experienced as a rejection. As Appleby et al. (1999) conclude: "The central role of deep emotional involvement in explaining the continued prevalence of unprotected intercourse is thus not surprising" (p. 339). Though those words were written 6 years before this book, they seem as applicable and on target now as they were earlier in the epidemic.

SECTION II: PARTNERS OF DIFFERENT HIV STATUS

In the case of seroconcordant couples the risks are often ambiguous. For men in mixed antibody status relationships the risk is obvious and ever-present. In addition there is an uneven risk. The HIV-negative partner faces more dire consequences than does the HIV-positive partner. Any existing power imbalances in the relationship will have some bearing on the way the issue of safety is negotiated, and such negotiations call for a whole different level of trust and understanding between the men.

RESEARCH ON DISCORDANT COUPLES

There is inconsistency in the research findings regarding the frequency of UAI by HIV-positive gay men in relationships with HIV-negative men. Doll et al. (1990), Remien, Carballo-Dieguez, and Wagner (1995), and Remien, Wagner, Dolezal, and Carballo-Dieguez (2001) found that higher levels of unprotected anal sex occur in relationships where strong emotional involvement is present. Hays, Kegeles, and Coates (1997) found that being in a relationship with a steady boyfriend was not predictive of not using condoms among young seropositive men. Kalichman et al. (1997) reported high rates of sex without condoms by HIV-positive men both in exclusive and non-exclusive relationships. Fischer, Wilcutts, Misovich, and Weinstein (1998) suggest that HIV-positive men in sexually exclusive relationships with uninfected men are more likely to consistently use condoms for anal sex. Approximately 25 percent of the seropositive men in another study reported having condomless anal sex with their uninfected steady partner (de Vroome, de Wit, Stroebe, Sandfort, & van Griensven, 1998). That means that one quarter of HIV-infected gay men who are in an ongoing relationship are having unprotected sex with their HIV-negative boyfriends.

Obviously, it is impossible to generalize about the kinds of dynamics that play out in negotiations among men in HIV mixed antibody status relationships with regard to unprotected or unsafe sex. But I can say that after observing more than two decades of gay men demonstrating trustworthiness by using condoms, it is an interesting paradox that we are at a moment when more than a handful of men may feel that the only way to prove either how much they trust a romantic partner or how trustworthy they are is to have unprotected sex with a man to whom they are growing closer. There are also personal intrapsychic issues that lead both partners to want to engage in sex without condoms, and we have to listen carefully and openly to each story to unravel the psychology behind the behavior. In the case of Joe and Henry (described below), a factor that I have not yet discussed much will become clear. That is how the unconscious, intrapsychic content of each man affects his decision-making process. In the case that follows, Joe felt a pressure to dispense with condoms as a way to try to test Henry's feelings about him and the relationship. For men who are in therapy, conversations about what trust is, how it develops, what their feelings are about trusting another person, how to pace a growing sense of trust, what the appropriate limits of trust are, and what past experiences each has had where trust was ill founded or well deserved may all provide very fertile areas for exploration in conjunction with an exploration of their past family and relationship history. Individual issues and personal history cannot be separated from motivations to take sexual risks.

SEXUAL RISK-TAKING AS A TEST OF LOVE

Joe was a 30-year-old HIV-negative gay white man who originally entered therapy to deal with having an alcoholic and violent father. He has a history of depression that is mostly alleviated with prescribed antidepressants. During the third year of therapy, Joe courted and began a relationship with Henry, a 44-year-old white gay man who was a prominent and affluent health care professional within the gay community. On their first date, Henry shared that he was an HIV-positive, long-term nonprogressor. Joe was not concerned since they had agreed about the precautions they would take sexually.

The relationship was problematic from the beginning, as Joe felt that he was much more in love with Henry than Henry ever was with him. This made him feel insecure and sad, especially since he considered Henry to be a "catch," even though Henry was still mourning the death of his lover 3 years earlier. About 6 months into the relationship, Joe reported that the previous night while he was the inserter in anal intercourse he pulled out, took the condom off, and continued until both men had reached orgasm. In discussing what had occurred they both felt excited as well as concerned. Neither of the men considered the "top" in UAI with an HIV-positive man to be completely free of risk, even if the receptive partner's viral loads were beneath the level of detection.

While exploring this situation in therapy, Joe said that in addition to the improved sensation that not using a condom provided, it made him feel more spontaneous. I urged him to dig a little deeper to understand what motivated this behavior. He described having researched available medical literature and, despite finding a few medical journal articles that reported the presence of HIV in the semen of positive men with undetectable levels in their blood, he felt this was low-risk to him. Since he had obviously been thinking about this enough to do the research, I asked what had prevented him from discussing it in therapy? He described feeling ashamed and embarrassed about wanting to have unprotected sex and fearful of what my reaction would be. After validating that it was normal and understandable for him to want to have sex without a condom, I reflected back to him that it seemed as if he might be projecting his own ambivalence about having unsafe sex onto me by worrying about my reaction, when it was really his own response that was disturbing him. He agreed and owned that he had not actually planned on when he would stop using a condom. Since he and Henry had not discussed it in advance, it was an impulsive behavior and something that we needed to continue to explore. The relationship remained rocky, and they even broke up once during a weekend trip.

Joe entered one session visibly unhappy. When I commented on this he responded: "Over the weekend, while Henry was fucking me, I thought that if Henry took off the condom it would feel better, and he would feel closer to me. So I told him to take it off." Henry complied, continued, but withdrew prior to orgasm. Afterward, they both talked about how hot this had been, but how nervous it made them. Joe said he hoped that having anal intercourse without a condom would help Henry feel closer to him. I began to ask questions about the emotional climate of the relationship, and Joe sadly admitted that he did not feel as close to Henry as he wished. As Joe began to cry, he admitted feeling desperate about wanting to make the relationship work. Despite even dispensing with condoms, he sensed a reluctance on Henry's part to allow the relationship to grow. Henry had no interest in having Joe move into his large apartment, even though Joe had spent almost every night there for the past 18 months.

The dynamic of using sex as a commodity to barter within a relationship, whether consciously or unconsciously, is obviously not limited to same-sex partnerships. People use sex for all kinds of things — physical pleasure and intimacy; to feel admired, loved, wanted, and validated; and to express love, admiration, desire, and validation of others. It can also be used as a kind of currency between partners — I will give you sex and you give me (take your choice). But when the aspect of sex that is offered as barter is UAI by an HIV-negative man in a serodiscordant relationship, the emotional as well as physical implications become complex and alarming. Because he based a large part of his identity and self-worth on being found sexually desirable, Joe felt that the currency of his sexual attractiveness was a defense against depression and painful feelings of not being lovable.

As tensions with Henry escalated, Joe became depressed. They continued to have unprotected anal sex with Henry withdrawing prior to orgasm. After a follow-up HIV test confirmed that Joe remained uninfected, he called for an emergency session. Instead of feeling relieved, Joe reported feeling despondent and even more desperate. He said that no matter what he did to try to please Henry, he always wound up feeling the way he did as a child when his father was drinking and completely unavailable to him. He recognized that part of his attraction to Henry had been his fantasy of having this older, attractive man take care of him and love him in a way that he had never experienced from his father. He realized now that this would never happen. I asked him what he thought the solution was. Without skipping a beat, he said: "I need to get out of this before I do something even crazier than I have been doing."

I had been working very hard to remain neutral with Joe and conceal my assessment that he had been working much harder in this relationship than Henry was, and I did not know why he was so desperate to keep the relationship with Henry going. These were my reactions long before Joe ever told me that he had begun to have condomless sex with Henry.

Joe seemed ready now to dig deeper and look at the meanings of his actions with Henry. Every time he and Henry had unprotected sex, he felt bad about himself and worse about the relationship. He was angry that Henry had gone along with his suggestions to dispense with condoms. His secret fantasy was that Henry would have a high enough degree of loving concern for him that it would outweigh his own pleasure, but that never happened. Before our next session, Joe ended the relationship with Henry. Though sad, Henry was not greatly distressed and did not try to convince Joe to reconsider. This confirmed Joe's confidence in his decision. Within a week of the breakup, Joe's depression began to lessen without any increase in the dosage of antidepressant.

In discussions following the end of his relationship with Henry, Joe admitted that what he felt Henry most valued in him was his youth and sexual energy. He had hoped that if he dispensed with condoms and offered Henry something unique and special within the sexual realm of their relationship, Henry's feelings for him would grow more intense. Perhaps he even hoped that Henry would start to need him. When I questioned him about this he shrugged and said that he would have to think about it. Joe described that historically, he felt most strong, powerful, and in control only during sexual encounters where his partner expressed a strong intensity of desire for him. Joe often doubted that he had anything else to offer a potential partner. This was as true during recreational sexual encounters as when he was seriously dating someone. As he began to recognize that Henry was not deeply interested in him beyond their sexual connection, he felt that engaging in unsafe sex was the only option open to him to get Henry to see how special he was. When the UAI had failed to deepen their relationship, Joe became more depressed and finally was confronted with his own longings to be seen as much more than a "hot, young sexual commodity," both by himself and by the men he partnered with. Joe used the end of the relationship with Henry as an opportunity to begin to explore this issue in depth.

Joe's case illustrates how high-risk sex can be a means of attempting to ameliorate feelings of powerlessness and helplessness and may appear to the sexual risk-taker to be an adaptive option. Clearly, Joe's family history and depression contributed to his decision to place himself in a potentially risky situation, as so much of his sense of self-worth was bound up in having confused feeling sexually desirable with being loved and valued as a whole person.

LOVE, TRUST, AND DISCLOSURE

Most couples on some level want to believe that falling in love encompasses being with someone they can trust completely and without question. As was discussed in Chapter 6, we are all bombarded with the popular myth that love and trust are indivisible. Frequently I suggest to patients in both individual and couples sessions that trust has to be earned over time and reearned in order to truly grow into an emotional foundation on which a relationship can really grow and flourish.

Jerry and Art, white gay men in their forties, first met while Art was in a long-term relationship with another man. Art was HIV-negative, as was his previous partner. Jerry had seroconverted a few months prior to first meeting Art. Jerry entered therapy for help in adjusting to his HIV diagnosis. A lot of our early work in therapy explored Jerry's feelings about disclosing his HIV status to men he met. Whenever Jerry told me about meeting a man in a bar and going home with him to have sex, I always asked him the same question: "Did you tell him that you're positive?" We talked at length about how he might find an appropriate time to disclose his HIV status. I always counsel HIV-positive patients that in situations with a new romance, the longer they wait to share this information, the more difficult it will be to do so. Additionally, an HIV-positive man runs the risk of his new boyfriend experiencing him as not being trustworthy even if they did not do anything sexually high risk. Jerry spent hours describing his fears and anxieties about disclosing to someone he cared about that he was HIV-positive. He never tried to rationalize not telling people and always said that he knew it would be better to tell people before he went home with them, but he rarely could bring himself to do so. Even when men wanted him to bareback, he refused. The issue was very new to him, and the prospect of telling a man he liked that he was HIV-positive made him extremely nervous. This anxiety was the reason that except for Art, Jerry had been limiting himself to what he called "hit and run" sex since his diagnosis. Jerry was predominantly a sexual top and had become strict about always using condoms after learning that he had become infected.

When Art and Jerry met, Jerry was single and Art was in an open relationship. They met for sexual liaisons every few weeks, which grew in intensity as the men's dates began to include deep, revealing conversations. Over time, they became more emotionally vulnerable with each other; 18 months after they met, they both realized that they had begun to fall in love and wanted to explore building a life together. Jerry explained to me during a session that he and Art had realized that there was a major obstacle that had to be dismantled before they could move ahead and explore partnering: Art needed to end his former relationship and move into his own apartment. Since I had often asked Jerry whether he had disclosed his HIV status to Art and at the time he had not done so, I queried Jerry about whether this was the only obstacle. He acknowledged that he still needed to tell Art that he was HIV-positive. We worked on his feelings about this, which largely centered on his fear that this man he now was in love with would be angry at him for not having told him sooner and would end their relationship upon learning that he was infected both because he would not want to be in a relationship with an HIV-positive man and because Jerry had withheld the information. Jerry was amazed that Art had never asked him about his HIV status, but he figured that the reason that Art had never asked about this was because they were "just" having an affair. He had told me on previous occasions that had Art ever asked him, he would not have lied.

In the session following Jerry's disclosure, he reported that Art was indeed upset that Jerry had not told him sooner. As Jerry had suspected, Art was upset for both of the reasons that he had thought. What would it mean for Art to share a long life with someone who had HIV? Jerry had told Art he was completely asymptomatic and on combination therapy and had given Art several HIV/AIDS-related Web sites so that he could educate himself about what this meant. As to Art's hurt feelings and concern that Jerry had not trusted either him or their growing bond enough to have told him sooner, the men spent days talking through all of their feelings about this. Jerry said he began to cry when he told Art he was afraid he would have lost him if Art learned he was HIV-positive. This caused Art to begin to cry also and became one of the foundations of sensitivity and trust that enabled their love to grow even stronger. Jerry had asked Art if Art felt betrayed by his not having told him that he was HIV-positive sooner. Art explained that he was hurt, angry, and upset, but since he had never asked Jerry about his HIV status and had not been lied to he did not feel as if there had been any betrayal on Jerry's part.

They had never had UAI, but unprotected fellatio was a regular part of their lovemaking. On rare occasions, Jerry had ejaculated in Art's mouth at Art's insistence. The next concern that Art expressed was his desire to be retested to ensure that he was still uninfected. Jerry was anguished over the even remote possibility that he may have infected Art and was highly anxious until Art's test came back negative. Art was concerned that the oral sex they had might have put him at risk, but since he had been the one who had pushed to have Jerry ejaculate in his mouth despite Jerry's reluctance to do so, he was not angry and this did not have a negative impact on their sexual trust. They agreed that Jerry would continue to use condoms when he was the inserter during anal sex. Art said that he was comfortable continuing to perform oral sex on Jerry and even wanted Jerry to ejaculate in his mouth. Jerry felt comfortable about the unprotected oral sex but refused to ejaculate inside of Art's mouth.

HOW SAFE IS UNPROTECTED ORAL SEX?

This brings us to a discussion of the degree of risk when an HIV-negative man performs unprotected oral sex on a man who is HIV-positive. Since the start of the AIDS epidemic, there has been no clear resolution of this issue. It is now documented that the vast majority of HIV seroconversions in gay and bisexual men has been through UAI. Yet unprotected oral sex is not without risk, as demonstrated by a limited number of documented cases of HIV transmission via unprotected oral sex worldwide (Lifson, O'Mally, Hessol, & Buchbinder, 1990; Chen & Samarasinghee, 1992). Seroconversion rates from unprotected receptive oral sex that ends in an ejaculation are estimated to occur at about one tenth the rates of UAI (Vittinhoff, Douglas, & Judson, 1999). As Halkitis and Parsons (2000) state, "Perhaps as a result of the conflicting data, messages about the transmission of HIV through oral sex without a condom from AIDS service organizations have been varied" (p. 3). These inconsistent messages from community-based AIDS organizations have contributed to the ambiguity and confusion surrounding the safety of unprotected oral sex.

COMBINATION ANTIVIRAL THERAPIES AND INFECTIVITY

The advent of combination antiretrovirals has further contributed to the uncertainty pertaining to the safety of both UAI and unprotected oral sex. Today, many men believe that if the level of HIV is undetectable in a person's blood then the same holds true for that individual's semen. As a result of this belief, they engage in high-risk behaviors, thinking that being on combination therapy makes a person less infectious (Kalichman et al., 2002). Research has shown, however, that when an HIV-positive man is on combination therapy he is still able to transmit HIV. In one study conducted in Brazil and the United States, approximately 10 percent of men on triple combination therapy who had undetectable viral levels in their blood still had a detectable level of virus in their semen (Barros et al., 2000). A Swiss study found that in men treated with combination therapy who had undetectable viral levels in their blood, less than 4 percent had detectable viral levels in their semen (Vernazza et al., 2000). These researchers concluded that antiviral therapy may help reduce the sexual transmission of HIV, but it does not eliminate the risk. Thus, there is no guarantee that engaging in unprotected oral sex is without some risk of spreading HIV. I shared this information with Jerry during a session and asked him to convey this to Art.

Art discussed the issue of sexual risk with his physician and decided that now that he knew Jerry was infected with HIV, he was not comfortable penetrating Jerry without a condom, which he had done prior to knowing this information. Hearing this reminded me of so many other men I had worked with who were willing to take greater sexual risks with men whose HIV status they did not know. It seems to reflect a combination of rationalizations, not all of which are conscious, including, "If he is letting me do this to him he must not be infected"; "If he is letting me do this to him and not asking me to use a condom he must already be infected"; "Even if he is infected I'm not at risk being the top"; and the magical thinking of "I've topped so many men before him without a using a condom and have not gotten infected so far so I won't get infected this time." Since Art was not a client of mine I could not explore any of these with him.

When I asked Jerry to inquire from Art why he was comfortable continuing to have unprotected oral sex, Art told him that for many years he had never inquired about a person's HIV status, as was most recently evidenced with Jerry. He had never stopped performing oral sex on men and sometimes allowed them to ejaculate in his mouth. While he never let men penetrate him anally without a condom except for his previous uninfected partner, he regularly had topped men bareback. He continued to remain HIV-negative, so he felt that if he had stayed uninfected so far, there was no good reason to change what he was doing with Jerry, especially since he enjoyed these things sexually so much. Now that he knew that Jerry was HIV-positive, he would always use a condom while topping him to decrease the chance of his becoming infected. From what Jerry told me, it seemed that by avoiding the highest-risk sexual behavior of being the receptive partner in UAI, Art had managed to greatly reduce his chances of becoming infected but still had taken some sexual risks. Two years later, Jerry's viral load remains beneath the level of detectability and Art continues to test HIV-negative.

This case illustrates several important points. The first is how fraught it still is, in the third decade of the AIDS epidemic, for many men to disclose their HIV status. The second is that despite understandable fears and concerns, many HIV-negative gay men are willing to have a relationship with someone who is HIV-positive. Art was not willing to allow Jerry's HIV status to impede their relationship from developing. Despite Jerry's intense desire to ejaculate in Art's mouth and having done so rarely in the past, he decided that he was not going to do so in the future. Art and Jerry are an example of what Remien et al. (2001) found in their study of 75 HIV mixed antibody status male couples. They found that UAI occurred more often among younger men, newer couples, Latino men, and men with less education. Art and Jerry were in the "newer couple" category. Art's decision to continue to perform fellatio without ejaculation on Jerry, whom he knew was HIV-positive, and past willingness to top him without a condom prior to knowing that Jerry was HIV-positive show how powerfully the combination of early love and sexual desire can cause men to engage in behaviors that are not entirely without risk.

NEW LOVE AND RISK-TAKING

A new romance is almost always intoxicating. Few drugs are as intoxicating as great sex, especially when it is within the context of a budding romance. Even when the men are not serosorting, as several of the research studies already cited demonstrate, this combination of sexual intoxication and romantic intoxication are very likely to lead to sex without condoms.

We will never know if all male couples go through a period of questioning and testing the boundaries of their sexual relationships.

Remien and colleagues' finding (2001) that being a newer couple was one contributing factor among mixed antibody status couples for taking sexual risks is not surprising when one reflects that most couples, gay and heterosexual, are in fact most sexually daring and experimental during the early courtship phase of their relationship. This is the period when two people are still most full of mystery to each other and are just exploring the potential to have two lives begin to overlap and merge. This is the period prior to when — contrary to most of the accepted wisdom in the American psychotherapeutic, sex therapy, and family therapy fields — the growth of intimacy and safety can have an anti-erotic impact on a couple's sex life (Perel, in press). Some couples may be perfectly happy and satisfied with safer sex, but the research seems to strongly suggest that most male couples are not using condoms during sex with each other.

SEXUAL SATISFACTION AND RISK-TAKING WITHIN RELATIONSHIPS

In their research, Remien et al. (1995, 2001) found that the need to always maintain safer sexual behaviors was a barrier to ongoing emotional intimacy for several reasons, including not being able to actually feel their lover's penis, representing more than a loss of physical sensation and the absence of semen being exchanged. These couples spoke of how condoms interfered with the development of sexual intimacy. Another rationale given for not using condoms was the reluctance on the part of the men to discuss their fears and concerns about HIV, and thus they avoided the topic, including avoiding talking about condoms. Men also reported that as the length of time that the relationship continued progressed, the perception of the possibility of being harmed by one's partner decreased and resulted in unprotected sex increasing (Remien et al., 1995). They report that men in these relationships perceive the risk to be an expression of intimacy, closeness, love, and commitment, and that, as in the cases of Art and Jerry and Joe and Henry, often it is the uninfected partner who pushes for increased levels of sexual risk-taking. Early on in the epidemic, these same researchers noted that rarely was unprotected sex considered to be an acceptable choice for couples of mixed HIV antibody status. But as the epidemic has dragged on, the number of serodiscordant couples has grown (Remien et al., 2001).

Many couples of mixed HIV antibody status engage in UAI (Remien, Carballo-Dieguez, & Wagner, 1995; Remien, 1997; Remien, Wagner, Dolezal, & Carballo-Dieguez, 2001). Appleby et al. (1999)[5] found that long-term male mixed antibody status couples were just as risky in their sexual behavior as were seroconcordant couples. There are a variety of ways these couples may relate sexually including: no longer being sexually active with one another; being sexually active but no longer having anal intercourse; having anal intercourse with condoms; or having UAI. If the couple includes UAI in their sexual repertoire there are a variety of ways they may minimize chances of infecting the HIV-negative partner, including the HIV-positive partner either not being the top or, if he is, not ejaculating inside his partner. The negative partner may or may not ejaculate inside of the positive man. Remien (1997) discusses that couples of mixed HIV status are confronted with numerous unique challenges and stressors increasing the vulnerability each man may feel. These include difficulty maintaining intimacy and sexual satisfaction.

RISK-TAKING AS A TURN-ON

In *The History of Sexuality* (1978), the late French philosopher Michel Foucault discussed that contemporary capitalistic societies had so com-modified sex that some people felt it was worth dying for. Sexual risk-taking speaks to part of what Foucault was talking about, which seems to be: how do modern people living in an age of a potentially threat-ening, sexually transmitted epidemic balance expressing our deepest desires and passions with our needs for safety and self-preservation? As anyone who has ever experienced a breathlessly exciting sexual experience can attest to, part of what makes any sexual exchange deeply satisfying is that on some level it is not totally safe, and that danger-ous edge expands our sense of ourselves sexually and in the best case scenarios, also emotionally. Sex is one of the most profound ways that our life force gets expressed. For many people, sex is actually equated with life. For most people, the difference between sex that is dull and routine is precisely venturing into a terrain that touches on a dark, dangerous, or "nasty" part of their psychic realm. It is the area of sexuality where fantasy overlaps with desire, and this is rarely a well-ordered, tidy, or safe experience. Barebacking and unprotected sex, especially between men in committed relationships, seem to occur precisely at this cutting edge where the comfort and safety of the known entity of a beloved partner converges with animal desire and the urge to have their limits expanded. One thing seems clear from the research on men in committed relationships having unprotected sex — the importance of the desire for unconstrained sex. It seems safe to say that for these men, raw sex and any of the risks entailed in having sex without condoms are a conscious effort to marry intimacy and sexual satisfaction with deep human needs for direct physical contact. Remien (1997) describes how for many mixed antibody status couples, condoms are perceived to be a barrier to intimacy. Using condoms is also a constant reminder that one of the men is infected with HIV and thus interferes with spontaneity and the pleasure of the couple expressing themselves sexually. Remien also reports that couples often feel that using condoms is like bringing death into the bedroom. Remien (1997) states: "not using condoms, or engaging in sex behavior that may be risky, can be perceived as exciting, passionate, and a true expression of love and commitment" (p. 167).

Obviously, for most couples, a satisfying and rich sexual life is an important aspect of their relationship. For couples where one or both are living with HIV or AIDS, sex can assume even a greater degree of importance. A satisfying sex life can become identified with life itself — and surely with being healthy. People who are very ill often do not have enough physical energy or stamina to have the same kind of sex they had before they became ill. So as long as both men can achieve erections and still ejaculate, a very primary and visceral bond is functioning between them that for many couples is part of the glue that holds them together. Yet when men in a serodiscordant partnership have sex with each other, it can also raise feelings of vulnerability and the possibility of impending loss.

For other couples, the increase in intensity and intimacy of having sex, some of it unprotected, when one man is living with a life-threatening illness flies in the face of a possibly looming disaster and adds to the excitement and uniqueness of their bond as they join together to live fully in the face of HIV and AIDS. There are unique tensions associated with mixed antibody status couples regarding how they express themselves sexually. A relaxed and healthy sex life can provide the mixed antibody status couple with a respite from the strains of dealing with the reality that one of them is living with a potentially life-threatening illness. Yet at the same time, tensions about whether or not to use condoms and the issue of the negative partner receiving the positive partner's semen have the potential to make couple's sexual play a source of anxiety, tensions, and fear. Those emotions need to be discussed and addressed as often as either member of the couple feels is necessary. As has been reported (Remien et al., 1995; Ramien, Wagner, Dolezal, & Carballo-Dieguez, 2003), very often all of the realities of the infected partner's health and related anxieties — as, for example, they relate to sex — are frequently not talked about and are the proverbial "pink elephant" in the room. If a couple does not learn how to introduce discussions about these topics into their relationship, they may be heading into difficulties that can be avoided by having conversations that have the potential to be highly fraught and thus are avoided.

SEXUAL AND EMOTIONAL SAFETY

It is probably safe to assume that the same couples who, for whatever reason, do not discuss whether to use condoms with each other are the same couples who do not share their deepest sexual fantasies with each other. Many men I have worked with fear that if they disclose their sexual fantasies they will be judged by their partners, and yet they complain of sexual monotony. Indeed, sometimes one partner's sexual desires are anywhere from repugnant to boring to the other. Yet it is crucial to remember that there is no good sex without risk-taking. Sometimes the risk is simply being more present and vulnerable to a person to whom one is making love. It seems completely understandable that one arena where the equation of love, trust, and risk is being played out is in the sexual realm and particularly around not using condoms. One way that therapists can be helpful is to encourage men to at least give voice to their desires and fantasies about sex without condoms and to help facilitate conversations between partners about this issue.

Remien (1997) describes how in any couples therapy, but especially when working with couples where one has HIV and the other does not, the therapist has the opportunity to raise issues that the couple has been avoiding as a way of normalizing thoughts and feelings that either or both may be having but have been avoiding speaking about. Remien suggests that there is enormous potential for healing when a therapist voices topics and issues that neither of the men has been able to raise on his own. Remien offers that one way he introduces topics into treatment that have not been spoken of so far is by saying something like, "I've often heard from other couples in your situation. . . ." This helps the couple by raising the topics they have been avoiding and giving them permission to talk about the painful and highly charged realities with which they are living.

One study conducted in New York City of male mixed antibody status couples found that when a couple did not have a high level of sexual satisfaction their distress as a couple was high. This study also suggested the importance of sexuality to the psychological well-being of the men in HIV-discordant relationships; among couples who had a satisfying sexual relationship, there was a high level of emotional contentment (Remien et al., 2003). These researchers found that "maintaining sexual satisfaction, pleasure, and intimacy is particularly challenging for serodiscordant couples" (p. 533). Dolezal, Remien, Wagner, and Carballo-Dieguez (1999) found that when mixed antibody status male couples did not use a condom they experienced greater sexual satisfaction, despite anxieties produced by the behavior. A study of 75 mixed antibody status couples found that the vast majority of unprotected anal sex occurred without ejaculation inside the rectum, and that this behavior did not increase the level of emotional distress of the partners (Wagner, Remien, & Carballo-Dieguez, 1998).

A study of serodiscordant male couples living in London[6] was conducted later in the epidemic. Each of these couples had developed a set of rules regarding the kind of sexual relationship they would have. This research included sexually exclusive and nonexclusive relationships, as well as those with no sexual activity since diagnosis

(Palmer & Bor, 2001). In the partnerships that had become asexual, it was usually the HIV-positive man whose sexual desire had evaporated, and this was not challenged by the uninfected partner but was either accepted without discussion or avoided. This study did not find any significant differences between the couples who had entered into the relationship knowing that the men did not share HIV seroconcordance and the couples where one partner had seroconverted after the men were partnered. The couples in this study who had unprotected anal sex did so often to maintain their preexisting sexual status quo; the idea of not using condoms was more likely to be instigated by the uninfected partner.

As Henry and Joe illustrate, the reality is that often partners play by different rules, which are based on power, privilege, who is more invested in the relationship, and numerous other factors. All of these differences have to be navigated and negotiated in order for the couple to overtly decide when, how often, and why they will have sex without condoms. How the issue of stopping using condoms played out for Henry and Joe is rife with all of these power differentials. One problem is that these issues were never directly spoken about by these men. Instead, each of their confusions about love, desire, and yearning for closeness was played out in the unprotected anal sex.

BAREBACKING AS A STRESS ON A RELATIONSHIP

Not all the couples I have worked with around this issue live "happily ever after." I remember Terry and Gary, a couple who had been together only 15 months, who came to me in a crisis following Terry's having found out that he was HIV-positive. When they first met both men were uninfected, and they began having unprotected sex with each other within a few dates. They had agreed that sex outside the relationship was fine, but if either did have sex with an outside partner they would always use a condom. Terry had gone to the baths one night, where he had gotten high on crystal and allowed the man who gave him the drug to have UAI with him without a condom. Terry had been penetrated by the man. He only told Gary about the incident several months afterwards, when a routine HIV test showed that he had seroconverted.

Gary was understandably furious that Terry had continued to have UAI with him, often penetrating him, without ever having admitted to the incident at the baths. Gary felt totally betrayed by Terry's cavalier attitude toward his health. He wished that Terry had only come clean and told him what had happened so that he would have had a chance to reevaluate his decision about having anal sex without condoms. Hearing this, Terry admitted that he had been cowardly, selfish, and more importantly, reckless. Gary agreed but was still furious that Terry had been so irresponsible and put him at risk. After three sessions Gary informed Terry that the relationship was over. Terry said, "But you didn't even get infected! You're still negative!" To which Gary replied: "No thanks to you!" He told Terry that he no longer trusted him, and trust was the basis of any good relationship. Inside I was cheering Gary on and was thrilled that he said all of this to Terry. Terry looked wounded and said he loved Gary very much. Gary shot back that Terry sure had a bizarre notion of demonstrating his love by putting him at risk for HIV and AIDS.

Another couple, Mike and Steve, came to see me after learning that Steve had become infected. They have been a couple for 3 years and had just bought an apartment together. They had both been HIV-negative when they first met and after talking about wanting to have condomless sex for a few months they went to get tested together. The test confirmed that they were both still uninfected, so they stopped using condoms. They had discussed monogamy and had agreed that at least for the time being they would not have sex with anyone else. It was not until Steve was turned down for a life insurance policy that they discovered he had become HIV-positive.

When they came to see me the week after getting this news, both men were in shock. Mike appeared more devastated at Steve's diagnosis than Steve did. During our first session Mike could not stop crying. When I asked him to try to put into words what he was feeling he explained, "I finally found the man I wanted to spend the rest of my life with and now this happens." I asked him to elaborate. "I know that with current treatments being positive is not what it was in the early 1990s, but the drugs don't work for everyone. Even if we are lucky and they work for Steve, most likely this means that he will get sick and die before me," he sobbed. I spent the first few sessions urging them to talk to each other about their shock and grief and then educating them about the disease.

During the fifth session, I asked a question that seemed to be hanging in the air. "Steve, can you tell me what happened that resulted in your getting infected?" He explained that one time when Mike had been out of town on business he had been chatting with a guy online who suggested they hook up. After initially declining this offer, telling the man that he was in a sexually exclusive relationship, he eventually acquiesced. They had a few drinks together and smoked a bit of pot. When they started to play around he had not intended to have intercourse, but one thing led to another, and condoms had not been used during anal intercourse. He felt terrible, but just kept hoping for the best. Between the time this incident happened and his finding out he was infected, he had exclusively been the bottom during UAI with Mike and had not ejaculated in his boyfriend's mouth. I asked them both if this had been their normal sexual pattern. Mike told me that they were usually flexible, but he had really enjoyed Steve's being so sexually submissive and it had been great. He had never thought it might signify that Steve had taken sexual risks outside their relationship.

When I asked how this news had affected their sex life, they told me that they were cuddling more than ever but had not had sex in the 6 weeks since finding out the news. When I inquired about the reasons for this, Steve explained that he had not felt very sexual since learning that he was infected. I asked Mike how this made him feel. "It scares the shit out of me and saddens me as it feels like he is either pushing me away or drifting away from me now when I need to feel reassurance from him." "Reassurance?" I asked. "Yes, I'm feeling so vulnerable on so many fronts right now. We had agreed to be monogamous, and obviously I wasn't hot enough for Steve. I really worry that this means he wants to leave me for someone else." Hearing this Steve moved closer to Mike, held his hand and said, "Oh, baby, you're worrying about my leaving you. I'm terrified that you would want to leave me after you found out that I had cheated on you and brought this damn thing into our lives." This began a conversation about how neither wanted the relationship to end. Eventually, as Mike felt reassured that Steve was not going to dump him for some hotter man, he got in touch with some of his anger and mistrust of Steve for having played around and not having been safe. Therapy focused on helping them try to figure out what had caused Steve to do what he did and how they might move beyond this. Several months later they are still together but struggling to figure out how to regain their balance as a couple and negotiate how the trust might be rebuilt. During one session, Mike voiced his sadness, anger, and sense of loss at no longer being able to have condomless sex with Steve — or because of their agreement to be monogamous, with anyone else, either. Steve continued to express feelings of guilt and sadness and once flared up at Mike and said, "I miss it too, Mike. I miss what we had too!"

CONCLUSION

Love, desire, trust, intimacy, and commitment create a powerful mix that affects the choices men in partnerships make regarding condoms. No matter whether or not these men choose to use condoms, when they are able to discuss their feelings and desires, intimacy and trust between them has the opportunity to grow. If they shy away from these often difficult and potentially powerful conversations, they are creating limits about how authentic and safe either can be within his partnership.

Part Three

THE ROLE OF THE PROFESSIONAL AND THE COMMUNITY

CHAPTER EIGHT

Can Barebacking Be Curbed? What (If Anything) Works?

CHAPTER OVERVIEW — INTERVENTIONS WITH BAREBACKERS

The feelings associated with barebacking may range from eager and thrilled to dread-filled. Motivations range from sexual desire to emotional drives and even to desire for self-harm. Each and every case has to be assessed individually. We simply cannot work with preconceived ideas about what drives men to risk either transmitting or contracting HIV when we treat men having condomless sex. One of the most succinct ways to put it, as Yep, Lovaas, and Pagonis (2002) write, is that "Barebacking may be viewed as reinforcement of sexual identity, resistance to imposed behavioral norms, creation of a new sexual and political identity, or a continuation of practices unaffected by organized messages aimed at stopping such practices" (p. 1). Any one of these dimensions makes it a daunting challenge to try to reduce the incidence of sexual risk-taking by gay men.

This chapter asks whether the behavior can be curbed, and if it can be, is that desirable? Rarely has a client disclosed during the initial consultation that he was not using condoms for anal sex and wanted help to change this behavior. Very likely, it is not therapists, but physicians, nurse practitioners, and counselors at HIV testing sites and clinics that treat sexually transmitted diseases (STDs) who are seeing the bulk of gay men who are concerned about the physical results of condomless sex. Those men come to clinics seeking tests or treatment for STDs and HIV or looking for postexposure prophylaxis. Wolitski, Parsons, and Gomez (2004) discuss how important opportunities for risk reduction are being regularly missed. Almost one quarter of their research subjects reported that their current health care provider had never spoken to them about safer sex, and these are all men who are HIV-positive. This is no small matter. We "helping professionals" want to help, but what do we do if these men are not asking us for help? What can we do if these men do not view barebacking as problematic? If men don't ask for help regarding barebacking that does not necessarily mean that they don't view it as a problem.

Admittedly, if barebackers themselves are not reporting being upset, frightened, or worried about their sexual risk-taking, it is problematic for therapists and other health care professionals to engage with these men and help them. We have to examine what we mean by "helping." Is our goal to try to get men to stop having sex without condoms? Are we trying to help stem the tide of new HIV infections and keep uninfected men HIV-negative? Or are we trying to help men reduce the risks to themselves or others? This chapter brings together a number of innovative approaches to addressing barebacking, first exploring clinical options and then describing innovative community health approaches — essentially, AIDS prevention approaches for the new century. Barebacking will not go away, but we can become more effective at capturing barebackers' attention and helping them make choices that reduce their risk. That, I believe, is the best that can be hoped for.

This chapter explores a variety of innovative approaches to working with men who take sexual risks, within the context of therapy as well as meeting men where they are within the virtual and actual gay men's communities. Traditional AIDS prevention programs may still have some value for people who do not know the basics of how HIV is transmitted and what each person needs to do in order to protect himself and his partners. Most gay men who are having sex without condoms are already familiar with these basics. This is why extraordinary creativity is required on the part of AIDS prevention efforts and health care professionals. The rest of the chapter explains why an eclectic approach is required in order to get the attention of men who are sexually active and at risk for not using condoms. An understanding that most men who don't use them are not seeking to contract or spread HIV is the basis for employing harm reduction in most current AIDS education and prevention efforts that come out of AIDS service organizations. A variety of community-based harm reduction approaches will be described as will a case that illustrates how using harm reduction and motivational interviewing was an effective strategy for working with a barebacker who was a therapy client.

THERAPISTS' LIMITATIONS

While it is true that a single incidence of high-risk sex can result in infection, or possibly reinfection with HIV, the painful but realistic fact of the matter is that each individual has the right to make his or her own choices in life. Therapy may be able to guide clients to more self-nurturing decisions, but there is no guarantee that even using a thoughtful combination of treatments that incorporates harm reduction, motivational interviewing, and motivational enhancement therapy can have an impact on getting a barebacker to take fewer sexual risks. I was aware of this in every fiber of my body when clients would walk out the door after another therapy session, and I knew that they would be barebacking with strangers whose HIV status was unknown to them. But I had to remind myself that it was not ethical or good therapy to attempt to control or infantilize these men. They had to make their own decisions, and I could only gently try to coach them to be as fully mindful and aware of the decisions they were making and hope that they would someday choose to make decisions that would not have long-term negative consequences for the rest of their lives.

Most theoretical frameworks for addressing gay men who take sexual risks have come from preexisting psychological models that attempt to either address an individual's attitudes or change his behavior. The models most frequently drawn upon in developing AIDS prevention programs are the Health Belief Model (Becker, 1984) and the Theory of Planned Behavior (Ajzen & Madden, 1986). Thomas and Ratigan (2005) suggest that the majority of models of risk reduction largely concentrate on combining the following aspects: attempting to promote positive attitudes toward safer sex, encouraging change from high-risk behaviors by teaching behaviorial risk-reduction skills (e.g., condom use and sexual negotiations), and reinforcing the desired behavior changes. They state that these models are based on the assumption that behavior represents conscious activity that is based on reason and logic. They astutely note that sexual risk-taking often "represents an area of human behavior that may not always be under the conscious control of an individual. It may frequently conflict with his or her stated intentions and espoused beliefs. Given the irrational nature of such behavior it is not surprising that models of prevention based on the assumptions of a rational self have been found to be of limited value in reducing HIV-related risk-taking behavior" (In press, no page numbers available at publication time).

These authors argue that an often-overlooked aspect of risk reduction is the need to apply a psychodynamic model that will help individuals search for the meanings of their actions by helping them explore both the conscious and the unconscious processes that are the basis for so much human behavior. They offer clinical examples of how to use a psychoanalytic approach to work with sexual risk-takers who have been unresponsive to traditional behavioral-based interventions. Ostrow and Shelby (2000) discuss how it is useful to integrate a psychoanalytical and behaviorial approach to doing psychotherapy with gay and bisexual men who are having high-risk sexual encounters while under the influence of drugs and alcohol.

One way that professionals can begin to attend to the psychodynamics inherent in an individual's sexual risk-taking is by learning to listen carefully and ask questions that provide opportunities for the client to explore all aspects of his sexual risk-taking. Walker and Roffman (2004) explain: "When the client's motivation is mixed, ambivalence is often voiced through the expression of both the positive and negative aspects of the behavior, for example, 'I know using condoms is safer, but it's hard to do in the heat of the moment'" (p. 1). To me, this sounds like the basics of any good therapy, but I appreciate the reminder in the case of working with men who take sexual risks because it is so easy for us as clinicians to lose our clinical neutrality and impose our own values and judgments on the client.

It is hard to suspend our judgment when we feel anxious about a client's potentially life-threatening behavior. I am by no means suggesting that it is inappropriate for a professional to feel discomfort with a client's barebacking. I am of the belief that it is highly unrealistic for people to assume that they will be able to control what they feel, especially if it is a situation where a professional is working with an individual who is taking sexual risks or behaving in a way that is likely to spread HIV. In these situations, the best that we can expect of ourselves is not to become preoccupied with our judgments about a client's behavior and to learn how to not communicate our judgment. I understand that this creates a reality in which the therapist is not being his or her "authentic self." But not expressing our own thoughts, feelings, or reactions to what a client is reporting becomes the central aspect of professional self-control and discipline so as not to pollute the client's treatment with our reactions. What I am suggesting is that the struggle is to control the way we respond to our judgments so as not to have them be communicated to the client. What good will it do to say to a client: "I wish you were not placing yourself at risk?" This statement of concern is really more about us than about him. Obviously, a client who is barebacking is potentially courting death. Of course I will have a judgment about this, especially if I like and care about this individual. But at the same time, I have to accept that when an individual is not psychotic and has all of his faculties, he has the right the make a choice that I judge to be self-limiting or self-destructive. Even when I feel very strongly that not being infected with HIV is better than becoming infected, and even when the client agrees with this, it is not clinically useful for me to tell the client that these are my beliefs and therefore I want to help him stop barebacking.

All therapists have to walk a tightrope between being authentic with our clients and being effective. There is no cookie-cutter way to successfully accomplish this. But it helps me to remember that I should never become more attached to the idea of my clients having safer sex than they are. For a therapist not to be appropriately detached from the outcome of his or her work with clients is to court therapeutic disaster. Additionally, I often have to remind myself that in situations where clients elect to continue to bareback (or use drugs or remain in unsatisfying or destructive relationships), it does not mean that I am a bad or ineffective therapist. These perspectives help me transform my feelings of alarm and concern into compassion and patience. I can use the therapy to help the client be conscious and mindful of what is driving him to make whatever choices he makes. I have to make sure that I do not judge or shame clients for being normal, imperfect human beings. The "use a condom every time" message demands a "perhaps unattainable and certainly unsustainable standard of behavior," according to Goodroad, Kirksey, and Butensky (2000, p. 34). I agree. These authors also suggest, "A widespread adoption of the harm reduction approach will allow for the realities of human nature and desire to be addressed . . . and most certainly provide a more therapeutic environment in which clients feel comfortable and able to discuss actual sexual behavior and acceptable sexual risk-reduction methods" (Goodroad et al., 2000, p. 34). I would rather we set up our clients for success and not impose impossible goals on them, leading to their feeling like failures when they cannot live up to goals that are ours and not theirs.

THE BEST CLINICAL INTERVENTION FOR BAREBACKING

It is important to keep in mind how sexual desire can complicate and interfere with rational decision making. We must be realistic and understand that sexual behaviors hold various meanings for individuals, which evolve over time. So far it sounds as though I am saying that the only thing a therapist can do is his or her own internal work so as not to have judgments, expectations, or desires to change the client's behavior. My position is that no matter what the client's issue is that the therapist is facing, this is simply good therapy. Once therapists have really mastered this internal stance, they will have a powerful clinical tool that helps clients examine their behavior and perhaps even make healthy changes.

In Chapter 4, I described harm reduction as a therapeutic intervention. It is now time-tested and has proven to be versatile and efficacious in helping people with addictions. Motivational interviewing, also discussed in Chapter 4, is likewise very helpful. Traditional approaches that include psychotherapy may also have some benefit when working with men who take sexual risks if the therapy encourages clients to explore their family histories, core values, beliefs, needs, and desires while also inviting them to delve into their unconscious. I have found that a hybrid approach that synthesizes all of these dimensions is the only way to help my barebacking clients examine their sexual risk-taking. Using this hybrid therapeutic approach successfully engages sexual risk takers in the process of figuring out whether they want to change their behavior, and the best way to help them see what practical steps they might take to do so. Motivational enhancement therapy (MET) is an amalgam of several useful clinical interventions including harm reduction, motivational interviewing, and traditional psychodynamic therapy.

MET[1] is one effective way of engaging with clients who bareback. It is an expanded way of incorporating motivational interviewing into ongoing therapy. MET is a brief treatment modality lasting one to four sessions that uses motivational interviewing skills, concepts, and style to create a completely collaborative relationship between the professional and client (Walker & Roffman, 2004). I have found that MET is easily incorporated into longer, ongoing psychotherapy with almost any client who is feeling stuck about changing some aspect of his life. It is also a set of skills and a therapeutic approach that is drawn upon and employed again and again at various points during long-term therapy.

When a clinician hears a client express ambivalence about his behavior, he or she has a perfect opportunity to employ the tools of motivational interviewing that I described in Chapter 4 because motivational interviewing is a style of counseling designed to assist individuals in working through ambivalence and increasing their readiness for change (Miller & Rollnick, 2002). A motivational interviewing approach to ambivalence serves at least two purposes:

> First, it communicates to the client that ambivalence is normal and not a character flaw, nor is it an example of some way in which he or she is damaged.

Second, acknowledging the ambivalence protects the client from prematurely committing to a change for which he is not yet ready or that is not felt to be right for him.

One underlying premise of motivational interviewing is that it is impossible for a person to change a problematic behavior that has been strongly reinforced until the psychological barrier of ambivalence has been explored and understood and the client feels he is ready to overcome it. When a clinician accepts and works with a client's ambivalence about taking sexual risks, this in itself is a way of communicating to the client the therapist's own acceptance that though the client expresses a desire not to become infected with HIV, he is not yet ready, willing, or able to take the steps necessary to reduce or prevent this risk. Often, AIDS prevention messages that stressed use of a condom every time have been criticized for mechanizing and dehumanizing sexual behavior (Odets, 1994, 1996; McKirnan, Ostrow, & Hope, 1996).

According to Walker and Roffman (2004), MET has three basic principles. First, it is collaborative, so the helping professional and client explicitly become partners in the client's mental or physical health care. "Clinicians view themselves as having expertise and knowledge about HIV, while viewing their clients as being the experts on their own lives who know if and how change will work for them and the best methods for achieving their personal goals" (p. 1). The second principle is that MET is evocative, meaning that the client and not the therapist has the required expertise to alter the problematic behavior. The job of the professional is to try to elicit from the client his ideas about how the behavior can be changed, then enhance the client's confidence in being able to make the desired change, while constantly attempting to help the client locate and express his own reasons for wanting to change. The third principle of MET is a basic principle of any good therapy: respect for the autonomy of the client and whatever decision he makes, even if the professional does not personally agree with it. The decision about whether or not to change, or what to change, lies completely within the client's control. "Risk perception and social norms are aspects of motivation that are linked with HIV risk reduction," write Walker and Roffman. "Risk of HIV infection is often found to be greatly underestimated by those who engage in behaviors that put them at greatest risk for contracting HIV. Motivational Enhancement Therapy, designed to provide accurate feedback about risk behavior, is one way to motivate change, and is ideally suited to respond to this situation" (Walker & Rothman, 2004, p. 1).

THE CHALLENGE OF CLINICAL NEUTRALITY

As I discussed in Chapter 4, using shame to deter a client who is barebacking is generally not effective in reducing either the behavior or the risk. It may simply chase the client away. Even if there was a good clinical reason for the therapist to express the opinion that out of concern and caring for a client who is putting himself at risk, the therapist would prefer that the client not bareback, this intervention is not going to get him to stop. MET asks helping professionals to suspend judgment and to be genuinely clinically curious about what the man thinks and feels about his having sex without condoms, and then to unambiguously communicate nonjudgmental neutrality around his behavior. That is a tall order for many helping professionals. While we want to be neutral and nonjudgmental, we are humans and we have ideas, beliefs, and feelings of our own. MET offers a road map for effective intervention with clients, but it is up to the practitioner to learn how to set aside personal feelings and truly attain a neutral, nonjudgmental perspective. It is not sufficient to pretend outwardly that one is not having personal reactions and feelings to highly charged content, such as a client taking sexual risks or putting others at risk for becoming infected with HIV. Too often we communicate our reactions through facial expressions, body language, and the tone of voice with which questions are asked.

Since even the most exquisitely trained and experienced therapist can never be wholly judgment-free or value neutral, especially about something as controversial and emotional as people taking sexual risks, how do we manage whatever judgments we have so that they do not contaminate the therapy? A constructive way of managing our judgments is by listening for any ambivalence the client might be expressing about the high-risk behavior. For example, "I hear that you have concerns about the possibility of contracting HIV. You don't want to become infected and yet you also feel that there are real benefits for you when you don't use condoms. Is that right? Okay, so please tell me what those benefits are. I'm asking because once you are clear about what needs you're meeting by barebacking, maybe we can see if there are other ways of having those obviously very important needs met without placing yourself (or others) at risk." At times, it is useful to reflect back to a client who is exploring his ambivalence about sex without condoms, "I hear very clearly from you why you're drawn to barebacking for a variety of reasons, most important is that the kind of connection you make with other men by not using condoms is tremendously meaningful. Therefore, it seems as if your not using condoms is one way you are actually trying to take care of yourself, even though you have said that you know that in the long run, if you become infected, this might be problematic. Is that an accurate summary of what you are saying?" This kind of reflective listening transmits to the client that I am right there with him and understanding what he has been telling me, yet there is no overlay of my own thoughts and feelings about barebacking intruding on his therapy.

MET CASE EXAMPLE – ENGAGING WITH A CLIENT'S AMBIVALENCE

The following is an example of how I used MET, motivational interviewing, and harm reduction with Mario, the client I described in Chapter 5, to help him make better choices to mitigate his risk of contracting HIV.

> **MS:** So you've told me that you don't want to become infected with HIV, yet you don't ask any of your sexual partners about what their HIV status is — do I have that right?
>
> **M:** That's right. But remember that I also told you I never start to chat online with anyone whose profile describes him as HIV-positive.
>
> *In response to this I wanted to tell him that I thought this was great. But to have done so would have communicated to him a judgment on my part. So I only responded with the following.*

MS: This seems to be clearly an indication that you're not trying to get infected.

I had to restrain myself from saying what I was thinking, which was, "That's a great place for us to build on." Had I said that it would have told Mario that I was assuming that he wanted to stop barebacking, something I had not heard from him. Instead I asked him the following.

MS: Are you ever tempted to chat with an infected guy if he is hot and really turns you on?

M: Of course I'm tempted, but there are so many other guys who either identify as being HIV-negative or who just don't say what their HIV status is that I figure why play with fire?

MS: I just want to make sure that you know that there are some guys who either know that they are infected and don't put that information out there or who just might not know that they've got HIV, right? Additionally I also want to remind you that as reprehensible as it is, there are some men who are HIV-positive who lie about their status, even when they are directly asked.

I used the MET goal of ensuring that this client had accurate information about the possible risks he was taking, without trying to tell him what to do.

M: Of course I know that. I'm not stupid, you know.

MS: I know you're not stupid. I apologize for having said something that led you to think that I believed that you were.

I refuse to engage in either a power struggle or opposing whatever resistance he might be expressing.

MS: So I hear you saying you don't want to become infected. Yet, you know that when you have anal sex without condoms with men whose HIV status you don't know, or who say that they are uninfected, there is still a possibility that you might get HIV. I also hear you saying that you feel anxious about that possibility. Is that right?

M: I'm sick of being so fucked up by anxiety that every month I run to my doctor to get another HIV test. That's why I'm here talking about this with you. But honestly, short of only screwing with condoms every time, which I am not willing to do — at least not at this time — I don't know what else I can do.

The client has now clearly expressed a motivation to reduce his risks in order to reduce the anxiety he feels about possibly becoming HIV-positive. This is what is known in motivational interviewing as a "change statement."

MS: Let me see if I understand you. You're really fed up with feeling afraid that you might have gotten HIV. You are clear that at least for now, insisting that you and your sexual partners wear a condom is not an option. But you'd like other options for protecting yourself from getting infected. Is this an accurate summary of how you feel?

I am making certain that the client knows that I am with him about his not being open to using condoms, and I am verifying with him that he might be ready to try to instigate change.

M: Bingo. Do you have any other suggestions that might help?

Client is now unambiguously asking for a suggestion, which indicates that he may be ready to make some kind of change. At this point, exactly what suggestion he might be open to trying is still unclear.

MS: Well, short of using a condom, the best way you could protect yourself would be by not having sex with men who are infected. Right?

M: That's a no-brainer.

MS: Good, so we're on the same page there. Are you willing to try to increase the odds that the men you have sex with are not infected?

I'm working to reinforce the collaborative nature of this process and assess how ready, willing, and able he is to make a change.

M: I think so. What do you have in mind?

Client is now specifically asking me for my suggestion.

MS: One way a lot of HIV-negative guys who don't want to use a condom try to keep themselves uninfected is to directly ask every potential partner whether he is infected and when was the last time he was tested, and only have unprotected anal sex with other uninfected men. There is even a name for this now. It's called "serosorting." Another thing that many guys who are uninfected and want to stay that way do is that when they have anal sex without condoms, they are only the top. What are your thoughts about either of these as a possible prevention strategy for you?

I am making it clear that the choice is his and that I am only providing options, not giving advice.

M: Since everyone knows that there are way more bottoms in New York than tops, if I chose that route it might make me very popular.

We both laugh at this, reducing whatever intensity or tension had been infusing the session.

M: But seriously, I just don't think that I would feel comfortable asking guys, especially if I'm really turned on to them, whether they're POZ or not.

He looks a bit ashamed.

MS: Hey, I really respect you for knowing what your limits are and being able to tell me them so clearly. That's a really important part of our work together. I'm sure that we can come up with an alternative plan that feels do-able to you. We have never discussed whether you are more of a top or a bottom; what are your feelings about trying the second suggestion I mentioned?

I am not judging his limits and therefore not taking an oppositional stance that would almost invariably create a powerful resistance to any suggestions. I am also planting seeds of hope that there are other options we can explore.

M: Actually, I am truly versatile, and if I had to make a choice I'd probably rather bottom than top. But limiting my barebacking to just being top isn't a bad idea. But if a really hot butch guy wants to throw me on my back, I know I won't refuse.

MS: All right, so you have just figured out one way to try and reduce your risks, and also expressed some understanding about your own limits. That's important information for both of us to have.

When I inquired why Mario felt unwilling or unable to ask men he was attracted to what their HIV status was, he explained that he did not want to risk having men he chatted with on the Internet, to whom he was powerfully attracted, tell him that they were not interested in hooking up. I empathized with his fears and inquired about what need was being met by hooking up with hot men.

At this point, Mario began to disclose that even with his professional success, he often did not feel good about himself or sexually confident. He said that when a hot man expressed interest in him and they wound up having sex, it resulted in him feeling powerful and strong as well as desirable. I empathized with how important these feelings were for him and encouraged him to continue to talk about this. He said, "My whole life I felt like a frightened little faggot. I feel most like an adult man when I play with another man who I find strong and powerfully sexy. Even the fact that I may be taking a risk sexually contributes to my self-confidence and sense of adventure. This infuses my life for days and sometimes even weeks after a great romp."

Mario was beginning to get to the root of the need he was addressing through barebacking. I used this conversation to introduce the topics of control and power, and we began to talk about other ways he might experience these feelings and integrate them into his sense of self. I suggested that one way of feeling powerful and in control was to take responsibility for his well-being. In response, he looked at me blankly, an indication that my remark had not gone over well. When I asked him bout this, he said it sounded like I thought he was not already doing t, explaining further that he saw his pursuit of sex with attractive nd his willingness to assume the risks of unprotected sex as ways control. I acknowledged my blunder and we moved on.

Mario and I spent weeks discussing all of these issues, but I refrained from making additional suggestions as to how he might change his risky sexual behaviors. I was waiting for him to provide me with an opening. Eventually, he did so, raising the question of the HIV status of the men he chatted with online. He still felt worried that they might reject him. Hearing this, I suggested that there were ways he could increase his tolerance for this kind of discomfort, and that raising the HIV question involved skills so as to develop the necessary psychic muscle that he could learn. I also assured him that I was not proposing that he stop barebacking while he was developing these skills and suggested that he might be able to find "something else" to do to increase his safety. By joining with him in this way, I let him know that I understood the importance to him of sex with attractive men. This strengthened our therapeutic alliance, thereby increasing the odds of his later asking about additional prevention measures. I had grave concerns about Mario's behavior, but my main priority was to keep him engaged in therapy, which held out the possibility of further risk reduction efforts on his part.

In our next session, he asked me directly what I had meant by "something else." This was another opening. I suggested that, as an experiment, he might try putting the HIV status question to men to whom he was not attracted. Mario's first response was this would be a waste of time. After noting that I understood why he might feel that way, I explained that this would make it possible for him to develop his confidence and raise his comfort level regarding the process without having to worry about missing out on hooking up with any men he might be interested in. Note that, as an intervention tactic, this had one clear advantage: it avoided creating an all-or-nothing situation that would likely result in Mario's feeling hopeless about the prospect of his ever being able to make any change. But even at this point, it was key that he not think I was pressuring him into doing anything. Only after he told me unambiguously that he was sure that he could do this did I ask him to explicitly acknowledge his willingness to try this strategy. "So that's the plan for now?" He said that it was to strengthen his resolve. I reinforced that this was a first step toward his alleviating his anxiety about becoming infected. It took Mario a few weeks to warm up to the idea, but eventually he reported back that he tried the experiment and had succeeded a few times. He made a point of telling me that he appreciated that the suggestion had felt "risk-free": In other words, that it minimized the chance of his feeling rejected.

Once Mario reported that he had successfully asked men he was not attracted to about their HIV status, I asked him how long he felt he needed to practice this step before moving on to the next phase. After he inquired about what the next phase was, he told me he wanted a month. After a month had passed, during which he reported that he practiced asking men he was not attracted to their HIV status while chatting online, I asked if he was ready to try something that would build on the emotional muscle he had developed over the past month. He said he was. I next suggested he try inquiring about the HIV status of men to whom he had only a moderate attraction. He agreed to try this. Eventually, after about 3 months, he was able to ask all the men he flirted with online about their HIV status.

The next step was to explore with him his feelings about not agreeing to hook up with people who did not answer him or those who identified as HIV-positive or did not know their HIV status. (I am aware that there will be some HIV-positive men who upon hearing this will angrily accuse me of perpetuating what has been called "viral apartheid." My response to this as someone who himself is HIV-positive is that anybody has a right to refuse to have sex with anyone for any reason.)

We also discussed Mario's feelings about telling prospective partners that he wanted to use condoms. He was unsure that he wanted to take this step, so we let it rest for a few months until he said that he would feel more comfortable if, when he bottomed, the man used a condom no matter what he said his HIV status was. He was nervous about taking this step but eventually decided to try. The first three people who did not identify as HIV-negative did not balk when he said he wanted to play safely, and he had fun hooking up with them. The big test came the first time that a hot man who identified as HIV-negative wanted to top him. Following this incident he came to therapy and reported that he had ɔt been able to ask the man to put a condom on but had not enjoyed experience as fully as he had hoped because he had been preoccu- ʏ thinking how much more relaxed he would have been had he not bottom during bareback sex. This led to his deciding that he felt ready to commit to asking everyone he was interested in about their HIV status, and to continue to bareback as a top with men who reported being HIV-negative, but to use condoms with anyone else, and to ask men who wanted to top him to use a condom. Clearly, this is not a foolproof method for remaining HIV-negative, but Mario had taken an important step toward reducing the possibility of seroconverting.

COMMUNITY-BASED HARM REDUCTION INTERVENTIONS

Both on a conceptual level and in therapy itself, harm reduction must be value-neutral. In 1994, San Francisco Bay area psychologist Walt Odets discussed how futile it was for AIDS prevention programs to suggest an absolutist sexual message of "use a condom every time," and how this unrealistic message created a sense of hopelessness for gay men who occasionally had high-risk sex. This sense of hopelessness, Odets suggested, may actually have contributed to these men taking increased sexual risks. Odets (1994) was the first person to explicitly suggest that incorporating a harm reduction approach into AIDS education and prevention efforts might actually help reduce the number of new HIV infections among gay men. The primary goal of harm reduction is to reduce potential harm while encouraging safer behaviors. This makes it an ideal approach not only for clinical work with gay men who bareback but also for AIDS prevention campaigns. "A harm reduction approach to sex would suggest alternative risk-reduction strategies that may afford minimal protection (e.g., early withdrawal and vaccinations for hepatitis) or less-than-optimal protection (engaging in unprotected anal intercourse [UAI] only as the insertive partner)" (Suarez & Miller, 2001, p. 294).

Odets was the forerunner of advocating realistic and practical approaches to gay men having sex without condoms; several of these approaches have been developed in the San Francisco area. Harm reduction approaches have been attempted in the gay community, with some controversy. Community activist and writer Michael Scarce (1999b) created an uproar when he published "Safer Bareback Considerations" in *POZ* magazine. Scarce's ideas included the following practical information and suggestions. He mentioned that drugs like poppers, which dilate blood vessels in the rectum, can make bareback sex more risky.

He counseled using plenty of lubricant so as to reduce the risk of anal trauma from intercourse. He also urged barebackers to pull out prior to ejaculation and limit how often they engaged in bareback sex.

In response to data indicating that most gay men have sex without condoms at some point in their lives, the London organization GMFA (Gay Men Fighting AIDS) developed a set of practical harm reduction guidelines (GMFA, 2003; published here as Appendix 2). In my view, this is an exemplary public intervention, mobilizing hard information in the public interest, but under the guise of realism. Its most important recommendations are serosorting (although the term is not used) and withdrawal prior to ejaculation. Over the years, some AIDS service organizations have maintained that oral sex is safer sex (AIDS Action Committee, 1995) or low-risk sex (San Francisco Department of Health, 1996; Gay Men's Health Crisis, 1996). At least partly in response to these messages, many men have sought to reduce their vulnerability to infection, as well as the odds of their spreading the virus themselves, by substituting unprotected oral sex for unprotected anal sex (Halkitis & Parsons, 2000; Kalichman et al., 2002).

HARNESSING THE IMPULSE FOR SELF-PRESERVATION

The vast majority of men who are having sex without condoms are not seeking to get infected, nor are they trying to infect others (Wolitski & Bailey, 2005). By making small adjustments in their sexual practices, the members of this majority can greatly reduce the risk of their spreading or contracting the virus. This may seem like common sense, but it is also confirmed by data gathered by the social scientists studying the phenomenon. Below I provide a list of these behavior modifications, incorporating the labels now used for some of them:

- "Negotiated safety," which is an agreement between two gay men in a HIV-negative seroconcordant relationship to go through the process of getting ready to stop using condoms when they have anal sex.
- "Serosorting," which refers to the practice of men having UAI with other men of the same HIV status (Pinkerton & Abramson, 1996; Hoff et al., 2004).

- "Strategic positioning," which is used by both HIV-positive and HIV-negative gay and bisexual men and refers to the practice of infected men adopting the receptive role during UAI with HIV-negative men (Van de Ven et al., 2002b; Wolitski, 2005).
- "Dipping," which refers to anal insertion for just one or two strokes without wearing a condom (Parsons, Wolitski, Purcell, Gomez, Schrimshaw, Halkitis, Hoff, & The SUMIT Team, 2004).
- Withdrawal prior to ejaculation.
- Using information that they or a partner have undetectable viral loads to make decisions about whether or not to bareback.
- Substituting unprotected oral sex for UAI.

The precise degree of strategic positioning's effectiveness as a risk reduction tactic is not currently known (Wolitski, 2005). There can be no question about its favorable impact, for reliable research indicates that, of the two partners in anal intercourse, it is the receptive one who is most vulnerable to HIV infection (Vittinghoff, Douglas, & Judson, 1999; Wolitski & Branson, 2002). But it bears repeating: while all risk reduction strategies reduce the odds of transmission, none of them provide full protection. Consistent condom use remains the most effective way of preventing the spread of HIV.

A study conducted in Sydney revealed that, among men in serodiscordant relationships, UAI was more likely to occur when the HIV-positive partner reported having a viral load beneath the level of detectability (Van de Ven et al., 2005).[2] A parallel study in the Netherlands yielded similar results (Stolte, deWit, van Eeden, Coutinho, & Dukers, 2004). Van de Ven and colleagues are wise when they note that, despite the existence of data confirming that combination antiretroviral therapy can reduce the viral loads and infectiousness of HIV, it remains problematic to base risk reduction decisions upon this effect. Yet most of the participants in another study, conducted in San Francisco and New York, thought that UAI always entailed significant risk to themselves and/or their partner, even when one or both of them were on HAART (Remien, Halkitis, O'Leary, Wolitski, & Gomez, 2005).[3] As might be expected, awareness of the general health risks (including HIV transmission) entailed by UAI was lower among those participants who were practicing it — 16 to 18 percent of the group — than among those who were not. The authors conclude that the decision to engage in UAI often correlates with the degree of risk one perceives in it, suggesting that advances in medical treatments for HIV have led some gay men to minimize the dangers of the practice, and thus has made them more likely to engage in it.

The human implications of these findings, on a one-on-one scale, were brought home to me during a session with Ron, a 49-year-old white, HIV-positive man with a long-term partner who was also positive. Ron had long been suffering from chronic diarrhea, and his doctor had recently suggested that he try a structured treatment interruption — a temporary cessation of his AIDS medications — in the hope of stopping the medication side-effect, thereby confirming that his meds were the cause. Ron had agreed to the treatment interruption, and he wanted to discuss the impact this would have on his personal life. Due to 100 percent adherence to his AIDS regimen, his viral load had long been below the level of detectability. On this basis, he and his partner had been having unprotected sex, including intra-anal ejaculation, for six years. Ron told me that since stopping antiretroviral therapy he had decided not to ejaculate inside his partner while he was not taking his medications. Despite the impact this precaution would have on their lovemaking, he felt this was the right way to go.

Viral loads only have the potential to remain undetectable when there is an extremely high level of adherence to the therapeutic regimen. This is difficult for most people to sustain over extended periods. Thus viral loads and the potential for an individual to be infectious can be quite variable, especially during breaks in the antiviral treatment, regardless of whether they are supervised by a physician or just done by an individual on his own (Miller et al., 2000; Fagard et al., 2003). Thus when men in serodiscordant relationships have UAI based on undetectable viral loads of the infected partner, it is always advisable for them to opt for risk reduction strategies such as strategic positioning or withdrawal.

BAREBACKING ON A SEXUAL CONTINUUM

One advantage of incorporating a harm reduction approach into work with barebackers is that it has the potential to "provide tools for the individual to use if, and when, he does become motivated to change his behavior" (Suarez & Miller, 2001, p. 294). My work with Mario is one example of how this can play out. Goodroad et al. (2000) suggest that in order to take a harm reduction approach to gay men who bareback, it is useful to view bareback sex as part of the continuum of sexual behavior that includes the highest possible risk from frequent exposure to blood and semen through condomless sex, to the least risky, which is complete abstinence from sex with other people. They state, "The continuum approach allows for the development of interventions that are pragmatic rather than absolute, problem based" (Goodroad et al., p. 34). In other words, it enables the professional to help the client understand that the question of sexual risk-taking need not be framed in either/or terms, as if the only options were barebacking, with its enormously high level of risk, and consistent condom use, or abstention from anal intercourse. These are the two polar extremes, but they are linked by a continuum of intermediate behavioral options, all of which can reduce the risk of transmission. The same authors rightly emphasize the importance, again from a pragmatic standpoint, of the professional's not stigmatizing high-risk behavior. As when working with substance abusers, the odds of successful intervention improve markedly with a calm, temperate approach. When the client has failed in one or more attempts to modify the behavior, it is especially important to avoid making having high-risk sex into a crisis, for this tends to discourage him from making additional attempts. Whether it is having a drug- or alcohol-use relapse or resuming sex without condoms after a period of having protected sex, the therapist needs to view these behaviors as an expected part of human nature and of the therapy, and reflect this back to the client. He should be made to feel that compassionate health care is not conditional upon his adoption of safer-sex protocols. Otherwise, he will not feel sufficiently safe to discuss his sexual behavior frankly, and the window of potentially successful intervention will close.

INNOVATIVE AIDS PREVENTION PROGRAMS — THE USE OF HUMOR

"New and innovative ways are needed of delivering prevention messages that will excite and motivate those people who have thus far been unwilling to adopt safer sex practices or who have returned to condomless sex after years of safer sex," write Suarez and Miller (2001). They state, "A hybrid approach to prevention that includes elements of harm reduction, motivational interviewing, and traditional approaches may prove most fruitful" (p. 294). I agree. In fact, I know of no alternative approach that is effective for working with gay men who take sexual risks.

Psychologist Jeffrey T. Parsons is the Director of the Center for HIV Educational Studies and Training (CHEST) at Hunter College in Manhattan, one of the leading HIV/AIDS research and prevention centers in the world. Parsons (2005) has argued that "it is time to think outside the box of traditional individual and group-level interventions, as well as to be more creative in our approach" (p. 128). He and his team found that AIDS prevention interventions based on humor, as opposed to fear, have been particularly successful in engaging HIV-positive men in a risk reduction program. As these authors point out, their finding is consistent with earlier analyses of fear-based campaigns meant to discourage smoking and to encourage cancer screening: over the long term such campaigns are of limited efficacy. They found that a humor-based initiative often engaged men when fear-based initiatives had ceased to be effective (Parsons et al., 2004a). They discuss that AIDS prevention programs that are based on scaring men into safer-sex practices focus on the risks inherent in UAI and then offer a solution (i.e., abstain from anal intercourse or use a condom every time). As I mentioned in Chapter 2, the long-term efficacy of fear-based campaigns has been shown to be limited. The public becomes inured to the messages and blocks them out.

Humor, as opposed to fear, is more likely to appeal to men, and being able to initially capture their attention is crucial to the success of a prevention campaign. Parsons and his colleagues are also community activists who base their work at least in part on the theoretical foundations of Conway and Dube (2002), who wrote, "Humor can be used in persuasion on threatening topics, specifically on the promotion of preventive behaviors to alleviate health threats" (p. 863). One of the most entertaining examples of the use of humor by a safer-sex campaign is a program developed in New York City, by the staff at C.H.E.S.T., which is aptly named the DIVAs. It stands for Drag Initiative to Vanquish AIDS. In this outreach effort, community educators dressed in brightly colored wigs and matching outfits approach men in bars and at community events with safer-sex kits, engaging them in lighthearted conversation peppered with HIV prevention information. For example, a DIVA might say to someone, "Honey, syphilis is back and she's sore!" (Parsons, Bimbi, Grov, & Nanin, 2004b).

Another creative humor-based intervention originates out of San Francisco and is Internet based. It is called the "Healthy Penis" campaign. The Web site offers information about syphilis and other STIs using comic strips. One is entitled "Phil the Syphilis Sore" (www.healthypenis.org). Funding for this program comes from the San Francisco Department of Public Health and the Public Health Department of Seattle and King County in Washington state. Humor is a perfect way to lighten up the grave seriousness of the escalating syphilis and HIV epidemics while at the same time reaching men who otherwise might not have any interest in prevention messages.

ASSESSING SEXUAL HIERARCHIES

In order for a helping professional to become increasingly nonjudgmental — the bedrock of any successful harm reduction intervention — he or she must first be comfortable with the concept of human frailty and imperfection. Sexual desire can enormously complicate and interfere with rational decision making. We must be realistic about this, and understand that sexual behaviors hold various meanings for individuals, that evolve over time. According to Drescher (1998), the concept of sexual hierarchy can be potentially helpful to therapists when trying to help individuals assess the importance and nuances of specific sexual acts. Citing Schwartz (1995), he defines sexual hierarchies as "referring to the ordering of sexual practices as better or worse in terms of some implicit or explicit value system" (p. 217). In therapy with individuals who are taking sexual risks, I find it useful to ask explicitly about the person's sexual hierarchy and the meanings that each risky behavior holds for the patient, in terms of satisfying both intrapsychic and interpersonal needs and desires. (The concept of a sexual hierarchy refers to which specific behaviors an individual is most drawn to and finds most pleasurable and which ones hold less interest or desire for him or her to participate in. Thus, for an individual who most highly values either ejaculating inside someone or having someone ejaculate inside of him, it will be more difficult to stop barebacking than it might be for an individual who has generally always preferred mutual masturbation.) Yet, as Drescher (1998) notes in order to do this effectively: "the therapist must be aware of his or her own value system, including the kind of sexual hierarchy to which he or she adheres as well as the extent to which the theory he or she has learned has embedded within it sexual hierarchical judgments" (p. 217). He further cautions clinicians that it is often "not an easy matter to disentangle these different kinds of value judgments from each other, especially when the patient himself is in conflict about his own sexual practices (p. 217). Self-examination of this kind is likely to foster the empathic, nonjudgmental stance that is often a prerequisite for successful intervention with gay men engaging in UAI.

A POSITIVE SEXUAL HEALTH APPROACH TO PREVENTION

Sometimes, a variety of social factors can impede an individual's resolve not to engage in risky sexual behaviors. Researcher Rafael Diaz (1998) studied gay Latino men with HIV and found that among the men he surveyed, those who were best equipped to resist oppressive sociocultural realities like homophobia, anti-HIV biases, and antigay discrimination were more likely to be sexually self-protective. Diaz found that the men who reported a high level of sexual satisfaction — which was described as sex that was free from guilt, intolerance, and self-reproach — engaged less often in high-risk sexual activities than did men who were burdened by a high level of sexual guilt and a corresponding low level of sexual satisfaction.

Building on Diaz's findings, San Francisco social worker Kim Gilgenberg-Castillo (2004) suggests that utilizing a positive sexual health approach will be essential to increasing gay men's adoption of risk reduction behaviors. He cites a document prepared by the Department of Reproductive Health and Research at the World Health Organization, which defines sexual health as "a state of physical, emotional, mental, and social well-being related to sexuality; it is not merely the absence of disease, dysfunction, or infirmity. Sexual health requires a positive and respectful approach to sexuality and sexual relationships, as well as the possibility of having pleasurable and safe sexual experiences, free from coercion, discrimination, and violence. For sexual health to be attained and maintained, the sexual rights of all persons must be respected, protected, and fulfilled" (World Health Organization, 2002, retrieved online).

Gilgenberg-Castillo (2004) discusses that "sexual health includes self-acceptance, the capacity to communicate sexual needs, and define sexual boundaries" (p. 3). An increasing self-acceptance by HIV-positive men of their own health status can contribute to the harm reduction strategy around barebacking of always disclosing one's HIV status prior to having sex, even when a potential sexual partner has not asked. Disclosure is still an area where many HIV-positive men (like Jerry in the previous chapter) are, understandably, extremely vulnerable. Conversations with HIV-positive friends and clients, and my own memories of being an infected single man, all reinforce how difficult it is for people to disclose their HIV status, especially to someone new who is a possible sexual or romantic liaison.

Even helping professionals can be squeamish about raising the topic of HIV status. Wolitski et al. (2004) found that important opportunities for risk reduction are often missed. A quarter of their HIV-positive research subjects reported that their current health care provider had never spoken to them about safer sex. They also confirmed that disclosure of HIV was a difficult issue for many seropositive gay men. While most of the men in studies conducted by this team had disclosed being HIV-positive to their primary sexual partner, they had done so to less than half of their more casual partners prior to having sex. Clearly, there is a need for interventions to be developed that encourage all gay men to ask about the HIV status of all of their potential sexual partners prior to first having sex, and, especially for HIV-positive men to develop the emotional and social skills to volunteer their HIV status. Encouraging uninfected men to ask the question will distribute the heavy burden of initiating such conversations more widely, thereby fostering a more communal sense of responsibility for reducing HIV infection rates.

Professionals can encourage this behavior by raising the issue of disclosure and inquiring about HIV status with all of their gay male clients, not only the ones who are already infected. HIV status cannot be a taboo topic if we are seriously committed to reducing the number of new infections. We need to develop interventions likely to spur this major shift in community norms. Such a campaign will succeed only if uninfected men who choose not to have sex with infected men, or who opt exclusively for protected sex with them, make a commitment to being kind and gentle when they ask, as well as when they communicate their decision about whether and how to hook up. At its simplest this means treating all men with the same degree of sensitivity, regardless of your sexual intentions. Creating a community norm of discussing HIV status prior to having sex can help reduce instances of high-risk sex. Frank and honest conversations about HIV status could help barebackers negotiate sexual behaviors to minimize the risk of transmitting HIV. Wolitski et al. (2004) found that among the almost 2000 HIV-positive participants in their study, those men who did not consistently disclose being HIV-positive to uninfected potential partners or those whose viral status was unknown were more likely to have unprotected sex with these partners than were those who disclosed to all of their partners.

The positive sexual health approach to HIV risk reduction is "founded on the principle that sex is a basic human right," according to Gilgenberg-Castillo (p. 3). Although we were not aware of the theory of positive sexual health as an entity, in hindsight I see that my colleague Luis Palacios-Jimenez and I were using such an approach when, early in the epidemic, we tried to get gay men to eroticize safer sex. Gilgenberg-Castillo speaks about how the effort to help sexual minorities achieve sexual health is nothing short of a macro-level intervention that will require society-wide efforts to destigmatize all sexual activities and sexual diversity. He suggests that there are specific ways that professionals working with men who may take sexual risks can help promote positive sexual health in their clients, which hopefully will increase the likelihood of men taking fewer sexual risks. He urges health care professionals to communicate to their clients unambiguously, that regardless of their HIV status, that a fulfilling and safe sexual life is both possible and desirable. Professionals should then explain that they are willing to work with the client to help him discover ways to have a satisfying sexual life. He also suggests that it is helpful for providers to acknowledge to clients who are living with HIV, herpes, or hepatitis that they face special challenges in negotiating sexual activities and communicating their sexual desires. When a provider makes this kind of acknowledgment, it fosters discussions about an individual's fears and insecurities, as well as about his sexual practices and attitude toward viral-status disclosure.

INTERNET-BASED APPROACHES TO RISK REDUCTION

Since many gay men who engage in UAI meet online, it seems only logical to consider the Internet as a platform for harm reduction outreach to them. This approach is still in its infancy. So far, most such initiatives have been sponsored by local agencies, usually AIDS service organizations or community-based organizations. Health departments in Europe and North America have also begun to venture into cyberspace, delivering HIV prevention efforts via men who have sex with men (MSM) oriented chat rooms (Douglas-Brown, 2001; Turner, 2001; Seeley, 2002; MacMaster, Aquino, & Vail, 2003; Acosta, 2004; Rhodes, 2004; Tuller, 2004). "Many health workers say these programs can be particularly useful in reaching men in rural areas, young gay men, and others who may not want to identify themselves or visit a gay community center" (Tuller, 2004, p. F8). "I think the anonymity is extremely helpful," said Lyndon Cudlitz, a 21-year-old who is the education and outreach coordinator for Outright, a Maine gay rights group that posts profiles of peer counselors who can answer questions about safer sex and other health-related issues online (quoted in Tuller, 2004, p. F8).

One notable Internet-based intervention was developed in Philadelphia in 2000, when the Department of Health approached five community-based organizations in that city in an attempt to reduce the number of new syphilis infections among men who had sex with men. The catalyst was a city-wide rise in cases of syphilis, and many of the newly infected had met one another in online chat rooms. Of course for syphilis to be transmitted, there must be skin-to-skin contact, so the fact that this campaign pushed the use of condoms meant that it also functioned as a barebacking intervention. The protocols that guided the campaign were developed by David Acosta, a public health consultant with the Philadelphia Health Department. The goal was not to interfere with what men were talking about or planning online but to be a real-time, online resource regarding HIV and STD prevention. From December 2001 to June 2004, outreach workers engaged 1459 men in MSM chat rooms in individual chats. This collaborative effort included the AIDS Office, Disease Control Office, and community-based organizations working with gay, bisexual, and MSM populations (Acosta, 2004). At the same time, there were syphilis prevention messages in group chats that were observed by other men who chose not to engage the outreach workers in private chats. Each agency that participated in the program chose a distinct chat room in which to make its workers available as a prevention resource.

The outreach workers used consistent screen names like "Safe Buddy." The profiles for these screen names stated clearly that the person worked for such-and-such agency, and that anyone with questions about preventing HIV or other STDs, was welcome to IM (instant message) him directly. Sometimes, the workers also created an additional screen name and persona and made up both sides of a supposed real chat in order to draw the interest of other men in the chat rooms. Perhaps surprisingly, they found that aggressively engaging men in the chat rooms was a productive tactic, one that often led to intended online conversations.

The diversity of the agencies taking part in this effort greatly increased its breadth and effectiveness. The lesbian, gay, bisexual, and transgender (LGBT) specific agencies were able to reach people that the Department of Health alone could not. All of the online workers were themselves MSM, so they could speak to the men in the chat rooms in commonly understood vernacular. Two of the benefits of using this form of Internet outreach are:

1. The prevention message reaches everyone in the chat room even if they do not engage the outreach worker directly.
2. It reaches MSM on the "down low." (This refers to African American men who have sex with other men, but who do not identify as gay and therefore may not frequent gay-identified spaces.)

The drawbacks of this kind of Internet outreach are (Acosta, 2004):

1. Men who chat on the Internet are difficult to engage, probably because they are online to meet men for either social or sexual contact.
2. There is less incentive to talk online to outreach workers as compared to talking to outreach workers on the street, because on the street people can obtain free condoms from the workers.
3. Outreach workers, especially those who have been successful in street outreach, are often frustrated, since the immediate results of the online work are not as tangible.

MacMaster et al. (2003) discuss how the Internet is a venue where disenfranchised groups in general have the means to connect with other members of their group, noting and that this tends to foster a community of acceptance. They elaborate on how this dynamic is especially important for members of sexual minorities who may not have the means to identify or connect with similar people. When the sexual minority men, also doubly stigmatized, as members of a racial or ethnic minority, connections made on the Internet may be even more important to them. These authors describe a program that began in 2002 in San Jose, California, where Asian and Pacific Islander MSM were specifically targeted. This was a peer-driven model that used nonprofessional volunteers to target chat rooms designed for or frequented by Asian and Pacific Islander MSM throughout Santa Clara County in California.

To generate interest in the topic of AIDS prevention, two outreach team members would engage in a conversation about the specific topic chosen for that evening's intervention, in the hope of enticing other chatterers into the conversation. The lunch hours during the week and the hours between 12 and 5 P.M. on weekends were identified as the times when outreach efforts were most productive. They conjectured that the reason for this was that prevention messages were more easily ignored at night when the people who were online were focused on actually hooking up for sex. One of the successes of this program was its ability to provide consistent and accurate information to men who might not otherwise have received such information (MacMaster et al., 2003).

Another online outreach campaign was launched in North Carolina. The health educators entered chat rooms, announced their purpose and made themselves available to answer questions and offer referrals about HIV and AIDS. This intervention used the following discussion topics to engage chatters: Sexual risk reduction strategies (e.g., safer barebacking); HIV testing options; local alternative for nonsexual social support; referrals for youth; resources related to coming out and access to risk reduction materials and supplies. The educator's leading messages read "In the room to answer questions about HIV/AIDS," "I can answer questions about HIV and AIDS," and "Need condoms? I can tell you where to get them" (Rhodes, 2004, p. 317).

Rhodes (2004) reports that many respondents requested information about how they might lower their sexual risk, especially with regard to UAI. He describes one individual who wrote that he engaged in receptive anal intercourse with a regular partner and wanted to know how to make it safer. He told the health educator that he did not want to become infected with HIV, but he and his partners did not want to use condoms for anal sex. He wrote: "Do you know of a way not to get AIDS without using a condom? Me and my boyfriend hate condoms" (Rhodes, 2004, p. 319). Rhodes did not say what specific counsel was offered to this particular man. But he relates how the health educator led discussions about using condoms and risk reduction. The online conversation included various individual experiences and strategies engaged in by chatterers, including one man describing how he withdraws prior to ejaculating, and another advising that someone adverse to condoms should try them again and "put lots of lube on next time. Smear it on. I take it that way" (p. 320). When the men in the chat room shared their experiences of successfully broaching the topic of safer sex and doing it with their own sexual partners, the health educator provided additional information and corrected misconceptions about what constituted risk behavior.

Another online program, called CAMPsafe, is run out of Rehoboth Beach, Delaware. This program began in 2001 and mostly reaches men who live in rural areas as well as the seasonal summertime community. Salvatore Seeley, the program director of CAMPsafe, estimates that a majority of questions his online outreach workers get are about the safety of unprotected oral sex, and that 30 percent are about barebacking. Many of those who write are men who define themselves as "straight" but who are experimenting with anal sex and who have no information about the risks associated with barebacking. In this case, the Internet has proven to be a good tool to provide outreach to those men who may not go to traditional cruising places to look for sex but instead use online chatrooms, Web sites, and listserves (S. Seeley, personal communication, October 7, 2004).

Both public and private agencies in San Francisco have been at the vanguard of developing the most varied and innovative approaches to online prevention of HIV. The Healthy Penis campaign described earlier in this chapter is an example of creative use of the Internet to reach men with risk reduction information. It has never been easy for a man to let a sexual partner know that he may have infected him with something or caught an STD from him. One difficulty in stemming the tide of new infections of HIV and other sexually transmitted infections (STIs) or STDs is that with an increasing number of men engaging in anonymous sexual hookups with men they meet on the Internet, they may not have the name or even phone number of a recent sexual partner. Yet, they may know the e-mail or screen name and be able to contact their partners that way. An effort funded by the San Francisco Department of Public Health to use the Internet to help reach men who may have been exposed to a STI is www.Inspot.org, which is the STD Internet notification service for partners or "tricks." Men who have been diagnosed with an STD or even HIV can anonymously e-mail a postcard from the Inspot Web site to inform sexual partners that they need to go for STD or HIV testing (Inspot.org, 2005)

If someone receives an Inspot card letting him know that he may have been exposed, the Web site provides information about where he can go for screening and treatment. There are six different cards that a man can choose from to inform someone that he needs to get screened for an STD. One card that has a photograph of two screws reads, "I got screwed while screwing and you might have too. Get checked for STDs if you haven't recently," and provides the Inspot Web site. Another states, "You're too hot to be out of action. I got diagnosed with an STD since we played. You might want to get checked too." Both cards leave room for a personal message if the sender chooses to add one (www.inspot.org).

Despite this abundance of efforts, in San Francisco and elsewhere, health educators acknowledge they are uncertain what might be most effective, or even whether online prevention efforts work at all. "We really don't have any specific interventions we can hang our hats on and say, 'This is what works,'" said Dr. Jeffrey Klausner, director of the STD clinic at the San Francisco Department of Public Health (quoted in Tuller, 2004, p. F8). These sentiments were echoed by Scott Rhodes of the Department of Public Health Sciences, Wake Forest University School of Medicine in Winston-Salem, North Carolina: "Currently, no peer-reviewed published research exists that describes and evaluates a chat room-based HIV/AIDS prevention intervention for MSM" (Rhodes, 2004, p. 316). This lack of empirical research data should not interfere with ongoing efforts to develop online HIV and STD prevention efforts, for it is clear that they are providing accurate information and referrals to men who need them. In the words of CAMPsafe's Seeley, "Online prevention work is a good way of reaching married men and other MSM who don't identify as being gay. Many closeted men are drawn to chat rooms since they offer an extra level of anonymity and fantasy. Because these men are not involved in the gay community, they have not heard prevention messages targeting gay men" (Seeley, 2002, p. 60).

There are understandable tensions between the ways in which health officials and helping professionals would like to be able to reach out to men who are online and limitations imposed by the operators of the Web sites where online interventions have been conducted. On the one hand, San Francisco's Dr. Klausner and other health officials discuss how they try to work with the owners of popular Web sites but do not always find the owners to be cooperative. In response, the managers of the Web sites feel that the officials are not understanding the needs of the customers and have wound up sometimes lecturing men in chat rooms rather than simply providing information (Tuller, 2004). "A lot of our customers want to know, if they've decided to take a risk, here's how to minimize the risk of transmission," said a spokesman for Advanced Membership Services, which runs the M4M-USA.com Web site. "But a lot of public health agencies just want us to be a stern parent and to preach to our customers" (quoted in Tuller, p. F8). Some site owners have decided to impose limits on such interventions. For instance, the outreach or public health workers who visit chat rooms for professional reasons have been given permission to respond to questions posed to them but are not allowed to contact members first, even if they observe that members are preparing to engage in unsafe activities. "If our customers feel as if their right to practice sex as they chose is infringed upon, it endangers the whole program," said Stephen Adelson, director of operations for Online Buddies, which runs Manhunt. "We're really trying to find a balance between providing health education and outreach and respecting members' freedom of speech and choice" (quoted in Tuller, p. F8).

It may be that for large numbers of gay-identified men, the era of effective safer-sex programs has passed. As Wolitski et al. (2004) say — and I agree — "Many men are already sophisticated consumers of information about the risk of specific sexual practices, and programs that address only safer sex may not offer much that is new or appeal to these men (those who already know that they are infected with HIV)" (p. s107). They suggest that while a majority of HIV-positive men are interested in messages that promote the adoption and maintenance of safer sexual practices, these messages may need to be part of other information that these men feel is of greater importance to them, such as general health and well-being and new HIV treatments. This is probably true for the majority of gay men in general, whether or not they have been infected. If all community forums about issues important to gay men included a component on risk reduction and HIV prevention, they would probably reach a broader audience. For instance, the Centers for Disease Control and Prevention (2002)[4] issued guidelines for physicians treating HIV-positive individuals that offer specific suggestions for how to counsel infected patients regarding risk reduction during routine medical care. I suggest that these same guidelines be expanded so that every health care provider asks all men they are seeing about whether they have sex with men. Regardless of the response, physicians, nurse practitioners, physician's assistants, and all other health care professionals need to use each contact with a man as an opportunity to initiate conversations about HIV risk reduction techniques that go beyond "use a condom every time."

CONCLUSION

Human beings are complex and quirky, especially when it comes to changing an aspect of their lives that not only gives them pleasure but is also often an attempt to satisfy a variety of emotional and social needs. Even when the pleasurable behavior has the potential to be harmful, people find it extremely difficult to break longtime patterns and change, reduce, or give up their pleasures. When the pleasure in question is sex, creative and innovative combinations of approaches are required.

I am certainly not the first person to suggest that traditional AIDS prevention strategies are no longer enough to help stem the tide of new HIV infections. Nor am I the first to recommend using a diverse treatment approach that incorporates health education, harm reduction, motivational interviewing, and motivational enhancement therapy — for that matter, any innovative but sensitive technique likely to be an effective way to help gay men reduce the risks when they are ambivalent about having UAI. Gerhart (1999) suggests that in order to be effective, attempts to address UAI must change from an approach that stresses one solution (e.g., use condoms every time or do not have anal sex) to one that enhances an individual's sense of freedom and personal responsibility for his sexual decision making. Most men who are having risky sex have some degree of ambivalence about it. Only when this ambivalence is addressed and dealt with directly by the individual himself can there be any hope of his effecting the desired changes. Ambivalence about UAI is made more difficult to assess and address as it converges with internalized homophobia. Since many of the men who have unprotected or unsafe sex are out and, at least on the surface, proud, self-affirming gay men, it might seem strange to suggest that they suffer from internalized homophobia. But messages about gays being abnormal, unwelcome in the human family, are often introjected in pernicious and subtle ways. Such messages influence even the most self-actualized gay men's unconscious and can result in their feeling on some level that the way they have sex is unhealthy and abnormal. This can lead to a de facto devaluation of those with whom they have sex as well as of their own sexual desires. Society's messages about gay men can become internalized as an unexamined and deep distrust of other gay men and the gay community, resulting in a feeling that the queer community is not intrinsically valuable or deserving of respect, nor an entity within which one can truly feel comfortable and at home.

One macro level intervention that can help reduce self-destructive behavior by gay men is to dismantle societal homophobia. But in a world where the Pope says that the trend toward legal recognition of gay relationships is part of "a new ideology of evil" that undermines society (Humm, 2005) and where there is a consistent effort by officials in the U.S. government to make gay and lesbian people invisible by banning any mention of them on official government Web sites (Styrsky, 2005) and to roll back whatever gains and rights have been achieved, this is a daunting prospect, especially since antigay prejudice remains the last socially sanctioned form of bigotry. One crucial way that gay men can combat societal and internalized homophobia — which are inextricable — is to learn to take better care of themselves and others. Gay men may never find a safe haven within mainstream society. But there is no reason why we cannot diligently work toward creating a community that will be a safe home for all queers.

That said, there remain some men who have no ambivalence about sex without condoms. What, if anything, can helping professionals and the gay community do to address them? This leads us to the next chapter and the book's conclusions.

CHAPTER NINE

Conclusions: Sexual Freedom and Sexual Responsibility

One of my goals in writing this book has been to make it harder for readers to hold to a simple or essentialist position about barebacking and other forms of sex without condoms. The only definitive thing we can say about barebacking is this: it is not one behavior but a variety of behaviors that take place in many configurations among a wide range of men. There is no one social or sexual situation that leads to barebacking. If we want to understand the behavior, and reduce its frequency, we must come to terms with this complexity.

Our society likes to simplify and sensationalize controversial issues, especially when they pertain to sex. A painful example of this is the question of abortion. Barebacking is poised to become similarly controversial, especially in the wake of the apparent emergence of a new, even more dangerous strain of HIV (Santora & Altman, 2005). In the aftermath of news reports about this multidrug-resistant and fast-progressing strain of HIV, the level of rhetorical intemperance ratcheted up within days. "Gay men do not have the right to spread a debilitating and often fatal disease," Charles Kaiser, New York historian and author of *The Gay Metropolis,* was quoted as saying. "A person who is HIV-positive has no more right to unprotected intercourse than he has the right to put a bullet through another person's head" (Kaiser, quoted in Jacobs, 2005, p. A1).

In the same article in the *New York Times,* others proposed "tracking down those who knowingly engage in risky behavior and trying to stop them before they can infect others" (Jacobs, 2005, p. A1). One way of accomplishing this, it was suggested, was to "show up at places where impromptu sex parties happen and confront the participants. Or it might mean infiltrating Web sites that promote gay hookups and thwarting liaisons involving crystal meth" (Jacobs, 2005, p. A1). These last two proposals make me uncomfortable. I could never support creating any kind of sex police. There is no telling how far social censure would go — into the bedrooms of consenting adults?

THE NEED FOR SHARED RESPONSIBILITY

Of course I understand the basis of the outcry against barebacking — I do not want to see more human beings become infected with HIV. While I certainly agreed with Kaiser's concern, his tone troubled me. Kaiser seems to place all of the blame on the shoulders of HIV-positive men, implying that they are irresponsible and sociopathic. This is simplistic and inaccurate. We must remember that it takes two people to have unsafe sex. One man, even if infected, cannot pass the virus to a partner if that partner insists on using condoms. It would be a grave mistake, and counterproductive to public health, for the discourse around barebacking to become sensationalized and framed by a rhetoric of shame, blame, and moralizing. In my view, the most constructive framework within which to discuss barebacking, at least within the therapeutic context, is that of risk reduction. The alternatives could lead to clients fleeing our offices and potential clients never seeking help around this behavior.

SEXUAL FREEDOM AND PERSONAL RESPONSIBILITY

Is barebacking wrong? Is it immoral? After pondering these questions for a long time, I have concluded that it is neither morally appropriate nor politically desirable for anyone to decree universally that sex without condoms is bad or even that it needs to be stopped. This is not in contradiction with my strong feeling that ways need to be developed to reduce the rates of sexually transmitted diseases (STDs), including HIV, among gay men. How can one suggest that there may be responsible ways to bareback yet still advocate for the need to reduce disease transmission?

The answers to this extremely complex question originate in normalizing the desire to have sex without condoms, even in the face of a life-threatening epidemic. Men must not feel shame for desiring condomless sex. The vast majority of gay, bisexual, and straight men would prefer never to use a condom as most if not all men find that condom use substantially reduces the pleasure, intimacy, and spontaneity of sex (Dilley et al., 2002). I think that we also just have to accept the reality that there is no way to stop or even to reduce the amount of sex that takes place without a condom. The issue then is are we able to help reduce the frequency of sexual risk-taking within this understanding?

Part of the answer to reducing the spread of HIV, if not barebacking, lies in the gay men's community not blindly taking the position that anything that anyone does is beyond reproach or criticism. This is in stark conflict with some of the core principles of the early gay rights movement, which equated unbridled sexual freedom with gay liberation. The most constructive debates we can have as a community and society about barebacking need to focus on sexual responsibility. Feminist theory taught decades ago that sexual freedom needs to be in balance with individual sexual responsibility (Califia, 1983; Vance, 1984; Nichols, 1987; Ogden, 1999; Munson & Stelboum, 1999). All members of a community need to factor in the impact of their individual behavior on the community as a whole. Some gay men who bareback seem to be acting out traditional male privilege without giving a thought to the impact of their behavior either on their sexual partners or on society at large. It is also useful for the gay community to question whether we, as a community, use our status as members of an oppressed minority as an excuse to justify to ourselves high-risk behaviors, for example, "society tells me I shouldn't want to have sex with men. Screw society. I'll have whatever kind of sex I want, and that includes barebacking." It is not healthy or appropriate to leave unchallenged the mentality of being a victim as an excuse to rationalize engaging in dangerous behaviors.

I have had clients ask me if there is any way that they can exercise their freedom to have sex without condoms yet still behave responsibly. I tell them that I am unable to answer that for anyone but myself, but I can open up these kinds of conversations about freedom and responsibility and help my clients explore these issues during our therapy sessions. I can also suggest tactics for reducing risk if they choose to bareback and initiate conversations about reducing the risk from sex without condoms.

APPROACHING BAREBACKING REALISTICALLY

While I hope that everyone who reads this book will take up the challenge of raising the community's consciousness about sexual responsibility, I also believe that we have to work on prevention efforts that are forged with the understanding that barebacking will inevitably continue, at least on some scale, among segments of the gay population. Therefore, we need to develop even more radical approaches to risk reduction. One focus, as I discussed in the last chapter, would be to develop a community-wide effort to remove the stigma of being HIV-positive. This will help encourage the development of the broad cultural norm of "Do ask (about HIV status), and do tell (that you are HIV-positive)" prior to first having sex. This would greatly help to reduce the rates of sexual risk-taking. We know this to be true from Wolitski's research (2004), which demonstrated that when people either disclose that they are HIV-positive or know that their sexual partner is HIV-positive, they are significantly less likely to take sexual risks.

VIRAL STATUS

As an HIV-positive man, I can hear the critics of this suggestion, accusing me of advocating a kind of "viral apartheid," where men who might have had sex with someone if they did not know that he was HIV-positive might elect not to if they knew he was infected. An op-ed piece in the New York weekly *Gay City News* speaks to this issue. "The reality is that infected men have little to gain by exposing their status, and when they do it is an act of altruism, which should be appreciated" (Riley, 2005, p. 13). Disclosing one's HIV status prior to having sex with someone is indeed an act of altruism, an expression of caring about the greater good that can lead to improved public health, and reducing new HIV infections. If men only barebacked with others of the same HIV status, there would be far fewer HIV seroconversions. Those barebackers would still have to worry about other STDs, but the risk is greatly reduced for spreading HIV.

"An added complication in the effort to stop the spread of HIV is the number of negative people who say they don't care and enthusiastically participate in barebacking. It's one thing to say that you should inform your partner, but what seems simple becomes complicated when the partner says, 'let's do it anyway'" (Riley, 2005, p.13). In a situation like this, it is incumbent upon the infected man to try to discourage barebacking. But if barebacking does happen, then the infected man would be well advised to do one of two things:

1) Position himself strategically at the bottom; failing that,

2) Withdraw prior to ejaculating inside of his partner.

Either of these behaviors (or a combination of them) will minimize the odds of his partner's receiving infected semen, and possibly becoming infected. It is true that many uninfected gay men will choose not to have sex with someone upon learning that he has HIV or will only want to have sex with condoms. A serious public health situation requires some tough decisions and potentially difficult accommodations. I am aware that the concept of serosorting is controversial, and that it may be difficult for some men — at least initially. But the ultimate gains far outweigh the initial discomfort.

STRATEGIES FOR INFECTED MEN

Knowing that a potential sex partner has HIV, some men will still want to have unprotected sex with him; therefore, I urge positive men who bareback to position themselves strategically as indicated above. If these recommendations take hold, larger numbers of gay men would be taking active responsibility for reducing the chances of spreading HIV. Gay men would basically be saying "AIDS stops with me." This powerful slogan was used by New York's Gay Men's Health Crisis as the theme for one of their AIDS prevention campaigns. Prevention campaigns early in the epidemic did urge gay men to have sex in ways that assumed that all of their partners were infected. This remains excellent advice, especially for men who bareback, unless two people are sexually exclusive and have gone through the process of getting tested for HIV together.

However misleading, the announcement of a "new strain" of HIV in February 2005 (Santora & Altman, 2005), was a useful wake-up call. Had the case in question been the harbinger of many such, as opposed to the freak occurrence it now seems to have been, the consequences could have been dire. As we breathe a sigh of relief, however, we should remember that the outcome could have been different, and we need to renew our sense of urgency about HIV-related education and prevention. Community programs should help gay men to understand that it only takes one man committed to having protected sex to prevent HIV from being spread, and the responsibility for doing this starts and stops with him. Every man who commits to having protected sex and protected sex only stops the virus in its tracks. This is a difficult pledge to keep in any case, and that is why I put forth the options of "safer" but not ever completely "safe" ways to have sex without condoms as an alternative. The epidemic of crystal use among gay men has made the restraint of safer sex always, virtually impossible for some individuals.

DRUG USE

The widespread abuse of drugs may be an expression of communal pain gay men experience as an oppressed minority. Walt Odets suggests that many crystal users employ it as an antidepressant (quoted in Jacobs, 2005). He also notes, aptly: "that it would be more effective to try and identify the underlying causes of drug abuse and self-destructive behavior, including the difficulty of living in a society that rejects committed gay relationships while condemning homosexuals for having sex outside those relationships" (quoted in Jacobs, 2005, p. A1).

ETHICS AND BAREBACKING

Some gay men do place a higher value on hot sex than on personal safety. Social constructionists would explain this by saying that it must be interwoven with the historic realities of societal pressure for men who desired other men. For most of history, the message in industrialized countries was that there was something wrong, dangerous, immoral, sick, and illegal about two men acting on shared consensual erotic desires. This overt sexual oppression resulted in generations of men with same-sex desires who were too intimidated, frightened, or isolated to openly accept their own feelings and discover how these feelings could blossom into a rich and fulfilling expression. Therefore, social constructionist theory might suggest gay men may be more forceful about their right to take sexual risks as a reaction to homonegativity.

Throughout history, there were men who could not be at peace with their own homoerotic desires. Even if they managed to sometimes act on these feelings, they did so in a manner that resulted in their living furtive lives often split between their public selves and the authentic selves they kept hidden. The secret and hidden lives some of these men lived caused pain and harm to both themselves and their loved ones. Men who were trapped and compartmentalized by their secret lives frequently felt they had no choice but to live a lie that was inextricably bound to their inability to comfortably integrate the reality that they desired or loved other men. So if one were to take an ethical position that argued for each individual's right to sexual self-determination by being able to freely express his own sexual orientation and act on these feelings, how does that ethical position reconcile a parallel position that privileges hot, unconstrained sex over other values such as preservation of health and possibly life? Part of the problem is that for some men the freedom to express their sexual orientation becomes confused with the license to bareback freely. Just because someone was or is oppressed does not mean that anything they do as a result of this oppression is acceptable.

CHALLENGES FOR THERAPISTS

After doing therapy with many men who bareback, immersing myself in the research and literature about barebacking, and writing this book, I find myself profoundly ambivalent about barebacking. I can understand and empathize with the rationales for why men are not wearing condoms. I feel sad and deeply concerned that men who do and should "know better" are contracting HIV, syphilis, and other STDs in record numbers. By this point it should be obvious that I hold the bias (as an HIV-positive man) that it would be better and more desirable if gay men were to remain uninfected with HIV. I feel this way despite recognizing, as was discussed in Chapter 5, that for some men there are advantages to having high-risk sex and becoming HIV-positive.

It was extremely difficult to work with large numbers of young men who were dying earlier in the epidemic. But that work did not raise contradictions for me, just enormous sadness and frustrations. The most difficult clients I am working with currently are those who are wrestling with their use of crystal and/or those who are barebacking. It is always a challenge for me to contain the contradictions and inconsistencies that I experience working with men whose crystal use is creating havoc in their lives and who are unwilling, unable, or not ready to face how problematic their drug use has become. I face similar challenges when working with uninfected men who are having unprotected sex that is frequently high-risk. In my practice, it is more often than not men who are using crystal who are having high-risk sex. With every fiber of my intellect and the whole of my professional training, I know that only by remaining nonjudgmental and engaging with these men using a harm reduction approach can I have any hope of helping them. I spend hours in my own supervision developing ways to contain my anger, fear, and concern. It is frustrating to watch gay men put themselves and others on the fast track to doing permanent and lasting harm to themselves as well as to the larger society.

CLINICAL DETACHMENT

I know the mechanics of change — that only if and when someone is ready to change will it ever happen, no matter how deeply I may wish for it on their behalf. It has to come from within my clients. Dangerous drug-taking combined with sexual risk-taking is a powerful hook that still raises some discomfort in me, even after some 30 years as a practicing therapist. I need constantly to remind myself that clients who are discussing these issues will elicit strong feelings in me. I prepare myself before a session, I calm my racing pulse and move into a more curious, patient, and clinically detached mental state to ensure that I will not respond in inappropriate ways during a client's session. It is not about detaching from my caring and concern for my client. To the contrary, I detach from becoming more invested in having the client change than he is. I need to detach from any investment I might have that the client will begin to address his crystal use or high-risk sexual behavior. Of course, I hope that our work can help him move toward change, but I must accept that I am powerless to make this happen, while being mindful of whatever power I do have to try to encourage my client to move toward change. If I am not careful, by remaining inappropriately attached to my goals or treatment plan rather than the client's, I can actually be an impediment to the kind of change I wish for him.

I see that I cannot simply condemn these behaviors or the people who engage in them. Rather, I have to resolve to acknowledge and reconcile how dangerous certain behaviors are, not only for the individual but for the gay community as a whole and for the broader society as well. I try to create a community ethic that stresses that each person has a sense of responsibility not only for his own well-being, but for the well-being of all others. Everything is impacted by everything else, and therefore what an individual does affects every one of us on some level. This ecological view runs counter to the deeply entrenched American ideals of staunch and rugged individualism, which bolsters a lack of awareness of, or respect for, the interconnections that bind together societies and is one basis of civilization.

A FEMINIST PERSPECTIVE

What has been conspicuously absent from much of the discourse surrounding barebacking is any inclusion of feminism's historical insistence on talking about both sexual freedom and responsibility (Califia, 1983; Vance, 1984; Nichols, 1987; Ogden, 1999; Munson & Stelboum, 1999). On the sexual freedom part of the equation, even with the myriad risks associated with barebacking, the policing of sexual behaviors and desires is not warranted and is full of dangers to a free society. On the sexual responsibility side, ways must be found so that each individual takes more responsibility for protecting himself from becoming infected and, if he is already infected, takes responsibility for preventing the virus from being transmitted. The world has lost innumerable, irreplaceable, precious human resources — hundreds of thousands dead from AIDS. The gay community's struggle for recognition, acceptance, and equality within American society was derailed by the reprioritization of leadership, money, and energies into caring for sick and dying people and building vital community-based AIDS service organizations. When a client states that it is his right to do what he pleases, I do not argue with him, but these days I explore his understanding of a social contract where people have a mutual responsibility for one another within the community and society. I also ask him to think not only emotionally but critically about why he wants to bareback. Is it really just about hot sex? Could it also be a response to experiencing pressure from other gay men to bareback? Could his motivation to take risks be linked to his need to be desired, to be valued, to fit in and feel part of the community? As his therapist, I search for ways that I may be able to help this individual develop his inner core of strength and self-confidence to become conscious of these pressures and explore what options he may develop in response to them.

In an open letter to gay and bisexual men in response to the news of the new strain of HIV, the Institute for Gay Men's Health asked some very pertinent questions about what steps can be taken to help strengthen the mutual responsibility and ties that gay men need to feel in order to reduce the spread of HIV. This letter is a social planning and public health document, which suggests: "Whether over a dinner table with friends and family or in bed with a boyfriend or trick, we must have difficult conversations about why we should matter to ourselves, each other, and the world." The document goes on to suggest that, to facilitate this conversation, gay men could talk about a number of specific issues, including the following (GMHC & APLA, 2005):

- Why should gay men matter to each other?
- How do we extend consideration and concern to other men with whom we have sex?

This letter goes on to suggest specific actions that can be taken. Two of the actions are:

- Insist that every sex act be an expression of consideration as well as desire.
- Resist urges to police other men, but instead surprise your friends, lovers, sex partners, family members, and acquaintances with conversations about sex, love, crystal use, relationships, homophobia, HIV/AIDS, racism, work, art, and the million other things that matter to you (GMHC & APLA, 2005).

This document, although a political manifesto and call to action on the part of each gay man, is also a visionary challenge for each gay man to look inside himself and take personal responsibility for what he can do to help transform the gay community into a more loving and safe environment. If increasing numbers of gay men will heed the call of this letter, we can work together effectively to create a climate where HIV and other diseases are spread less often.

Scholar, writer, and AIDS activist Cindy Patton cut through the knot of ambiguities and conflicts attached to barebacking: "It is simple, but must be stated over again that sex is not murder, even if we have not yet created a culture in which each person will be equally responsible toward every other person, even if we have not yet created a culture in which every person will have the power (or self-esteem) to take care of him/herself" (1991, p. 385). Her concerns were framed within a radical critique of both the larger erotophobic and misogynist society that does very little to empower anyone's sexuality, particularly that of women and sexual minorities. Yet her critique was also of aspects of the gay male sexual subculture that privileged individual sexual expression above any considerations of interpersonal or broad responsibilities. Patton's comments about sexual risk-taking were written more than a decade before I wrote this book, and the scene has changed radically from those days. Today, for many men who engage in it, barebacking is a subculture of its own, and barebacking has become part of the gay male Zeitgeist. Patton's comments are still relevant insofar as they speak to gay men having to explore ways they can meet the needs that barebacking fulfills in order to take care of themselves while simultaneously assuming a mutual responsibility for the men with whom they have sex.

ETHICS AND HIV INFECTION

It is sometimes implied that a majority of men who bareback are recklessly spreading HIV, but research does not bear this out. Only a minority of HIV-positive men bareback with HIV-negative partners or partners whose status is unknown. Two studies, conducted in San Francisco and New York, suggest this (Wolitski, Parsons, & Gomez, 2004).[1] But the willingness of even a small number of gay men to allow another person to contract a serious and potentially life-threatening illness, even when he willingly accepts that risk, raises public health and ethical issues. A majority of HIV-positive subjects in the Wolitski, Parsons and Gomez (2004) studies used condoms (though not consistently, even with HIV-negative partners or men whose HIV status they did not know). Most men employed a variety of harm reduction strategies that they thought likely to reduce the risk of transmitting HIV, including serosorting; strategic positioning (where HIV-positive men engage in UAI only when they are the bottom); withdrawal prior to ejaculation; and "dipping," or anal insertion for just one or two strokes without wearing a condom (Hoff et al., 2004).

It is a relief to know that the vast majority of HIV-positive men are not actively trying to infect uninfected men, and that the majority of uninfected men are not consciously trying to become infected, even if large numbers are willing to take a degree of risk by having anal sex without condoms. Wolitski et al. (2004) found that most participants in their two studies of HIV-positive men felt they had a personal responsibility to protect sex partners from becoming infected with HIV, and this belief had a strong effect on what they did sexually.

But, as I explored in Chapter 5, a small number of men actually do seek to become infected with HIV. The men who spoke in the film *The Gift*, who were either willing to infect others or seeking to become infected, never expressed any awareness of, or concern about, the ethical issues or long-term consequences arising out of an intentional infection with HIV. In order not to deteriorate from HIV disease, most people will eventually have to begin an inordinately expensive regimen of antiretroviral treatment for the rest of their lives. If they do not have health insurance, entitlement programs will assume the burden of these costs, which can exceed $15,000 a month. If they become too disabled to work, they will need to be maintained on one form or another of public assistance.

Cost is by no means the only problem, or even the most serious one, associated with people becoming newly infected with HIV. There is the physical impairment, discomfort from medications, vulnerability to other infections and illnesses, and the social and emotional toll that becoming infected causes in an individual and his loved ones. Many, and perhaps most people who are willing to spread HIV, fail to consider the cost to society as a whole, from lost productivity to government subsidies. It is not difficult to see how one man's asserting his right to his sexual freedom to become infected leaves the rest of us to pay for the very serious, long-term consequences — to all of us. The gay community, which acted with remarkable compassion and effectiveness at the onset and height of the AIDS epidemic, will again be burdened by the need to care for more men with HIV. Perhaps understandably, some will question how deserving of compassion and care these men are if they actively sought to become infected with HIV.

POLITICAL CONTRADICTIONS

When asked his opinion about whether he felt that the trend to bareback was growing, the host of one of the leading bareback Web sites, barebackjack, gave the following explanation (2003):

> Yes I see it growing. I think that there are several reasons. Of course, the Internet has sparked a renewed interest. But that's the vehicle by which the "movement" (and I really dislike calling it that) is growing. The reasons behind it most likely include the obvious. First, the safe-sex movement was doomed to fail from the start. Historically, it couldn't work. Prohibition didn't stop people from drinking even though it was made a criminal offense. It was repealed after 10 years. That was booze. This is sex. And the safe-sex movement has been asking men to compromise their pleasure in sex voluntarily for the last 15+ years. Second, there's the defeat of the Gay Marriage Bill. While it may not be directly tied in to

the upsurge of barebacking in this country, the defeat of the bill seems to have kicked barebacking out of the closet. The opponents to the Gay Marriage Bill expected too much. They didn't want gays to enter into legally binding relationships, and at the same time they didn't want us to be promiscuous. Realistically, it isn't going to work both ways.

The political and social climate in the United States is illustrated by the ascendancy of the religious right and the Bush administration's global, domestic, and environmental policies. People who were disenfranchised previously are only more so now, both within the United States and abroad. Within a political climate where a woman's right to choose is threatened, where the teaching of evolution in schools is being challenged, where federally funded sex education teaches "abstinence only," and where, under pressure from religious conservatives, any mention of the fact that condoms can help prevent HIV is removed from the Web site of the Centers for Disease Control and Prevention (CDC), honest conversations about sex and the balance between sexual freedom and sexual responsibility will not be encouraged as part of official, government-approved AIDS prevention programs. This is why private citizens, both gay and straight, including men, women, and transgender people, need to speak out regarding the need for open public debate of these issues.

Many disenfranchised gay men, especially those who are economically disadvantaged and/or men of color, are not receiving the mental-health care that can be one important component of stopping high-risk sexual behaviors. Part of this is a direct reflection of the American health care system, where health insurance is not universally available, so poor people or those who do not have health insurance often do not obtain vital nonemergency health care, in this case psychotherapy. Additionally, for those who either are able to afford to purchase private health insurance or who obtain it as a benefit of their employment, with the onset of managed health care, most health insurance policies now limit the number of sessions covered for psychotherapy. The current trend in health care in the United States is for a model based on brief treatment that only seeks to reduce or eliminate an individual's symptoms and not pay for a longer-term therapy. Gay men who take sexual risks need the opportunity to delve into how their internalized homophobia, alienation, rage, and feeling invisible and devalued in contemporary American society all contribute to high levels of depression, drug use, barebacking, and other destructive behaviors. In order to do this effectively, they need access to affordable mental-health treatment with gay-sensitive providers.

MORAL CONTRADICTIONS

The public controversy about barebacking was reignited when openly gay, HIV-positive, right-wing writer and former editor of *The New Republic* Andrew Sullivan was outed as a barebacker by journalist Michelangelo Signorile (2001). According to GAYBC Radio, Sullivan, under an assumed screen name, placed profiles at Bareback City and in an AOL M4M chat room seeking partners for bareback sex. He listed himself as HIV-positive and expressed a preference for bareback sex with other HIV-positive men (though he did not say that he would *only* have bareback sex with other infected men). GAYBC verified that these profiles were Sullivan's when two different people met him through these profiles and confirmed that the individual who placed these particular profiles was indeed Sullivan (Signorile, 2001). Sullivan confirmed Signorile's report on his own Web site a few days after it appeared on the Internet (Sullivan, 2001), and Sullivan's screen names and Web sites were shut down shortly thereafter.

What is of interest here is that a conservative, proudly practicing Catholic public figure who purports to play the role of the moral conscience of the gay community was drawn to barebacking. He sought sex that some feel is at the absolute limit of the sexual spectrum. Obviously, Sullivan is not the only individual who is socially conservative, actively religious, and inclined toward sex that is on the edge. Sullivan is like many of my clients who bareback. They often experience a disconnection between public positions they hold dear and their own private sexual conduct. In his book *Love Undetectable* (1999), Sullivan describes his sexual behavior after the onset of AIDS as "an unrepentant assertion of freedom, an assertion that the deepest personal struggles do not end in the middle of a crisis. Indeed, in the middle of a crisis, refusal to end them is a mark of the ultimate resistance."

One sad and enervating piece of the Sullivan episode is that he repeatedly lambasted AIDS researchers who publish studies showing that rates of unsafe sex and new HIV infections among gay men in the United States had increased (Sullivan, 1996). He did this even after he himself became HIV-positive in 1993 (Kurtz, 1996). Like many other barebackers, Sullivan seems to have a conflicted relationship to barebacking — drawn to it, yet publicly attempting to downplay its dangers.

An article published in *The Nation* reflects my feelings about this episode. "It's not so much Sullivan's sexual practices that are irresponsible as his policing of other people's sex lives in such a way that preserves his own sexual privilege" (Kim, 2001, retrieved online). According to this author, the stir generated by the exposure of Sullivan's barebacking exemplifies the extent to which what passes for public discourse about the issue is governed by a "politics of sexual fear and revulsion." I can only agree. It is my hope that this book will bring us closer to the reasoned, respectful, and frank public conversations about pleasure and safety that we now so sorely need. Health care professionals who work with gay men would do well to initiate such discussions among themselves, as well as with their clients. Gay men have an ethical and public health responsibility to have these conversations among ourselves. The failure to do so will bring dire consequences, but the courage to engage honestly with one another about these difficult issues will result in a stronger and healthier community, and will serve the public good.

Negotiated Safety Agreement Questionnaire

Developed by www.freedoms.org.uk
©2002 freedoms.org
(Reproduced with permission.)

"Negotiated safety" is an agreement between two gay men in a relationship to go through the process of getting ready to stop using condoms when they have anal sex. The basis is an explicit understanding that both know each other's HIV status and both are uninfected. The only time they don't use condoms is when they have sex with each other, making this an acceptable safer sex option. There must be no unprotected sex outside the relationship; if either partner does so, then he must immediately inform his partner prior to their having sex again. Then, they have to resume using condoms until subsequent HIV tests prove that the partner who had unprotected sex is still negative.

The Negotiated Safety Agreement Questionnaire has four sections, which each contain questions and discussion points that you and your partner should talk about when working out your agreement.

Try not to rush the process of making an agreement. Be forthright about your needs and expectations, and respect your partner's.

Writing down some notes might help you to keep track of your discussion.

Use your notes to help you build up a clear agreement on what you want and how it will work.

And after you have completed the questions in each section, try to write down a statement that sums up your discussion and what you have agreed on.

Start with About Us, then work your way through Our Expectations, then Practical Steps, and finish with A Few Months from Now.

If you find you are having difficulty agreeing on any of the discussion points, you can make an appointment with a sexual health adviser at a sexual health clinic and take it from there.

THE AGREEMENT QUESTIONNAIRE: PART ONE

About Us: What Sort of a Couple Are We?

If you and your partner are thinking about making an agreement not to use condoms in your relationship, the following questions will help you to work out how well you really know each other:

- How would you describe your relationship?
- In what areas of your lives do either of you have an advantage over the other?
- What has been your past experience of making agreements with each other?
- How do you usually talk to each other about important things or uncomfortable situations?
- What do you know about each other's HIV status, drug-taking, and sexual history?
- How well informed are you about sexually transmitted infections (STIs) like gonorrhea, herpes, hepatitis, or HIV? Herpes is a distinct illness so I added a comma after it.

To sum up your discussions, write a statement beginning: We are a couple who...

THE AGREEMENT QUESTIONNAIRE: PART TWO

Our Expectations: What Do We Want from Each Other?

The following questions will help you work out what you are expecting each other to do and not to do if you make an agreement about not using condoms in your relationship:

- Under what circumstances would you consider allowing your partner to have sex with other people in the future?
- What risks are you prepared to take when you have sex with other people?
- What risks do you accept that your partner is allowed to take? Under what circumstances will you use condoms with other sex partners in the future?
- What will you tell each other about sex outside the relationship?
- How confident are you that you could tell your partner that something had happened that may have exposed you to HIV or a sexually transmitted infection?

And to sum up your discussions, write a statement beginning: We want. . .

THE AGREEMENT QUESTIONNAIRE: PART THREE

Practical Steps: How Will It Work?

If you and your partner are making an agreement not to use condoms in your relationship, there are some practical things you need to agree on. And it's better if you don't just assume that you will agree with each other. You need to be explicit. Say it out loud to each other, or write it down if that makes it clearer to both of you:

- **HIV Testing**
  - Depending on the level of risk you both accept, you will need to consider how often you have HIV tests in the future. Do you both agree?
- Sexual health checkups
  - If either of you has sex outside the relationship, you will need to have regular checkups for sexually transmitted infections. Do you both agree?

- Communication
  - Any agreement you make will increase the need to talk openly about sex and your relationship. Do you both agree?

And to sum up your discussions, write a statement beginning: We will...

THE AGREEMENT QUESTIONNAIRE: PART FOUR

A Few Months from Now: What Will We Do If Things Go Wrong?

Sometimes people do things they didn't plan. So despite your commitment to the agreement you are making now, it's possible that in the future you or your partner will have to disclose something that's embarrassing or difficult to talk about.

The following questions will help you both be prepared for that eventuality and make it easier for you to admit mistakes:

- Reporting slip-ups
  - How would you tell your partner if you broke the agreement?
  - How would you respond if your partner told you he had done something which broke the agreement?
  - How would you tell your partner if a condom broke while you were having sex with someone else?
- Changing the agreement in the future
  - Relationships change over time, so it's realistic to expect that you will need to consider changing your agreement in the future. If you agree to do that together when the time comes, you're less likely to break the first agreement or to feel your trust has been betrayed. Setting a time at some point in the future to review your agreement is a good way to make sure it remains a workable agreement. Do you agree?

And to sum up your discussions, write two statements, the first beginning: If we have any slip-ups we will. . . and the second beginning: We will review our agreement...

Safer Barebacking Procedures

Developed by
GMFA (Gay Men Fighting AIDS), London, U.K.
©2003 GMFA
http://www.metromate.org.uk/
(Reproduced with permission.)

Most gay men fuck without a condom at some point in their lives.

If you fuck without a condom, there are still ways you can reduce the chance of HIV being spread. These vary depending on your HIV status.

The more times you fuck without using a condom, and the more men you fuck with, the greater the chances you will infect someone with HIV or that he'll infect you.

NEGATIVE

If you are HIV-negative and have sex without a condom, there is less chance of getting HIV if:

- You do the fucking rather than getting fucked.
- You don't let your partner come inside you if he does the fucking.

• You use plenty of lube.
• You have regular tests for other sexually transmitted infections.

UNTESTED

If you don't know your HIV status, and you have sex without a condom, you don't know if it's you or your partner who risks catching HIV.

If you fuck without a condom, there is less chance of HIV being spread if:

• You don't cum inside him or let him cum inside you.
• You use plenty of lube.
• You have regular tests for other sexually transmitted infections.

POSITIVE

If you are HIV-positive and have sex without a condom, there is less chance of passing on HIV if:

• You get fucked by him.
• You don't come inside him if you fuck him.
• You use plenty of lube.
• You have a low viral load.
• You have regular tests for other sexually transmitted infections.

CARRY ON SCREENING

It is possible to have HIV without knowing it. In the same way, there are other sexually transmitted infections (STIs) that you may not know you have. Fortunately most STIs can be treated so long as they are detected soon enough. How often you get checked out probably depends on how many men you have sex with and the kind of sex that you have. An STI checkup every 6 months is enough for most gay men.

Sexually transmitted infections (such as syphilis, NSU [nonspecific urethritis], gonorrhea, herpes, and hepatitis) make HIV-positive men more infectious and HIV-negative men more vulnerable to infection.

COME OUTSIDE

If you do not use a condom for fucking the risk of HIV being transmitted is less if you pull out before you cum. There is less chance of HIV being transmitted if he pulls out and cums over your back, chest, or face. However, withdrawing before cumming is safer, it is not safe as pre-cum may contain HIV. Some men choose to withdraw before cumming even when they use condoms in case of condom failure. Withdrawing before cumming makes little difference to the chances of catching other sexually transmitted infections (such as syphilis, NSU, gonorrhea, herpes, and hepatitis). These STIs make HIV-positive men more infectious and HIV-negative men more vulnerable to infection.

VIRAL LOAD RANGE

Viral load is the term used to describe the amount of HIV a person has in their blood. People who have been diagnosed as having HIV will be encouraged to have their blood tested regularly. Looking at viral load and CD4 (T-helper cells) in the blood helps doctors monitor an individual's progress, for example to see if the drugs are working for him. Modern anti-HIV drug therapies mean that many people with HIV have a very low, or even undetectable, viral load. Most doctors believe that viral load has a large impact on how infectious a person is. A person with a low viral load will be less likely to transmit HIV. It is very difficult to know exactly what your viral load is. Viral load tests usually take more than a week to process, so by the time you get your result the information is already out of date. Viral load can alter dramatically in a short period of time, especially if you pick up any other infections, including the flu. Sexually transmitted infections (such as syphilis, NSU, gonorrhea, herpes, and hepatitis) can make your viral load shoot up. The viral load level in your blood is probably not the same as it is in your semen. In some men viral load is usually higher in the blood than in the semen, but in other men it is higher in the semen than in the blood. Tests at an HIV clinic are usually only on the viral load in your blood.

TO FUCK OR BE FUCKED

Gay men are more likely to catch HIV from being fucked (being bottom) than from fucking (being top).

Men who do not have HIV have less chance of becoming infected if they do the fucking (are top).

If you have HIV, there is less chance of you passing it on to your partner if he fucks you. If you are both HIV+, and you fuck without condoms, you both risk picking up a drug-resistant strain of HIV, which may limit your treatment options. Using plenty of water-based lube means that there is less chance of damage to your cock or arsehole, which makes it safer for both of you.

Whoever is doing the fucking, it makes little difference to the chances of catching other sexually transmitted infections (such as syphilis, NSU, gonorrhea, herpes, and hepatitis). These STIs make HIV-positive men more infectious and HIV-negative men more vulnerable to infection.

TOYS FOR BOYS

Here are some things you can shove up your arse (other than a cock):

- Vegetables (e.g., carrots, courgettes, even cucumbers if you like).
- Sex toys like dildos and butt plugs (these come in all shapes and sizes).
- Fingers and hands (just because it's called fisting doesn't mean it has to be a fist).

Lots of the things that men have shoved up their arse can damage the arse lining. This means that infections, such as HIV, are more likely to be transmitted. The lining of the arse is very delicate and can be damaged easily, even if there are no signs of bleeding. Fucking someone who has just been fisted or had sex toys shoved up his arse makes it more likely that HIV will be passed on.

When you fuck, fist, or use sex toys, it is best to use plenty of lube. This reduces the damage to the arse which makes it safer for both of you. If you like long arse sessions you should reapply the lube about every 20 minutes. Water-based lubes, especially, tend to dry out after 20 minutes of hard grinding.

WET AND WILD

Whether or not you use condoms, using plenty of lube makes it less likely that HIV will be transmitted. Lots of lube when you fuck means that there is less chance of damage to your cock or arsehole, which makes it safer for both of you.

The amount of lube you use is more important than the thickness of the condom. A kitemark-approved standard condom should be fine for anal sex so long as you use plenty of water-based lube (such as KY or any lube that you find with free condom packs). Oil-based lubes (such as baby oil, massage oil, or any moisturizer) have a damaging effect on condoms and can cause them to fail.

Both the cock and arse should be well lubed before you fuck. If you lube your cock before you put a condom on there is more chance that the condom will slip off when you're fucking.

If you like long fuck sessions you should reapply the lube about every 20 minutes. Water-based lubes, especially, tend to dry out after 20 minutes of hard pounding.

Squashing the "Super-Bug": An Open Letter to Gay and Bisexual Men

The Institute for Gay Men's Health
A collaboration of GMHC www.gmhc.org (1-800-243-7692) &
APLA www.apla.org (213-201-1600)
(Reproduced with permission.)

FEBRUARY 2005

In the United States, recent media attention about a multi-drug resistant HIV (the "super-bug") couldn't come at a worse time — when HIV prevention efforts are both increasingly censored and underfunded. Unfortunately, many public health officials are currently relying on a one-size-fits-all approach to preventing further transmission of HIV. Abstinence is promoted over more comprehensive sex education approaches that address contextual as well as individual-level factors. There is plenty of research showing the strong link between important contextual factors — HIV/AIDS stigma, homophobia, class, racism, community cohesion, depression, substance use, etc. — and individual-level HIV risk.

FACTS:

HIV infections with drug resistance (and even multi-class drug-resistant HIV) are not a new phenomenon. In the U.S. and in Europe 8–20% of all new infections are one-class drug resistant, and 1–4% are multi-drug resistant (it is higher in men who have sex with men).

It's well established in large studies that although "average" time of progression to AIDS after initial infection is 10–12 years, there are many cases where people progressed rapidly (within 2 years). Without additional case validation, it is impossible to scientifically conclude that increased viral virulence, and not host immune factors or some combination of the two, is responsible for rapid progression.

Three conditions must be met before there is serious cause for alarm: multiple cases have to be shown to be virologically related; rapid progression must be linked to the virus itself and not host genetics or weakened immune system (i.e., due to drug use); and the virus must be readily transmitted.

REFLECTION:

Fear campaigns launched on the backs of gay men are not new in the 24-year history of the HIV/AIDS epidemic. What remains crucial is that we retain control over our bodies and health during these times. Men who have sex with men, gay-identified or not, must be supported in our efforts to live satisfying and healthy sex lives, which must include consistent employment of effective safer sex and risk-reduction strategies. We must work to reinforce as social norms in our community both sex with the minimal exchange of bodily fluids and condom use whenever possible.

For those of us living with HIV, it is vital that we have access to and adhere to treatment. For those of us who are HIV-negative, routine STI and HIV screening must be a part of our regular health care regimen.

Sex while under the influence of any substance greatly increases the chance of HIV transmission because a person's ability to negotiate safer sex may be impaired. We must support efforts by men to minimize or eliminate their use of alcohol and/or drugs especially before and during sex. Treatment of addictions must be viewed as integral to our STD and HIV prevention efforts.

DIALOGUE:

Dialogue is also critical during these times. Whether over a dinner table with friends and family or in bed with a boyfriend or trick, we must have the difficult conversations about why we should matter to ourselves, each other, and the world. Here are some questions to get the discussion going:

- Why should gay men matter to each other?
- How do we extend consideration and concern to other men with whom we have sex?
- How do we feel about our bodies as gay men and how do those feelings influence the decisions we make about the sex we have or the drugs we use?
- What motivates some gay men's abuse of crystal?
- Is self-policing a viable strategy for gay men?
- What will self-policing really mean inside of gay communities that are already highly divided by race, class, and serostatus?
- How can we promote a progressive gay men's health agenda in a socially and politically conservative environment?
- How can we respond to questions about complacency among gay men?
- What are the long-term psychological and social consequences of prolonged periods of HIV vigilance?
- Where is the outrage over depictions of gay men as the embodiment of terror as government officials and some elements of the mainstream media continue to portray us, especially those of us living with HIV as walking time bombs ready to explode HIV all over the concerned public?

ACTION:

There has never been room for complacency or resignation in our fight to end the HIV/AIDS epidemic. We must remain deliberate in our organizing efforts. Here are some organizing principles to be mindful about as we ready ourselves for the continued work which lies ahead:

- Understand and reject HIV/AIDS stigma. Stigma can serve as the basis for discrimination. Its sole function is to exclude. Exclusion will not work as an STD/HIV prevention strategy.
- Insist that every sex act be an expression of consideration as well as desire.
- Resist urges to police other men, but instead surprise your friends, lovers, sex partners, family members, and acquaintances with conversations about sex, love, crystal use, relationships, homophobia, HIV/AIDS, racism, work, art, and the million other things that matter to you.
- Request participatory, open-ended, and community-level interventions aimed at signaling to all gay men that we matter — to each other and to the world. These can range from pot-luck dinners to 12-step programs; from story-telling circles to interactive Internet-based programs; from personal art projects to large-scale home-grown social marketing campaigns; from reading groups to community forums.
- Demand gay-sensitive, culturally relevant mental health programs, addiction services, and treatment strategies for men who have sex with men.
- Establish alliances that are unexpected and that break from HIV/AIDS industry convention (civil rights groups, anti-hate crime advocates, art organizations, antipoverty coalitions, etc.) as a strategy for addressing the contextual factors underlying heightened risk for STD and HIV.
- Work to end homophobia, racism, sexism, HIV/AIDS stigma, transphobia, and poverty as part of a broader health and wellness agenda for men who have sex with men.

Sadly, there is no cure for AIDS. Nor is there a magic bullet to prevent the transmission of HIV. If nothing else, the media attention about multi-drug resistant HIV reminds us about the seriousness of HIV/AIDS disease. We must move past the trivialization of HIV, because living with AIDS is neither glamorous nor easy. Now more than ever, we must reaffirm with dignity the many expressions of love and pride we extend to ourselves and to each other. We must continue to advocate for comprehensive and creative prevention approaches that are multi-pronged and sustained over time. In the current challenging political and fiscal environment, this will require our collective, unrelenting, and steady resolve.

Endnotes

CHAPTER ONE

1. Homophobia has been defined in a variety of ways. The term was first coined by Dr. George Weinberg (1983) and initially referred to the irrational dread and loathing of homosexuals and homosexuality. Others have made the analogy between homophobia and racism or sexism with an emphasis on negative attitudes of all kinds (Weinberger & Millham, 1979). Internalized homophobia represents an internalization of negative attitudes and assumptions concerning being homosexual by gay and lesbian individuals themselves (Herek, 1998).

2. The ambiguity about what constitutes "safer sex" is ongoing. For example, there is continued confusion in the gay community about precisely how risky oral sex is with regard to the spread of HIV (Vittinghoff et al., 1999). The article by Vittinghoff and colleagues provides scientific documentation of a few cases where gay men contracted HIV through oral sex but that this is not an easy method for transmitting the virus.

3. Mansergh et al. (2000) found that simply knowing a person or people with HIV or AIDS did not affect whether or not people had unprotected anal intercourse (UAI). But greater emotional closeness to an HIV-positive person without AIDS was associated with reduced UAI among participants in this study. An important area of research would be to determine whether or not this still holds true for gay men in the third decade of the AIDS epidemic.

4. The introduction of a second class of drugs that acted directly upon the human immunodeficiency virus (HIV) itself ushered in an era of combination therapies (also known as HAART) to treat HIV and AIDS. This had

a revolutionary impact upon the health and medical care of people with HIV and AIDS. Many seriously ill people with HIV disease experienced a serious and dramatic improvement in their health from being treated with the new drugs. Large numbers of individuals who had been approaching or were near death were able to regain their health and vitality due to these new treatments.

5. The term "bottom" refers to the man who is the receptive partner in anal intercourse, and a "top" refers to the man who is the insertive partner.

6. This article describes findings from the Seropositive Urban Men's Study (SUMS), which had 456 participants, and the Seropositive Urban Men's Intervention Trial (SUMIT), which had 1168 participants. The studies were conducted from 1996 to 2002 (Wolitski et al., 2004).

7. Twenty-seven percent of the SUMIT participants identified as barebackers, and 57 percent of these men did not limit bareback sex to seroconcordant partners (Wolitski et al., 2004).

CHAPTER TWO

1. The names and identifying information of all individuals, have been changed to respect their anonymity.

2. Introjection can be defined as the process of taking on another person's ideas, opinions, values, or even information, without either fully understanding it or otherwise making it our own.

CHAPTER THREE

1. Negotiated safety is an agreement between two gay men in a relationship to go through the process of getting ready to stop using condoms when they have anal sex. The basis is an explicit understanding that both know each other's HIV status and are both uninfected. The only time they do not use condoms is when they have sex with each other. This risk reduction strategy was first reported among gay men in Sydney, Australia (Kippax et al., 1993), and will be discussed in depth in Chapter 6.

2. An Axis II psychiatric diagnosis is where the presence of personality disorders or mental retardation is indicated.

3. HIV "superinfection" is defined as a second infection with HIV after a primary infection has been established. This is distinct from "coinfection," which is defined as the simultaneous transmission of two or more subtypes of HIV (Blackard et al., 2002).

CHAPTER FOUR

1. To address the reality that not everyone wants to or can stop using drugs, a new approach was developed that has become known as the harm reduction approach. Harm reduction is a philosophy and a set of practical and effective strategies originally designed to help drug users reduce the potential risks of using drugs when they have no desire for abstention. Harm reduction differs from an abstinence-based approach in that it is not judgmental about the individual's use of substances. It will be described in more detail later in this chapter.

2. For professionals who seek resources about working with sexual minority clients who have problems with substance abuse, two of the best books are: *Addictions in the Gay and Lesbian Community*, edited by J. Guss and J. Drescher, 2000, published by Haworth Press, and *Counseling Lesbian, Gay, Bisexual and Transgender Substance Abusers: Dual Identities*, by D. Finnegan and E. McNally, 2002, Haworth Press. The National Association of Lesbian and Gay Addictions Professionals has a Web site (www.nalgap.org) that has links to resources both for professionals seeking readings, conferences, and training and for individuals seeking gay-friendly recovery facilities and professionals.

3. Sixty-four percent of the 456 men in this study had drunk alcohol at some point in the 3 months prior to the study. Of the men who drank alcohol, 80 percent drank before or during sex. Fifty-five percent of the men who used alcohol before or during sex used it "frequently," as defined as more than three times a week (Purcell et al., 2001).

4. In this study of 202 gay and bisexual men to assess the extent of noninjection drug use, more than half of their sample reported using more than one drug in the 3 months prior to this study, and one third reported the use of three or more drugs. Of the 172 participants who reported using some drugs during the past 3 months, more than 140 reported having UAI while under the influence of alcohol and inhalants (Halkitis & Parsons, 2002)

5. In this study of 463 men in San Francisco and New York, 367 reported sex with nonprimary partners; slightly more than half had UAI with the nonprimary partner (Parsons et al., 2003).

6. This study was of 258,567 men and women who were surveyed at HIV counseling and testing sites. More than 32,000 were gay or bisexual men and more than 2200 of the gay and bisexual men reported using methamphetamine. Of the men who used crystal, more than 80 percent reported having anal intercourse, and 60 percent said that they did not use condoms. Almost 12 percent of the gay men and almost 7 percent of the bisexual men whose UAI was linked to crystal use were HIV-positive (Molitor et al., 1998).

7. These researchers define "extreme" sexual behaviors as fisting, which refers to the practice of inserting a hand or arm into the anus or vagina.

8. Halkitis et al. define hypersexuality as an excessive interest or involvement in sexual behavior, which has also been characterized as sexual compulsivity (in press, a).

9. This summary of the stages of change is based on work by Edith Springer (2004).

CHAPTER FIVE

1. Cooper and Griffin-Shelley (2002) defined "online sexual activity (OSA) as use of the Internet for any activity (including text, audio, graphic files) that involves sexuality, whether for purposes of recreation, entertainment, exploration, support, education, commerce, or efforts to attain and secure sexual or romantic partners. Cyber sex is a subcategory of OSA and can be defined as using the medium of the Internet to engage in sexually gratifying activities, such as looking at pictures or videos, engaging in sexual chat, exchanging explicit sexual images or e-mails, and 'cybering' (i.e., sharing fantasies over the Internet that involve being sexual together while one or both people masturbate" (p. 3).

2. In this study, of the 832 individuals who reported having met a sexual partner on the Internet in the past 12 months, 335 (40.3 percent) reported having used a condom during their last sexual encounter (McFarlane et al., 2000).

3. "Bug chaser" is a term used to describe an HIV-negative man who is actively seeking to become infected with HIV by having unprotected sex. Other terms for this are "bug seeker" and "gift chaser." "Bug giver," "gift giver," or "bug breeder" are all terms that refer to an HIV-positive man who is willing to knowingly infect an HIV-negative man.

4. Tewksbury examined self-reported HIV status and the desired HIV status of potential partners (e.g., HIV-negative, HIV-positive, or no preference). His results indicated that 37 of the 139 HIV-positive men (almost 27 percent) stated in their profiles that they only wanted to bareback with other positive men, and only 2 (1.4 percent) stated that they were actively seeking uninfected men to bareback with. Of the 505 men who labeled themselves HIV-negative, only three (0.6 percent) had profiles stating that they were looking to bareback only with HIV-positive men, while 414 (82 percent) stated that they would only bareback with other uninfected men. Of the 71 men who either did not know their HIV status or refused to disclose it, 15 (21.1 percent) stated that they sought to bareback only with HIV-negative men (Tewksbury, 2003).

5. In Grov's sample of 81 men, 74 percent were seeking to be infected with HIV. Of these, 53 percent identified as HIV-negative, 17 percent reported not

knowing their HIV status, and 5.1 percent did not disclose their HIV status (Grov, 2004).

6. The results of my nonscientific sample from one of the bareback Web sites are as follows: Of the eight men who did not know their HIV status, six were willing to give semen anally and five were willing to receive it, obviously indicating a willingness to place themselves at risk for becoming infected or possibly infecting another person. The HIV-positive men who only wanted other infected partners were all willing to give or receive semen anally, thus indicating a willingness to risk the possibility of superinfection with a multidrug resistant strain of HIV. Fewer of the positive men who did not specify the HIV status of their partners or who said it did not matter were willing to give semen, but all were willing to receive it. Twelve of the 15 uninfected men who wanted or preferred another uninfected man as a partner were willing to give semen anally, and 14 of them were willing to receive it, thus again using serosorting as a means of trying to prevent themselves from becoming infected. The two uninfected men who stated a preference for an HIV-positive partner did not specify whether they were willing to give or receive semen anally, which can be interpreted as their being open to the possibility of becoming infected. Of the two uninfected men who did not specify a preference regarding HIV status of their partners, one was willing to give semen and neither indicated a willingness to receive it, indicating that they were not seeking to become infected with HIV. Of the three uninfected men who stated that the HIV status of their partner did not matter, two were willing to give semen anally and one was not, yet all three stated that they were willing to receive semen anally, thus suggesting that they were willing to intentionally place themselves at risk for becoming infected. None of the 16 men who did not specify their own HIV status or that of their partner specified whether or not they were willing to give or receive semen anally. This group is clearly the most ambiguous with regard to whether they are seeking to, or willing to, become infected or infect another person.

7. Blood samples I gave as part of the New York Blood Center's Hepatitis B study in 1977 were frozen, and after the development of the HIV test, were tested for HIV antibodies.

CHAPTER SIX

1. Hunt and colleagues (1992) found that among men they interviewed in 10 cities in England, UAI was nearly five times as common among men in ongoing relationships than among men with casual sexual partners. Similarly, McLean et al. (1994) found that 71 percent of the men they interviewed in the United Kingdom reported that their most recent incidence of UAI had been with a regular partner. In a survey of more than 2000 Danish gay men,

Schmidt et al. (1992) found that having a steady partner was the strongest predictor of men who have anal sex without condoms.

2. In this study, Elford and colleagues (1999) found that of the 140 men who reported only having UAI with their main partner, 62 (44 percent) did not know their own HIV status or that of their partner.

3. Of 4240 heterosexual couples whom Blumstein and Schwartz (1983) studied who were either married or living together, 26 percent of husbands and 21 percent of wives, and 33 percent of men living with a woman (unmarried couples) and 30 percent of women living with a man, reported not being monogamous.

4. A long-term study in Australia looked at 537 men who were in relationships from 1986 to 1991. When surveyed in 1986 to 1987, 80 percent were nonmonogamous. When surveyed again in 1991, 75 percent were sexually nonexclusive (Kippax et al., 1993).

5. In this study, Elford and colleagues (1999) found that of the 140 men who reported only having UAI with their main partner, 62 (44 percent) did not know their own HIV status or that of their partner.

6. "I have been in this field (sex research) for 30 years, and the level of fear and intimidation is higher now than I ever remember," said Dr. Gilbert Herdt, a researcher at San Francisco State University who runs the National Sexuality Resource Center, which is a clearinghouse for sexual information. "With the recent election, there's concern that there will be even more intrusion of ideology into science" (quoted in Carey, 2004). With the reality of increasing rates of sexually transmitted diseases including HIV, and teen pregnancies in the United States, the right-wing intrusion of ideology and conservative religious beliefs into science can have serious public health consequences that will prove expensive, and even deadly, to our society in general and to gay men in particular, though obviously women and all other sexual minorities are also negatively impacted by the current political climate.

7. In the 6 months prior to the interview, of the 181 men in relationships where both they and their partners were HIV-negative, 62 percent had engaged in UAI with their steady partner. Ninety-one percent (165) of these same men had not engaged in UAI outside their relationship. Of these 165 men, 82 percent had negotiated agreements about sex outside their relationship (Kippax et al., 1997).

8. A study conducted in Amsterdam surveyed 435 gay men under the age of 30. Of those, 285 reported having a steady partner in the 6 months prior to the beginning of the study, and 113 of the men who had a steady partner had engaged in UAI with their steady partner. Yet only 37 of those 113 men who had UAI with their steady partner reported being in an HIV-negative concordant relationship, and 35 of these 37 (95 percent) had a negotiated safety agreement. Twenty-one of the men who practiced negotiated safety agreed to

be sexually exclusive, and 14 allowed sex outside the relationship as long as condoms were always used during anal sex. These authors noted that at the time of their study, the term "negotiated safety" was fairly unknown outside social science circles and therefore the term was never used when asking men about their sexual behaviors (Davidovich et al., 2000).

9. Researchers have wondered whether age is a factor in how, why, and whether male couples negotiate unprotected or unsafe sex agreements. A study of young gay men aged 18 to 24 from three medium-sized cities on the West Coast of the United States, conducted in 1991, found that several characteristics of a couple's relationship — living together, greater length of time together, greater frequency of seeing each other, a higher amount of arguing, and being monogamous — predicted which couples engaged in UAI. These relationship traits were consistent, whether the couples were seroconcordant or serodiscordant (Hays et al., 1997). The authors suggest that these findings seemed to reflect relationships that were more intense or involved. Additionally, these researchers found that poor sexual communication skills, misperceptions about safer sex, and greater interpersonal barriers also contributed to why these men did not use condoms with their primary partners. They also suggest that "engaging in unprotected sex, for many couples, cannot be considered a rational decision, but rather one that is influenced by a variety of emotional and situational factors, such as enjoyment of unprotected sex, living together, and frequency of sex" (Hays et al., p. 327).

CHAPTER SEVEN

1. HIV "superinfection" is defined as a second infection with HIV after a primary infection has been established. This is distinct from "coinfection," which is defined as the simultaneous transmission of two or more subtypes of HIV (Blackard, Cohen, & Mayer, 2002).

2. In this study 91 HIV-positive men who were in a primary partner relationship with another man who was also HIV-positive were investigated, and 62 percent were found to have had unprotected sex with their partners because they did not believe that there was a significant risk of reinfection with a drug-resistant strain of HIV (Halkitis et al., 2004).

3. This study of 33 HIV-positive couples was conducted by the Gladstone Institute of Virology and Immunology in San Francisco; partners in 28 of the couples were infected with a strain of HIV that was genetically different from his or her partner's. Among those who engaged in frequent unprotected vaginal or anal sex with each other, no evidence of superinfection was found. In this study, in 28 of the 33 couples, each participant was infected with a strain of HIV-1B that was genetically different from that of the person's partner.

(HIV-1 is the particular strain of the virus that the vast majority of people in the developed countries are infected with.) (Gross, Porco, & Grant, 2004; Yerly et al., 2004).

4. The findings were presented at the XV International AIDS Conference in Bangkok on July 15, 2004 (Grant et al., 2004). They call into question the widely held perception that people with HIV-1 are highly susceptible to additional infection by other strains of HIV-1 that may be drug resistant or more virulent. This study is known as the "Positive Partners Study"; it began in 2001 and will eventually involve up to 200 HIV-1–infected couples. It is designed to investigate the incidence of superinfection in the HIV-positive population (Gross et al., 2004). The bottom line is that the issue of whether or not reinfection with an additional subtype of HIV-1 is possible is still uncertain, and if possible the frequency of HIV-1 superinfection is unknown (Yerly et al., 2004).

5. This study questioned 46 long-term male mixed antibody status couples (Appleby et al., 1999).

6. This study was of 10 serodiscordant sexually nonexclusive male couple relationships (Palmer & Bor, 2001).

CHAPTER EIGHT

1. So far, there is a small body of research literature that reports on using MET as an effective intervention to promote HIV risk reduction (Baker, Heather, Wodak, Dixon, & Holt, 1993; Baker, Kochan, Dixon, Heather, & Wodak, 1994; Catania, Kegeles, & Coates, 1990), and only one deals specifically with men who have sex with men (MSM). Picciano et al. (2001) showed that a telephone counseling–based motivational enhancement approach in Seattle helped white, black, and Latino MSM reduce their sexual risk-taking. Three studies also demonstrated that using MET was effective in helping low-income urban black women reduce their sexual risk (Carey et al., 1997; Belcher et al., 1998; Carey et al., 2000). The two published studies that discuss using motivational enhancement therapy with people on methadone maintenance or who were not in treatment for their injection drug use did not demonstrate that this modality was effective for helping this population reduce their sexual risk-taking behavior.

2. This study was conducted from July 2001 until December 2003 of 119 men in serodiscordant relationships of at least 6 months duration. Forty-five of the men were HIV-negative and 74 were HIV-positive. This study found that most of the serodiscordant couples did not have any UAI, but when it did happen, it was significantly more likely to occur when the HIV-positive partner had undetectable viral loads (Van de Ven et al., 2005).

3. This article is based on the Seropositive Urban Men's Study (SUMS), which had 456 participants (Remien, et al., 2005).

4. This document is available online at www.cdc.gov/mmwr/PDF/RR/RR5212.pdf.

CHAPTER NINE

1. This article summarizes findings from two studies conducted of HIV-positive men in San Francisco and New York City from 1996 to 2002. There were 456 participants in the Seropositive Urban Men's Study (SUMS) and 1168 participants in the Seropositive Urban Men's Intervention Trial (SUMIT). Sixty-three percent of the men interviewed expressed that the responsibility rested on them to ensure that their partners did not become infected. Only 24 percent felt that it was their partner's responsibility to ensure that he did not become infected, and 12 percent felt it was a shared responsibility to prevent HIV transmission (Wolitski, Parsons, & Gomez, 2004).

References

Acosta, D. (2004). *The power of collaboration: Internet outreach to MSM in Philadelphia.* Presentation at the Harm Reduction Coalition, NYC, October 15, 2004.

Adelson, S. (2005, February 28). A gay cruising site defends itself: The manager of Manhunt.net on the HIV superstrain, unsafe sex, crystal meth, and corporate and personal responsibility. *New York Magazine, 12.*

AIDS Action Committee. (1995). Oral sex is safer sex [poster campaign], Boston, MA.

Ajzen, I., & Madden, T. (1986). Prediction of goal-directed behaviour: Attitudes, intentions, and perceived behavioural control. *Journal of Experimental Social Psychology, 22,* 453–474.

Ajzen, I. (1991). The theory of planned behaviour: Some unresolved issues. *Organisational Behaviour and Human Decision Processes, 50,* 179–211.

American Psychiatric Association. (1994). *Quick reference to the diagnostic criteria from DSM-IV.* Washington, DC: American Psychiatric Association, 299.

American Psychiatric Association. (1998). Position statement on psychiatric treatment and sexual orientation. Retrieved from www.psych.org/news_stand/rep_therapy.cfm.

American Psychiatric Association. (2000). *COPP position statement on therapies focused on attempts to change sexual orientation (reparative or conversion therapies).* Retrieved from www.psych.org/psych/htdocs/practofpsych/copptherapyaddendum83100.html.

Ames, L., Atchinson, A., & Rose, D. (1995). Love, lust and fear: Safer sex decision making among gay men. *Journal of Homosexuality, 30,* 53–73.

Amirkhanian, Y. A., Kelly, J. A., Kukharsky, A. A., Borodkina, O. I., Granskaya, J. V., Dyatlov, R.V., McAuliffe, T.L., & Kozlov, A.P. (2001). Predictors of HIV risk behavior among Russian men who have sex with men: An emerging epidemic. *AIDS, 15,* 407–412.

Anapol, D. (1997). *Polyamory: The new love without limits.* San Rafael, CA: Internet Resource Center.

Appleby, P. R., Miller, L. C., & Rothspan, S. (1999). The paradox of trust for male couples: When risking is a part of loving. *Personal Relationships, 6,* 81–93.

Aspinwall, L., Kemeny, M., Taylor, S, Schneider, S. & Dudley, J. (1991). Psychosocial predictors of gay men's AIDS risk-reduction behavior. *Health Psychology, 10,* 432–444

Avery, A.M., Hellman, R.E., & Sudderth, L.K. (2001). HIV and sexually transmitted infection risk behaviors among men seeking sex with men online. *American Journal of Public Health, 91,* 988–991.

Baker, A., Heather, N., Wodak, A., Dixon, J., & Holt, P. (1993). Evaluation of a cognitive–behavioural intervention for HIV prevention among injecting drug users. *AIDS, 7,* 247–256.

Baker, A., Kochan, N., Dixon, J., Heather, N., & Wodak, A. (1994). Controlled evaluation of a brief intervention for HIV prevention among injecting drug users not in treatment. *AIDS Care, 6,* 559–570.

Ball, S. (1998). A time limited group model for HIV-negative gay men. In S. Ball (Ed.), *The HIV-negative gay man: Developing strategies for survival and emotional well-being.* Binghamton, NY: Haworth Press, 23–42.

Bancroft, J. (2002). Preface. In A. Cooper (Ed.). *Sex and the Internet: A guide for clinicians.* New York: Brunner-Routledge, ix–xii.

Bancroft, J., Janssen, E., Strong, D., Carnes, L., Vukadinovic, Z., & Long, J.S. (2003). Sexual risk-taking in gay men: The relevance of sexual arousability, mood, and sensation seeking. *Archives of Sexual Behavior, 32,* 555–572.

Barebackjack.com. (2004a). http://www.barebackjack.com/preview.html.

Barebackjack.com. (2004b). http://www.barebackjack.com/members/fuckbuds. html.

Barebackjack.com. (2004c). http://www.barebackjack.com/health.html.

Barros, P., Schechter, M., Gupta, P., Melo, M., Vieira, M., Murta, F., Souza, Y., & Harrison, L. (2000). Effect of antiretroviral therapy on HIV shedding in semen. *Annals of Internal Medicine, 133,* 280–284.

Bartolomeo, N. (1990, April 6). Study: One in five gay men sometimes slip into unsafe sex. *The Washington Blade, 21,* 6.

Bateson, G. (1972). *Steps to an ecology of mind.* New York: Ballantine Books.

Bauman, L. J., & Siegel, K. (1987). Misperceptions among gay men of the risk for AIDS associated with their sexual behavior. *Journal of Applied Social Psychology, 17,* 329–350.

Beachy, S. (April 17, 1994). 20+, HIV+. *New York Times Magazine,* 52–53.

Becker, M. (1984). The health belief model and personal health behaviour. *Health Education Monographs, 2,* 324–508.

Belcher, L., Kalichman, S., Topping, M., Smith, S., Emshoff, J., Norris, F., & Nurss, J. (1998). A randomized trial of a brief HIV risk reduction counseling intervention for women. *Journal of Consulting and Clinical Psychology, 66,* 856–861.

Bell, A. P. (1972). Human sexuality — a response. *International Journal of Psychiatry, 10,* 99–102.

Bell, A. P., & Weinberg, M.M. (1978). *Homosexualities: A study of diversity among men and women.* New York: Simon & Schuster.

Bell, A.P., Weinberg, M., & Hammersmith, S. (1981). *Sexual preference: Its development in men & women.* Bloomington, IN: Indiana University Press.

Benotsch, E., Kalichman, S., & Cage, M. (2002). Men who have met sex partners via the Internet: Prevalence, predictors and implications for HIV prevention. *Archives of Sexual Behavior, 31,* 177–183.

Bettinger, M. (2005). Polyamory and gay men: A family systems approach. *Journal of GLBT Family Studies: Innovations in Theory, Research and Practice, 1,* 97–116.

Blackard, J. T., Cohen, D. E., & Mayer, K. H. (2002). Human immunodeficiency virus superinfection and recombination: Current state of knowledge and potential clinical consequences. *Clinical Infectious Diseases, 34,* 1108–1114.

Blasband, D., & Peplau, L. (1985). Sexual exclusivity versus openness in gay male couples. *Archives of Sexual Behavior, 14,* 395–412.

Blechner, M.J. (2002). Intimacy, pleasure, risk and safety: Commentary on Cheuvront's "High-risk sexual behavior in the treatment of HIV-negative patients." *Journal of Gay and Lesbian Psychotherapy, 6,* 27–34.

Blumstein, P., & Schwartz, P. (1983). *American couples: money, work & sex.* New York: William Morrow.

Bochow, M. (2000). The response of gay German men to HIV: The national gay press surveys, 1987–96. In R. Rosenbrock & M. Wright (Eds.), *Partnership and pragmatism. Germany's response to AIDS prevention and care.* London: Routledge.

Boden, D., Hurley, A., Zhang, C. Y., Jones, E., Tsay, J., Farthing, C., et al. (1999). HIV-1 drug resistence in newly infected individuals. *JAMA, 282,* 135–141.

Bolton, R., Vincke, J., Mak, R., & Dennehy, E. (1992). Alcohol and risky sex: In search of an elusive connection. *Medical Anthropology, 14,* 323–363.

Bonnel, C., Weatherburn, P., & Hickson, F. (2000). Sexually transmitted infection as a risk factor for homosexual HIV transmission: A systemic review of epidemiological studies. *International Journal of STD and AIDS, 11,* 697–700.

Boulton, M., McLean, J., Fitzpatrick, R., & Hart, G. (1995). Gay men's accounts for unsafe sex. *AIDS Care, 7,* 619–630.

Brehm, S. (1985) *Intimate relationships.* New York: Random House.

Bringle, R. (1995). Sexual jealousy in the relationships of homosexual and heterosexual men: 1980 and 1995. *Personal Relationships, 2,* 313–325.

Bronski, M. (2004) Foreword. *Beyond shame: Reclaiming the abandoned history of radical sexuality.* Boston: Beacon Press.

Bryant, A.S., & Demian. (1994). Relationship characteristics of American gays and lesbians: Findings from a national survey. *Journal of Gay & Lesbian Social Services, 1,* 101–117.

Buchanan, D., Poppen, P., & Reisen, C. (1996). The nature of partner relationship and AIDS sexual risk taking in gay men. *Psychological Health, 11,* 541–555.

Bull, S., Reitmeijer, C., & Piper, P. (2001). Synergistic risk for HIV: The complexity of behavior among men who have sex with men and also inject drugs. *Journal of Homosexuality, 42,* 29–49.

Cabaj, R. P. (1992). Substance abuse in the gay and lesbian community. In J. Lowenson, P. Ruiz, & R. Millman (Eds.), *Substance abuse: A comprehensive textbook* (2nd ed.). Baltimore, MD: Williams & Wilkins, 852–860.

Caldwell, J. (2003, February 28). Chasing the bug chasers: Community leaders reflect on the controversial *Rolling Stone* article about gay men seeking HIV infection. *Frontiers Newsmagazine.* Retrieved from http://www.aidshealth.org/newsroom/news/news_archive/N022703d.htm.

Califia, P. (1983). *Sapphistry: The book of lesbian sexuality.* San Francisco: Naiad Press.

Callen, M. (1990). *Surviving AIDS.* New York: HarperCollins.

Canin, L., Dolcini, M. M., & Adler, N. E. (1999). Barriers to and facilitators of HIV-STD behavior change: Intrapersonal and relationship based factors. *Review of General Psychology, 3,* 338–371.

Carballo-Dieguez, A., & Dolezal, C. (1996). HIV risk behaviors and obstacles to condom use among Puerto Rican men in New York City who have sex with men. *American Journal of Public Health, 86,* 1619–1622.

Carballo-Dieguez, A. (2001). HIV, barebacking, and gay men's sexuality, circa 2001. *Journal of Sex Education and Therapy, 26,* 225–233.

Carballo-Dieguez, A., & Lin, P. (2003, October 10). Barebacking and the Internet: HIV Prevention failure or new opportunity. Panel presentation. *Barebacking: Research and Clinical Issues.* Forum held at the Lesbian, Gay, Bisexual, Transgendered Community Services Center, New York, NY.

Carballo-Dieguez, A., & Bauermeister, J. (2004). "Barebacking": Intentional condomless anal sex in HIV risk contexts. Reasons for and against it. *Journal of Homosexuality, 1,* 1–16.

Carey, M., Maisto, S., Kalichman, S., Forsyth, A., Wright, E., & Johnson, B. (1997). Enhancing motivation to reduce the risk of HIV infection for economically disadvantaged urban women. *Journal of Consulting and Clinical Psychology, 65,* 531–541.

Carey, M., Braaten, L., Maisto, S., Gleason, J., Forsyth, A., Durant, L., & Jaworski, B. (2000). Using information, motivational enhancement, and skills training to reduce the risk of HIV infection for low-income urban women. A second randomized clinical trial. *Health Psychology, 19,* 3–11.

Carey, B. (2004, Nov. 9). Long after Kinsey, only the brave study sex. *New York Times,* retrieved electronically, http://query.nytimes.com/search/restricted/article?res=FA0D11F638580C7A8CDDA80994DC404482.

Carnes, P. (1983). *The Sexual Addiction.* Minneapolis: CompCare.

Carter, D. (2004). Stonewall: The riots that shaped the gay revolution. New York: St. Martin's Press.

Catalan, J., Green, L., & Thorley, F. (2001). The changing picture of HIV: A chronic illness, again? *FOCUS: A Guide to AIDS Research and Counseling, 16.* San Francisco: UCSF AIDS Health Project, 1–4.

Catania, J., Coates, T.; Kegeles, S., Ekstrand, M., Guydish, J., & Bye, L. (1989). Implications of the AIDS risk reduction model for the gay community: The importance of perceived sexual enjoyment and help seeking behaviors. In S. Schneider, G. Albee, V. Mays, & S.F. Schneider (Eds.), *Primary prevention of AIDS: Psychological approaches.* Newbury Park, CA: Sage Publications, 242–261.

Catania, J., Kegeles, S., & Coates, T. (1990). Toward an understanding of risk behaviour: An AIDS risk reduction model. *Health Education Quarterly, 17,* 53–72.

Centers for Disease Control and Prevention. (1998). Gonorrhea — United States, 1998. *Morbidity and Mortality Weekly Report, 49,* 538–542.

Centers for Disease Control and Prevention. (1999). Increases in unsafe sex and rectal gonorrhea among men who have sex with men — San Francisco, California, 1994–1997. *Morbidity and Mortality Weekly Report, 48,* 45–58.

Centers for Disease Control and Prevention, Division of STD Prevention.(2000). *Sexually Transmitted Disease Surveillance, 1999.* U.S. Department of Health and Human Services. Atlanta, GA: Centers for Disease Control and Prevention.

Centers for Disease Control and Prevention. (2002). Unrecognized HIV infection, risk behaviors, and perceptions of risk among young black men who have sex with men: Six U.S. cities, 1994–1998. *Morbidity and Mortality Weekly Report, 51,* 733–736.

Centers for Disease Control and Prevention. (2002). Incorporating HIV prevention into the medical care of persons living with HIV: Recommendations of Centers for Disease Control and Prevention, the Health Resources and Services Administration, the National Institutes of Health, and the HIV Medicine Association of the Infectious Diseases Society of America. *Morbidity and Mortality Weekly Report, 52(RR-12),* 1–24.

Centers for Disease Control and Prevention. (2003). Increases in HIV diagnoses — 29 states (1999–2002). *Morbidity and Mortality Weekly Report, 52,* 1145–1148.

Centers for Disease Control and Prevention. (2003). HIV/STD risks in young men who have sex with men who do not disclose their sexual orientation — six U.S. cities, 1994–2000. *Morbidity and Mortality Weekly Report, 52,* 81–85.

Centers for Disease Control and Prevention. (2004). No need to wrap it: HIV gift-giver newsgroups, gift theory and exchanging HIV as a gift. WWW.cdc. gov/std2004stdconf/slides/D-sessions/D4/Graydon.pps.

Charny, I. W. (1992). *Existential/dialectic marital therapy: Breaking the secret code of marital therapy.* New York: Brunner Mazel.

Chen, W., & Samarasinghe, P. (1992). Allergy, oral sex, and HIV. *Lancet, 339,* 627–628.

Chesney, M. (1997). HIV postexposure prevention (PEP): Summary sheets on HIV treatment strategies. *San Francisco AIDS Foundation,* www.sfaf.org/treatment/factsheets/pep.html.

Chesney, M., Barrett, D., & Stall, R. D. (1998). Histories of substance use and risk behavior: Precursors to HIV seroconversion in homosexual men. *American Journal of Public Health, 88,* 113–116.

Cheuvront, J. P. (2002). High-risk sexual behavior in the treatment of HIV-negative patients. *Journal of Gay and Lesbian Psychotherapy, 6,* 7–26.

Cheuvront, J. P. (2004). Couples, imagined. In A. D'Erocle & J. Drescher (Eds.), *Uncoupling convention: Psychoanalytic approaches to same-sex couples and families.* Hillsdale, NJ: The Analytic Press, 43–68.

Clark, M. (2001, February 5). Gay men of the world, give up the Russian roulette. *New Statesman, 14,* 32–33.

Coates, T. (2004). Depression, gay men, and HIV acquisition. *FOCUS: A Guide to AIDS Research and Counseling, 19,* 5–6.

Coates, T. (2005). Foreword. In P. Halkitis, C. Gomez, & R. Wolitski (Eds.), *HIV+ sex: The psychological and interpersonal dynamics of HIV-seropositive gay and bisexual men's relationships.* Washington, DC: American Psychological Assn., xiii–xvi.

Cochran, S. & Mays, V. (1990). Sex, lies, and HIV. *New England Journal of Medicine, 322,* 774–775.

Coleman, E. & Rosser, B. (1996). Gay and bisexual male sexuality. In R. Cabaj & T. Stein (Eds.), *Textbook of homosexuality and mental health.* Washington, DC: American Psychiatric Press, 702–721.

Colfax, G. N., Mansergh, G., Guzman, R., Vittinghoff, E., Marks, G., Rader, M., & Buchbinder, S. (2001). Drug use and sexual risk behavior among gay and bisexual men who attend circuit parties: A venue-based comparison. *Journal of Acquired Immune Deficiency Syndrome, 28,* 373–379.

Conway, M., & Dube, L. (2002). Humor in persuasion on threatening topics: Effectiveness is a function of audience sex role orientation. *Personality & Social Psychology Bulletin, 28,* 863–873.

Cooper, A., & Griffin-Shelley, E. (2002). Introduction. The Internet: The next sexual revolution. In A. Cooper (Ed.), *Sex and the Internet: A guide for clinicians.* New York: Brunner-Routledge, 1–15.

Coxon, A. P. M., & McManus, T. J. (2000). How many account for how much? Concentration of high-risk sexual behaviour among gay men. *Journal of Sex Research, 37*, 1–7.

Crawford, J., Rodden, P., Kippax, S., & Van de Ven, P. (2001). Negotiated safety and other agreements between men in relationships: Risk practice redefined. *International Journal of STD & AIDS, 12*, 164–170.

Crenshaw, T. (1987, April). "AIDS update: Condoms are not enough," *American Association of Sex Educators, Counselors, and Therapists Newsletter 18*, 20.

Crimp, D. (1989). Mourning and militancy. *October, 15*, 3–18.

Crosby, G., Stall, R., Paul, J., Barrett, D., & Midanik, L. (1996). Condom use among gay/bisexual male substance abusers using the timeline follow-back method. *Addictive Behaviors, 21*, 249–257.

Crossley, M. (2001) Don't do it! Why health promotion messages fail. *Human Givens: Radical Psychology Today, 8*, 17–21.

Crossley, M. (2002). The perils of health promotion and the 'barebacking' backlash. *Health, 6*, 47–68.

Crossley, M. (2004). Making sense of barebacking: Gay men's narratives, unsafe sex, and the resistance habitus. *British Journal of Social Psychology, 43*, 225–244.

Csepe, P., Amirkhanian, Y. A., Kelly, J. A., McAuliffe, T. L., & Mosonoki, L. (2002). HIV risk behavior among gay and bisexual men in Budapest, Hungary. *International Journal of STDs and AIDS, 13*, 192–200.

Dahir, M. (1998). Hard to swallow: The morning after pill. *POZ, 72*, 60–63.

Davidovich, U., de Wit, J., & Stroebe, W. (2000). Assessing sexual risk behavior of young gay men in primary relationships: The incorporation of negotiated safety and negotiated safety compliance. *AIDS, 14*, 701–706.

Davidovich, U., de Witt, J., Albrecht, N., Geskus, R., Stroebe, W., & Coutinho, R. (2001). Increase in the share of steady partners as a source of HIV infection — A 17-year study of seroconversion among younger and older gay men. *AIDS, 15*, 1303–1308.

Davidovich, U., de Witt, J., & Stroebe, W. (2004). Behavioral and cognitive barriers to safer sex between men in steady relationships: Implications for prevention strategies. *AIDS Education & Prevention, 16*, 304–314.

Dawson, A., Ross, M., Henry, D., & Freeman, A. (2005). Evidence of risk in "barebacking" men who have sex with men: Cases from the Internet. *Journal of Gay and Lesbian Psychotherapy, 9*, 77–88.

Dean, T. (1996). Sex and syncope. *Raritan, 15*, 64–86.

Dean, T. (2000). *Beyond sexuality.* Chicago: University of Chicago Press.

DeCarlo, P., & Coates, T. (1997). What is postexposure prophylaxis? http://www.caps.ucsf.edu/PEP.html.

Denning, P. (2000). *Practicing harm reduction psychotherapy: An alternative approach to addictions.* New York: Guilford.

De Vroome, E., de Wit, M., Stroebe, W., Sandfort, T., & van Griensven, G. (1998). Sexual behavior and depression among HIV-positive gay men. *AIDS and Behavior, 2,* 137–149.

Diaz, R. (1998). *Latino gay men and HIV.* New York: Routledge.

Dilley, J., McFarland, W., Woods, W., Sabatino, J., Lihatsh, T., Adler, B., et al. (2002). Thoughts associated with unprotected anal intercourse among men at high risk in San Francisco 1997–1999. *Psychology and Health, 17,* 235–246.

Dolezal, C., Meyer-Bahlburg, H., Remien, R., & Petkova, E. (1997). Substance use during sex and sensation seeking as predictors of sexual risk behavior among HIV+ and HIV–gay men. *AIDS and Behavior, 1,* 19–28

Dolezal, C., Remien, R., Wagner, G., & Carballo-Dieguez, A. (1999). Psychosocial factors associated with unprotected anal sex among male couples of mixed HIV status. *Abstract book for the Twenty-Fifth Annual Meeting of the International Academy of Sex Research,* StonyBrook, NY, 26 June.

Doll, L., O'Mally, P., Perhsing, A., Darrow, W., Hessol, N., & Lifson, A. (1990). High-risk sexual behavior and knowledge of HIV-antibody status in the San Francisco City Clinic cohort. *Health Psychology, 9,* 253–265.

Doll, S., Byers, R., Bolan, G., Douglas, J., Moss, P., Weller, P., Joy, D., Bartholow, B., and Harrison, J. (1991). Homosexual men who engage in high-risk sexual behavior. A multicenter comparison. *Sexually Transmitted Diseases, 18,* 170–175.

Dollimore, J. (1998). *Death, desire and loss in western culture.* New York: Routledge.

Douglas-Brown, I. (2001, October 12). Prevention efforts are going online. *The Washington Blade, 32,* 1, 22, 24.

Drescher, J. (1998). *Psychoanalytic therapy and the gay man.* Hillsdale, NJ: The Analytic Press.

Drescher, J. (2001). I'm your handyman: A history of reparative therapies. In A. Shidlo, M. Schroeder, & J. Drescher (Eds.), *Sexual conversion therapy: Ethical, clinical and research perspective.* Binghamton, NY: Haworth Medical Press, 5–24.

Drug Enforcement Administration (DEA). Strategic Intelligence Section Domestic Unit, Washington, DC (1989). A special report on "Ice" (D-meth-amphetamine Hydrochloride), Proceedings of the Community Epidemiology Work Group Public Health Service, NIDA, 69-83.

Duberman, M. (1991). *Cures: A gay man's odyssey,* New York: Dutton.

Dukers, N.H., Goudsmit, J., de Wit, J.B., Prins, M., Wverling, G.J., & Coutinho, R A. (2001). Sexual risk behaviors relate to the virologic and immunological improvements during highly active antiretroviral therapy in HIV-1 infection. *AIDS, 15,* 369–378.

Eggan, F., Reback, C., & Ditman, D. (1996) Methamphetamine use among gay male drug users: An ethnographic study. Presented at the International Conference on AIDS (ICA Abstracts Tu.C.24117).

Ekstrand, M., Stall, R., Paul, J., Osmond, D., & Coates, T. (1999). Gay men report high rates of unprotected anal sex with partners of unknown or serodiscordant status. *AIDS, 13,* 1525–1533.

Elford, J., Bolding, G., Maguire, M., & Sherr, I. (1999). Sexual risk behavior among gay men in a relationship. *AIDS, 13,* 1407–1411.

Elford, J., Bolding, G., & Sherr, L. (2001). Seeking sex on the Internet and sexual risk behaviour among gay men using London gyms. (2001). *AIDS, 15,* 1409–1415.

Elford, J., Bolding, G., Maguire, M., & Sherr, L. (2001). Gay men, risk and relationships. *AIDS, 15,* 1053–1055.

Elford, J., Bolding, G., & Sherr, L. (2002). High-risk sexual behavior increases among London gay men between 1998 and 2001: What is the role of HIV optimism? *AIDS, 16,* 1537–1544.

Elford, J. (2002). Surfing for sex. *FOCUS: A Guide to AIDS Research and Counseling, 17,* 1–3.

Ellenhorn, M., Schonwald, S., Ordog, G., & Wasserman, J. (1997). *Ellenhorn's medical toxicology: Diagnosis and treatment of human poisoning* (2nd ed.). Baltimore, MD: Williams & Wilkins.

Ellis, D., Collins, I., & King, M. (1995). Personality disorder and sexual risk taking among homosexually active and heterosexually active men attending a genitourinary medicine clinic. *Journal of Psychosomatic Research, 39,* 901–910.

Exodus-International (2005). www.exodus-international.org.

Fagard, C., Oxenius, A., Gunthard, H., Garcia, F., Le Braz, M., Mestre, G. et al. (2003). A prospective trial of structured treatment interruption in human immunodeficiency virus infection. *Archives of Internal Medicine, 163,* 1220–1226.

Fishbein, M., & Ajzen, I. (1975). *Belief, attitude, intent, and behavior: An introduction to theory and research.* Reading, MA: Addison-Wesley.

Fischer, J., Wilcutts, K., Misovich, S., & Weinstein, B. (1998). Dynamics of sexual risk behavior in HIV-infected men who have sex with men. *AIDS and Behavior, 2,* 101–113.

Flichman, D., Cello, J., Castano, G., Campos, R., & Sookoian, S. (1999). *In vivo* regulation of HIV replication after hepatitis superinfection. *Medicina, 59,* 364–366.

Flowers, P., Smith, J. A., Sheeran, P., & Beail, N. (1997). Health and romance: Understanding unprotected sex in relationships between gay men. *British Journal of Health Psychology, 2,* 73–86.

Folkman, S., Chesney, M. A., Pollack., L., & Phillips, C. (1992). Stress, coping, and high-risk sexual behavior. *Health Psychology, 11,* 218–222.

Forstein, M. (2002). Commentary on Cheuvront's high-risk sexual behavior in the treatment of HIV-negative patients. *Journal of Gay and Lesbian Psychotherapy, 6,* 35–44.

Foucault, M. (1978). *History of sexuality. Volume 1: An introduction.* Translated by Robert Hurley. New York: Random House.

Fox, K. K., Whittington, W. L., Levine, W. C. et al. (1998). Gonorrhea in the United States, 1981–1996. Demographic and geographic trends. *Sexually Transmitted Diseases, 26,* 386–393.

Fox, K. K., del Rio, C., Holmes, K. K., Hook, E. W., Judson, F. N., Knapp, J. S. et al. (2001). Gonorrhea in the HIV era: A reversal in trends among men who have sex with men. *American Journal of Public Health, 91,* 959–964.

Freedoms.org.uk (2002). http://www.freedoms.org.uk/advice/air/air02.htm.

Freeman, G. (2003, February 6). Bug chasers: The men who long to be HIV+. *Rolling Stone,* http://www.rollingstone.com/news/newsarticle.asp?nid=17380.

Freese, T. E., Miotto, K., & Rebeack, C. J. (2002). The effects and consequences of selected club drugs. *Journal of Substance Abuse Treatment, 23,* 151–156.

Freud, S. (1917). Mourning and melancholia. J. Stratchey (Ed. and Trans.), *Standard Edition of the Complete Works of Sigmund Freud, 17,* London: Hogarth, 237–258.

Freud, S. (1920). Beyond the pleasure principle. J. Stratchey (Ed. and Trans.), *Standard Edition of the Complete Works of Sigmund Freud, 18,* 1–64, London: Hogarth.

Frieden, T. (2003). Methamphetamine and HIV: A dangerous combination. *Five Boroughs AIDS Mental Health Alliance, 5,* 2–3.

Fries, S. (1998). A place where no one knows your name. *The Advocate: The National Gay and Lesbian Newsmagazine, 752,* 24–31.

Frosch, D., Shoptaw, S., Huber, A., Rawson, R., & Ling, W. (1996). Sexual HIV risk and gay and bisexual methamphetamine abusers. *Journal of Substance Abuse Treatment, 13,* 201–216.

Frost, J. C. (1994). Taking a sexual history with gay patients in psychotherapy. In S. Cadwell, R. Burnham, & M. Forstein (Eds.), *Therapists on the front line: Psychotherapy with gay men in the age of AIDS.* Washington, DC: American Psychiatric Press, 163–183.

Frutchey, C. (1988, November 11). *AIDS prevention programs for gay men in four U.S. cities.* Presentation at 31st annual program meeting of The Society for the Scientific Study of Sex, San Francisco.

Gauthier, D. K. & Forsyth, C. J. (1999). Bareback sex, bug chasers, and the gift of death. *Deviant Behavior, 20,* 85–100.

Gawin, F. (1978). Drugs and eros: Reflections on eros. *Journal of Psychedelic Drugs, 10,* 227–235.

Gawin, F. & Ellinwood, E. (1988). Cocaine and other stimulants: action, abuse and treatment. *New England Journal of Medicine,* 319, 1173–1182.

Gay Men Fighting AIDS, (2003). www.metromate.org/.uk.

Gay Men's Health Crisis (1996). *To suck or not to suck?* New York: GMHC.

Gendin, S. (1997). My turn riding bareback; Skin-on-skin sex: Been there, done that want more. *POZ Magazine*, downloaded from www.poz.com/archive/june1997/columns/myturn.html.

Gendin, S. (1999a). They shoot barebackers, don't they? *POZ Magazine*. www.poz.com/archive/february1999/inside/theyshootbare.html

Gendin, S. (1999b). Both sides now. *POZ Magazine* online.http://www.poz.com/index.cfm?p=article&art_id=1329.

Gerhart, K. (1999, June). Beyond barebacking: The complacency crisis. *Genre Magazine, 7*, 47–51.

Germaine, C. B. (1978). General systems theory and ego psychology: An ecological perspective. *Social Service Review, 52*, 535–555.

Germaine, C. B. (1980). Social context of clinical social work. *Social Work, 36*, 7–11.

Germaine, C. B. (1981). The ecological approach to people–environment transactions. *Social Casework, 62*, 323–331.

Gerrard, M., Gibbons, F. X., & McCoy, S. B. (1993). Emotional inhibition of effective contraception. *Anxiety, Stress, and Coping. 6*, 73–88.

Gibson, P., Pendo, M., & Wohlfeiler, D. (1999). Risk, HIV and STD prevention. *FOCUS: A Guide to AIDS Research and Counseling, 14*, 1–4.

Gilgenberg-Castillo, K. (2004). Supporting positive sexual health among people with HIV. *FOCUS: A Guide to AIDS Research and Counseling, 19*, 1–4.

Gitterman, A. & Germaine, C. B. (1976). Social work practice: A life model. *Social Service Review*, 601–610.

Glass, S. P. & Wright, T. M. (1985). Sex differences in type of extramarital involvement and marital satisfaction. *Sex Roles, 12*, 1101–1120.

Glass, S. P. & Wright, T. M. (1992). Justifications for extramarital relationships: The association between attitudes, behaviors, and gender. *The Journal of Sex Research, 29*, 361–387.

GMHC & APLA. (2005). Squashing the "super-bug": An open letter to gay and bisexual men. The Institute for Gay Men's Health, received via the Internet from a listserv.

Gochros, H. (1988). Risk of abstinence: Sexual decision making in the AIDS era. *Social Work, 33*, 254–256.

Goodroad, B. K., Kirksey, K. M., & Butensky, E. (2000). Bareback sex and gay men: An HIV prevention failure. *Journal of the Association of Nurses in AIDS Care, 11*, 29–36.

Gorman, E. M., Morgan, P., & Lambert, E. Y. (1995). Qualitative research considerations and other issues in the study of methamphetamine use among men who have sex with other men. *NIDA Research Monographs 157*, 156–181.

Gorman, M. E., Gunderson, R., Marlatt, A., & Donovan, D. (1996). *HIV risk among gay and bisexual methamphetamine injectors in Seattle, Washington.* Presented at the International Conference on AIDS (ICA Abstracts Pub.C. 1257).

Gorman, M. (1998). A tale of two epidemics: HIV and stimulant use. *FOCUS: A Guide to AIDS Research and Counseling, 13,* 1–3.

Grant, R., McConnell, J., Boutelle, A., Hunt, E., Liegler, T., Tsui, R., Herring, B., & Delwart, E. (2004). *No superinfection among seroconcordant couples after well-defined exposure.* Presentation at XV International AIDS Conference, Bangkok, Thailand, July 15, Abstract ThPeA6949.

Green, J. (1996, September 15). Flirting with suicide. *New York Times Magazine,* 38–45, 54–55, 84–85.

Green, R., Bettinger, M., & Zacks, E. (1996). Are lesbian couples fused and gay male couples disengaged?: Questioning gender straightjackets. In J. Laird & R. Lifton (Eds.), *Lesbians and gays in couples and families.* San Francisco: Jossey-Bass, 185–230.

Greenan, D. & Tunnell, G. (2003). *Couple therapy with gay men.* New York: Guilford Press.

Greenan, D. & Shernoff, M. (2003). Do open relationships work? Gay couples and the question of monogamy. *Psychotherapy Networker, 27,* 71–75.

Gross, K., Porco, T., & Grant, R. (2004). HIV-1 superinfection and viral diversity. *AIDS, 18,* 1513–1520.

Grov, C. (2004). "Make me your death slave": Men who have sex with men and use the Internet to intentionally spread HIV. *Deviant Behavior, 25,* 329–349.

Guss, J. R. (2000). Sex like you can't even imagine: "Crystal," crack, and gay men. *Journal of Gay & Lesbian Psychotherapy, 3,* 105–122.

Halkitis, P. N. (2000). Redefining masculinity in the age of AIDS: Seropositive gay men and the "buff agenda." In P. Nardi (Ed.), *Gay Masculinities.* Newbury Park, CA: Sage Publications, 130–151.

Halkitis, P., & Parsons, J. (2000). Oral sex and HIV risk reduction: Perceived risk, behaviors, and strategies among young HIV-negative gay men. *Journal of Psychology & Human Sexuality, 11,* 1–24.

Halkitis, P. N., Parsons, J. T., & Stirratt, M. (2001). A double epidemic: Crystal methamphetamine use and its relation to HIV prevention among gay men. *Journal of Homosexuality, 41,* 17–35.

Halkitis, P. N. & Parsons, J. T. (2002). Recreational drug use and HIV risk sexual behavior among men frequenting urban gay venues. *Journal of Gay & Lesbian Social Services, 14,* 19–38.

Halkitis, P. N., Parsons, J. T., & Wilton, L. (2003). Barebacking among gay and bisexual men in New York City: Explanations for the emergence of intentional unsafe behavior. *Archives of Sexual Behavior, 32,* 351–357.

Halkitis, P. N. (2003, October 10). *Barebacking behavior. Barebacking identity. What it all means.* Panel presentation, Barebacking: Research and Clinical Issues. Forum held at the Lesbian, Gay, Bisexual, Transgendered Community Services Center, New York, NY.

Halkitis, P. N., & Parsons, J. T. (2003). Intentional unsafe sex (barebacking) among gay men who seek sexual partners on the Internet. *AIDS Care, 15,* 367–378.

Halkitis, P., Parsons, J., & Wilton, L. (2003b). An exploratory study of contextual and situational factors related to methamphetamine use among gay and bisexual men in New York City. *Journal of Drug Issues, 33,* 413–432.

Halkitis, P. N., Wilton, L., Parsons, J. T., & Hoff, C. (2004). Correlates of sexual risk-taking behavior among HIV seropositive gay men in seroconcordant primary partner relationships. *Psychology, Health, & Medicine, 9,* 99–113.

Halkitis, P. N., Greene, K., & Mourgues, P. (2005). Patterns, contexts, and risks associated with methamphetamine use among gay and bisexual men in New York City: Findings from Project BUMPS. *Journal of Urban Health, 82,* 18–25.

Halkitis, P., Green, K., Remien, R., Stirratt, M., Hoff, C., Wolitski, R., & Parsons, J. (2005b). Seroconcordant sexual partnerings of HIV-positive men who have sex with men. *AIDS (Supplement 1),* S77-86.

Halkitis, P., Wilton, P., Wolitski, R., Parsons, J., Hoff, C., & Bimbi, D. (2005c). Barebacking identity among HIV-positive gay and bisexual men: Demographic, psychological, and behavioural correlates. *AIDS (Supplement 1),* S27-36.

Halkitis, P., Wilton, L., & Galatowitsch, P. (2005). What's in a term? How gay and bisexual men understand barebacking. In P. Halkitis, L. Wilton, & J. Drescher (Eds.), *Barebacking: Psychosocial and public health approaches.* Binghamton, NY: Haworth Press, 39–52.

Halkitis, P., & Wilton, L. (2005). The meanings of sex for HIV-positive gay and bisexual men: Emotions, physicality and affirmations of self. In P. Halkitis, C. Gomez, & R. Wolitski (Eds.), *HIV+: The psychological and interpersonal dynamics of HIV seropositive gay and bisexual men's relationships.* Washington, DC: American Psychological Association, 21–38.

Halkitis, P. N., Fischgrund, B. N., & Parsons, J. T. (In press, a). Explanations for methamphetamine use among gay and bisexual men in New York City. *Substance Use & Misuse.*

Halkitis, P. N., Shrem, M. T., & Martin, F. W. (In press, c). Sexual behavior patterns of methamphetamine using gay and bisexual men in New York City. *Substance Use & Misuse.*

Halkitis, P., Green, K., & Carragher, D. (In press, d). Methamphetamine use, sexual behavior and HIV seroconversion. *Journal of Gay and Lesbian Psychotherapy.*

Hanson, G. R., Green, K., & Carragher, D. *NIDA research report series: Methamphetamine abuse and addiction* (NIH Publication No. 02-4210) 2000. Rockville, MD: National Clearinghouse on Alcohol and Drug Information, http://www.drugabuse.gov/PDF/RRMetham.pdf.

Harris, N. V., Thiede, H., McGough, J. P., & Gordon, D. (1993). Risk factors for HIV infection among injecting drug users: Results of blinded surveys in drug treatment centers, King County, Washington 1988–1991. *Journal of Acquired Immune Deficiency Syndromes, 6,* 1275–1282.

Hartmann, L. (1996). Foreword to *Textbook of homosexuality and mental health.* R. P. Cabaj & T. S. Stein (Eds.). Washington, DC: American Psychiatric Press, xxv–xxxii.

Hays, R. B., Kegeles, S. M., & Coates, T. (1997). Unprotected sex and HIV risk-taking among young gay men within boyfriend relationships. *AIDS Education and Prevention, 9,* 314–329.

Healthy penis campaign. (2005). www.healthypenis.org.

Hecht, F. M., Grant, R., Petropoulos, C., Dillon, B., Chesney, M., Tian, H., et al. (1998). Sexual transmission of HIV-1 variant resistant to multiple reverse-transcriptase and protease inhibitors. *New England Journal of Medicine, 339,* 307–343.

Heischober, B., & Miller, A. (1991). Methamphetamine abuse in California. *NIDA Research Monographs, 115,* 60–71.

Henderson, L., Keough, P., Weatherburn, P., and Reid, D. (2001). *Managing uncertainty: Risk and unprotected anal intercourse among gay men who do not know their HIV status.* London: SIGMA Research.

Hendrick, C., & Hendrick, S. (1983). *Liking, loving, and relating.* Monterey, CA: Brooks/Cole.

Herdt, G., & Boxer, A. (1993) *Children of horizons: How gay and lesbian teens are leading a new way out of the closet.* Boston, MA: Beacon.

Heredia, C. (2003, May 4). Dance of death: Crystal meth fuels HIV. *San Francisco Chronicle,* http://sfgate.com/cgi-bin/article.cgi?file=/c/a/2003/05/04/MN281636. DTL.

Herek, G. (1998). *Stigma and sexual orientation: Understanding prejudice against, lesbians, gay men, and bisexuals.* Society for the Psychological Study of Lesbian and Gay Issues, Thousand Oaks, CA: Sage.

Hicks, C., Eron, J., Lennox, C., Pilcher, C., Menenzes, P., Giner, J., et al. (2001). *Resistence to antiretroviral agents in a cohort of patients with acute HIV infection acquired in nonurban areas in the Southestern USA.* Paper presented at the 8th Conference on Retroviruses and Opportunistic Infections, Chicago.

Hickson, F. C., Davies, P. M., Hunt, A. J., Weatherburn, P., McManus, T. J., & Coxon, P. (1992). Maintenance of open gay relationships: Some strategies for protection against HIV. *AIDS Care, 4,* 409–419.

Hickson, F., Reid, D., Davies, P., Weatherburn, P., Beardsell, S., & Keough, P. (1996). No aggregate change in homosexual HIV risk behaviour among gay men attending the Gay Pride festivals, United Kingdom, 1993–1995. *AIDS, 10,* 771–774.

Hitzel, D. (2002). A boy's own story. *POZ.* www.poz.com/index.cfm?p=article&art_id=303.

Hoff, C., Coates, T., Barrett, D., Collette, I., & Ekstrand, M. (1996). Differences between gay men in primary relationships and single gay men: Implications for prevention: A review. *AIDS Education and Prevention, 8,* 546–559.

Hoff, C., Stall, R. D., Paul, J., Acree, M., Daigle, D., Phillips, K., Kegeles, S., Jinich, S., Ekstrand, M., & Coates, T. (1997). Differences in sexual behavior among HIV-discordant and -concordant gay men in primary relationships. *Journal of AIDS and Human Retrovirology, 14,* 72–78.

Hoff, C., Faigles, B., Wolitski, R., Purcell, W., Gomez, C., & Parsons, J. (2004). Sexual risk for HIV transmission is missed by traditional methods of data collection. *AIDS, 18,* 340–342.

Hooker, E. A. (1957). The adjustment of the overt male homosexual. *Journal of Projective Techniques, 21,* 17–31.

Horn, T. (1998, June) Party favors. *POZ,* 90.

Hort, H. K. (2000). *Barebacking domino.* Paper presented at the XIII International Conference on AIDS, Barcelona.

Hospers, H. J., & Kok, G. (1995). Determinants of safe and risk-taking sexual behavior among gay men: A review. *AIDS Education and Prevention, 7,* 74–95.

Hoyle, R., Fejfar, M., & Miller, J. (2000). Personality and sexual risk taking: A quantitative review. *Journal of Personality, 68,* 1205–1229.

Humm, A. (2005, February 24–March 2). Pope calls same-sex marriage "evil." *Gay City News, 4,* 4.

Hunt, M. (1974). *Sexual behavior in the 1970s.* Chicago, IL: Playboy Press.

Hunt, A., Davies, P., McManus, T., Weatherburn, P., Hickson, F., Christofini, G., Coxon, A., & Sutherland, S. (1992). HIV infection in a cohort of homosexual and bisexual men, *British Medical Journal, 305,* 561–562.

H. X. (2004, Sept 24) Issue 681.

Hyde, J. S. (1982). *Understanding human sexuality.* New York: McGraw-Hill.

Internet Notification Service for Partners or Tricks (2005). www.inspot.org., I.S.I.S., Inc.

Isay, R. (1989). *Being homosexual: Gay men and their development.* New York: Avon Books.

Jacobs, A. (2002, January 29). In clubs, a potent drug stirs fear of an epidemic. *New York Times,* B1.

Jacobs, A. (2004, January 12). The beast in the bathhouse: Crystal meth use by gay men threatens to reignite an epidemic. *New York Times,* B1, B5.

Jacobs, A. (2005, February 15). Gays debate radical steps to curb unsafe sex. *New York Times,* A1, B4.

Jacobs, A. (2005, April 3). AIDS fighters face a resistant form of apathy: Searching for ways to counter lax attitudes and risky behavior. *New York Times*, 29, 32.

Jacobseberg, L., Frances, A., & Perry, S. (1995). Axis II diagnosis among volunteers for HIV testing and counseling. *American Journal of Psychiatry, 152*, 1222–1224.

Johnson, T. W. & Keren, M. S. (1996). Creating and maintaining boundaries in male couples. In J. Laird & R. J. Green (Eds.), *Lesbians and gays in couples and families: A handbook for therapists*. San Francisco: Jossey-Bass, 231–250.

Joseph, J., Montgomery, S., Kirscht, J., Kessler, R., Ostrow, D., Emmons, C., & Phair, J. (1987). Perceived risk of AIDS: Assessing the behavioral and psychosocial consequences in a cohort of gay men. *Journal of Applied Social Psychology, 17*, 231–250.

Jost, S., Bernard, M. C., Kaiser, L., Yerly, S., Hirschel, B., Samri, A., et al. (2002). A patient with HIV-1 superinfection. *New England Journal of Medicine, 347*, 731–736.

Julian, P. (1997, February 27). Prevention may be getting wise. New study puts AIDS risk in the context of reality. *San Francisco Frontiers*, 11–13.

Kalichman, S., Kelly, J., & Rompa, D. (1997). Continued high-risk sex among HIV seropositive gay and bisexual men seeking HIV prevention services. *Health Psychology, 16*, 369–373.

Kalichman, S. C., Nachimson, D., Cherry, C., & Williams, E. (1998). AIDS treatment advances and behavioral prevention setbacks: Preliminary assessment of reduced perceived threat of HIV-AIDS. *Health Psychology, 17*, 546–550.

Kalichman, S. C., & Weinhardt, L. (2001). Negative affect sexual risk behavior: Comment on Crepaz and Marks (2001). *Health Psychology, 20*, 300–301.

Kalichman, S., Rompa, D., Cage, M., Austin, W., Luke, T., Barnett, P., Tharnish, J., Mowrey, R., & Schinazi, F. (2002). Sexual transmission risk perceptions and behavioural correlates of HIV concentrations in semen. *AIDS Care, 14*, 343–349.

Kaufman, D. (2002). *Ridiculous! The theatrical life and times of Charles Ludlam*. New York: Applause Theater and Cinema Books.

Kelly, J. A., Lawrence, J. S., Brasfield, T. L., Lemke, A., Amidei, T., Roffman, R. E., et al. (1990). Psychological factors that predict AIDS high-risk versus AIDS precautionary behavior. *Journal of Consulting and Clinical Psychology, 58*, 117–120.

Kelly, J. A., & Kalichman, S. C. (1998). Reinforcement value of unsafe sex as a predictor of condom use and continued HIV/AIDS risk behavior among gay and bisexual men. *Health Psychology, 17*, 328–335.

Kelly, J. A., Hoffman, R. G., & Rompa, D. (1998). Protease inhibitor combination therapies and perceptions of gay men regarding AIDS severity and the need to maintain safer sex. *AIDS, 12*, 91–95.

Kerr, M., & Bowen, M. (1988) *Family evaluation: An approach based on Bowen theory*. New York: W.W. Norton.

Kim, R. (2001). Andrew Sullivan, overexposed. *The Nation*, retrieved online at www.thenation.com/doc.mhtml%3Fi=2001061&s=kim20010605.

Kim, A., Kent, C., & McFarland, W. (2001). Cruising on the Internet highway. *Journal of Acquired Immune Deficiency Syndromes, 28*, 89–93.

Kinsey, A. C., Pomeroy, W. B., & Martin, C.E. (1948). *Sexual behavior in the human male*. Philadelphia: W.B. Saunders.

Kinsey, A. C., Pomeroy, W. B., Martin, C. E., et al. (1953). *Sexual behavior in the human female*. Philadelphia: W.B. Saunders.

Kippax, S., Crawford, J. M., Davis, M., Rodden, P., and Dowset, G. (1993). Sustaining safe sex: A longitudinal study of a sample of homosexual men. *AIDS, 7*, 257–263.

Kippax, S., Noble, J., Prestage, G., et al. (1997). Sexual negotiation in the AIDS era: Negotiated safety revisited. *AIDS, 11*, 191–197.

Kippax, S., Slavin, S., Ellard, J., Hendry, O., Richters, J., Grulic, A., & Kaldor, J. (2003). Seroconversion in context. *AIDS Care, 15*, 839–852.

Klausner, J., Wolfe, W., Fischer-Ponce, L., Zolt, I., & Katz, M. (2000). Tracing a syphilis outbreak through cyberspace. *Journal of the American Medical Association, 284*, 447–449.

Klausner, J., Kim, A., & Kent, C. (2002). Are HIV drug advertisements contributing to increases in risk behavior among men in San Francisco, 2001? *AIDS, 16*, 2349–2350.

Klitzman, R., Pope, H., & Hudson, J. (2000). MDMA ("ecstasy") abuse and high-risk sexual behaviors among 169 gay and bisexual men. *American Journal of Psychiatry, 157*, 1162–1164.

Koblin, B. A., Torian, L. V., Gulin, V., Ren, L., MacKellar, D. A.., & Valleroy, L. A. (2000). High prevalence of HIV infection among young men who have sex with men in New York City. *AIDS, 14*, 1793–1800.

Kramer, L. (1978). *Faggots*. New York: Random House.

Kramer, L. (1983a). 1112 and Counting. *New York Native, 59*. Reprinted in *Reports from the holocaust: The story of an AIDS activist*. New York: St. Martin's Press, 33–51.

Kramer, L. (1983b). The mark of courage. *New York Native, 67*. Reprinted in *Reports from the holocaust: The story of an AIDS activist*. New York: St. Martin's Press, 60–67.

Kramer, L. (1983c). 2339 and Counting. *Village Voice*. Reprinted in *Reports from the holocaust: The story of an AIDS activist*, New York: St, Martin's Press, 68–74.

Kurdek, L., & Schmitt, P. (1985/86). Relationship quality of gay men in closed or open relationships. *Journal of Homosexuality, 12*, 85–99.

Kurdek, L. A. (1988). Relationship quality of gay and lesbian cohabitating couples. *Journal of Homosexuality, 15,* 85–99.

Kurtz, H. (1996, April 13). Turning the page: *New Republic* editor ends rocky tenure. *The Washington Post,* B1.

Leigh, B. C. (1990). The relationship of substance used during sex to high-risk sexual behavior. *The Journal of Sex Research, 27,* 199–213.

Leigh, B., & Stall, R. (1993). Substance use and risky sexual behavior for exposure to HIV. *American Psychologist, 48,* 1035–1045.

Lenius, S. (1999, May 6). Barebacking: Stop the madness. It's not chic, it's rebellious: It's suicide. [Electronic Version] *Lavender Magazine, 102 (4).* www.lavendermagazine.com/102/102 out 56.html.

Lifson, A., O'Mally, P., Hessol, N., & Buchbinder, S. (1990). HIV seroconversion in two homosexual men after receptive oral intercourse with ejaculation: Implications for counseling concerning safer sexual practices. *American Journal of Public Health, 80,* 1509–1511.

Little, S. J., Daar, E. S., D'Aquila, R. T., Keiser, P. H., Conick, E., Whitcomb, J. M. et al. (1999). Reduced HIV drug susceptibility among patients with primary HIV infection. *JAMA, 282,* 1142–1149.

MacMaster, S. (2004). Harm reduction: A new perspective on substance abuse services. *Social Work, 49,* 356–363.

MacMaster, S., Aquino, R., & Vail, K. (2003). Providing HIV education and outreach via Internet chat rooms to men who have sex with men. *Journal of Human Behavior in the Social Environment, 8,* 145–151.

Madake-Tyndall, E. (1991). Sexual scripts and AIDS prevention: Variations in adherence to safer-sex guidelines by heterosexual adolescents. *The Journal of Sex Research, 28,* 45–66.

Mallinger, M. S. (1998, April 6). About anal sex, barebacking: Slogans aren't enough. http://gaytoday.badpuppy.com/garchive/viewpoint/040698vi.htm.

Malyon, A. (1982). Psychotherapeutic implications of internalized homophobia in gay men. In J. Gonsiorek (Ed.), *Homosexuality and psychotherapy: A practitioner's handbook of affirmative models.* New York: Haworth Press, 59–70.

Mansergh, G., Marks, G., Miller, L., Appleby, P., & Murphy, S. (2000). Is knowing people with HIV/AIDS associated with safer sex in men who have sex with men? *AIDS, 14,* 1845–1851.

Mansergh, G., Colfax, G., Marks, G., Rader, M., Guzman, R., & Buchbinder, S. (2001). The circuit party men's health survey: Findings and implications for gay and bisexual men. *American Journal of Public Health, 91,* 953–958.

Mansergh, G., Marks, G., Colfax, G., Guzman, R., Rader, M., & Buchbinder, S. (2002). Barebacking in a diverse sample of men who have sex with men. *AIDS, 16,* 653–659.

Martin, J. (1987).The impact of AIDS on gay male sexual behavior patterns in New York City. *American Journal of Public Health, 77*, 578–581.

Martin, J., & Hasin, D. (1990). Drinking, alcoholism and sexual behavior in a cohort of gay men. *AIDS Alcohol/Drug Abuse: Psychosocial Research, 5*, 49–67.

Martin, J. N., Roland, M. E., Neilands, T. B., Krone, M. R., Bamberger, J. D., Kohn, R. P., Chesney, M. A., Franses, K., Kahn, J. O., Coates, T. J., & Katz, M. H. (2004). Use of postexposure prophylaxis against HIV infection following sexual exposure does not lead to increases in high-risk behavior. *AIDS, 18*, 787–792.

Martinez-Bevin, A. (2004). *Playing it unsafe: Bareback parties, HIV and danger in numbers*. Retrieved online at: *Metrotimes*, www.metrotimes.com/editorial/story.asp?id=6953.

Mattison, A. M., Ross, M. W., Wolfson, T., & Franklin D., and the HIV Neurobehavioral Research Center (2001). Circuit party attendance, club drug use, and unsafe sex in gay men. *Journal of Substance Abuse, 13*, 19-126

Metrotimes, online version, www.metrotimes.com/editorial/story.asp?id=6953.

McCusker, J., Stoddard, A., Zapka, J., Zorn, M., & Mayer, K. (1990). Use of drugs and alcohol by homosexually active men in relation to sexual practices. *Journal of Acquired Immune Deficiency Syndrome, 3*, 729–736.

McDowell, K. H. (1999). Both sides now: Call this the seroconversion of a codependent. *POZ Magazine* online. http://www.poz.com/index.cfm?p=article&art_id=1330.

McFarlane, M., Bull, S. S., & Rietmeijer, C. A. (2000). The Internet as a newly emerging risk environment for sexually transmitted diseases. *Journal of the American Medical Association, 284*, 443–446.

McFarlane, M., Bull, S., & Reitmeijer, C. (2002). Young adults on the Internet: risk behaviors for sexually transmitted diseases and HIV. *Journal of Adolescent Health, 31*, 11–16.

McKirnan, D. J., & Peterson, P. L. (1989). Alcohol and drug use among homosexual men and women: Epidemiological and population characteristics. *Addictive Behaviors, 14*, 545–553.

McKirnan, D., Ostrow, D., & Hope, B. (1996). Sex drugs and escape: A psychological model of HIV-risk sexual behaviors. *AIDS Care, 8*, 655–669.

McKusick, L., Horstman, W., & Coates, T. (1985). AIDS and sexual behavior reported by gay men in San Francisco. *American Journal of Public Health, 75*, 493–496.

McKusick, L., Wiley, J., Coates, T., Stall, R., Saika, G., Morin, S., Charles, K., Horstman, W., & Conant, M. (1985). Reported changes in sexual behavior of men at risk for AIDS, San Francisco, 1982–1984 — The AIDS Behavioral Research Project. *Public Health Reports, 100*, 622–628.

McKusick, L., Hoff, C. C., Stall, R., & Coates, T. (1991). Tailoring AIDS prevention: Differences in behavior strategies among heterosexual and gay bar patrons in San Francisco. *AIDS Education and Prevention, 3*, 1–9.

McLean, J., Boulton, M., Brookes, M., Lakhani, D., Fitzpatrick, R., Dawson, J., McKechnie, R., & Hart, G. (1994). Regular partners and risky behaviour: Why do gay men have unprotected intercourse? *AIDS Care, 6,* 331–341.

McNall, M., & Remafedi, G. (1999). Relationship of amphetamine and other substance use to unprotected intercourse among young men who have sex with men. *Archives of Pediatrics and Adolescent Medicine, 153,* 1130–1135.

McNeal, L. (1997). The association of idealization and intimacy factors with condom use in gay male couples. *Journal of Clinical Psychology in Medical Settings, 4,* 437–451.

McVinney, L. D. (1988). Social work practice with gay male couples. In. G. P. Mallon (Ed.), *Foundations of social work practice with lesbian and gay persons.* Binghamton, NY: The Haworth Press, 209–227.

McWhirter, D., & Mattison, A. (1984). *The male couple: How relationships develop.* Englewood Cliffs, NJ: Prentice-Hall.

Mendes-Correa, M. C., Baronne, A. A., & Guastini, C. (2001). Hepatitis C virus seroprevalence and risk factors among patients with HIV infection. *Review of the Institute of Medicine San Paulo, 43,* 15–19.

Mendola, M. (1980). *The Mendola report: A new look at gay couples.* New York: Crown Books.

Mettey, A., Crosby, R., DiClemente, R., & Holtgrave, D. (2003). Associations between Internet sex seeking and STI-associated risk behaviours among men who have sex with men. *Sexually Transmitted Infections, 79,* 466–468.

Meyer, I. H., & Dean, L. (1998). Internalized homophobia, intimacy, and sexual behavior among gay and bisexual men. In G. M. Hereck (Ed.), *Stigma and sexual orientation: Understanding prejudice against lesbians, gay men and bisexuals.* Thousand Oaks, CA: Sage Publications, 160–186.

Miller, V., Sabin, C., Hertogs, K., Bloor, S., Martinez-Picado, J., D'Aquila, R., et al. (2000). Virologic and immunological effects of treatment interruption in HIV-1 infected patients with treatment failure. *AIDS, 14,* 2857–2867.

Miller, J., Lynam, D., Zimmerman, T., Logan, C., & Clayton, R. (2004). The utility of the Five Factor Model in understanding risky sexual behavior. *Personality and Individual Differences, 36,* 1611–1626.

Miller, W., & Rollnick, S. (1991). *Motivational interviewing: Preparing people to change addictive behavior.* New York: The Guilford Press.

Miller, W., & Rollnick, S. (2002). *Motivational interviewing: Preparing people for change* (2nd ed.). New York: The Guilford Press.

Mirken, B. (1999). Barebacking bickering: A rush to judgment hurts us all [Electronic version]. *The Guide: Gay Travel, Entertainment, Politics, & Sex.* http://208.249.122.222.

Misovich, S., Fischer, J., & Coates, T. (1997). Close relationship and elevated HIV risk behavior: Evidence and possible underlying psychological processes. *Review of General Psychology, 1,* 72–107.

Mnookin, S. (2003, February 17). Media: Using bug chasers. *Newsweek, 91,* 10.

Moderation Management (2004). http://www.moderation.org/whatisMM.shtml.

Molitor, F., Truax, S., Ruiz, J., & Sun, R. (1998). Association of methamphetamine use during sex with sexual behaviors and HIV infection among non-injection drug users in California. *Western Journal of Medicine, 168,* 93–97.

Moore, P. (2004). *Beyond shame: Reclaiming the abandoned history of radical sexuality.* Boston: Beacon Press.

Morales, E. S., & Graves, M.S. (1983). *Substance abuse: Patterns and barriers to treatment for gay men and lesbians in San Francisco.* San Francisco Department of Public Health.

Moreau-Gruet, F., Dubois-Arber, F., & Spencer, B. (2001). Management of the risk of HIV infection in male homosexual couples. *AIDS, 15,* 1027–1037.

Morin, J. (1999). When hot monogamy isn't happening, consider plan B. *In The Family, 4,* 12–15.

Morin, S. F., Vernon, K., Harcourt, J., Steward, W. T., Volk, J., Reiss, T. H., Neilands, T. B., McLaughlin, M., & Coates, T. (2003). Why HIV infections have increased among men who have sex with men and what to do about it: Findings from California focus groups. *AIDS & Behavior, 7,* 353–362.

Munson, M., & Stelboum, J. (Eds.). (1999). *The lesbian polyamory reader.* New York: Harrington Park Press.

Murray, J. (1998). Psychophysiological aspects of amphetamine–methamphetamine abuse. *Journal of Psychology, 132,* 227–237.

NARTH (2005). www.NARTH.com.

National Institute on Drug Abuse. (1996). Stimulants, Proceedings of the Community Epidemiology Work Group Public Health Service, NIDA, V. 1, 61-71.

Nary, G. (1998). Editorial. *Journal of the International Association of Physicians in AIDS Care.* Retrieved from www.thebody.com/iapac/edit698.html.

National Sex Panic Summit. (1997, November 13). http://www.managingdesire.org/sexpanic/sexpanicpressrelease.html.

Newcombe, R., & Parry, A. (1988). The Mersey Harm-Reduction Model: A strategy for dealing with drug users. Presentation at the International Conference on Drug Policy Reform, Bethesda, MD.

New York City Department of Health and Mental Hygiene. (2003). *NYC Vital Signs: A report from the New York City Community Health Survey, 2,* 1–4.

New York State Department of Health AIDS Institute. (2004). Recommendations for HIV Postexposure Prophylaxis (PEP). www.hivguidelines.org/public_html/center/clinical-guidelines/pep_guidelines/pep_card/pdf.

Nichols, M. (1987). What feminists can learn from the lesbian sex radicals. *Conditions Magazine, 14,* 152–163.

O'Brien, T. R., Kedes, D., Ganem, D., Macrae, D., Rosenberg, P., Molden, J. et al. (1999). Evidence of concurrent epidemics of human herpes virus 8 and human immunodeficiency virus type 1 in US homosexual men: Rates, risk factors and relationship to Karposi's sarcoma. *Journal of Infectious Diseases, 180,* 1010–1017.

Odets, W. (1994). AIDS education and harm reduction for gay men: Psychological approaches for the 21st century. *AIDS & Public Policy Journal, 9,* 3–15.

Odets, W. (1994). Seronegative gay men and considerations of safe and unsafe sex. In S. Cadwell, R. Burnham, M. Forstein (Eds.), *Therapists on the front line: Psychotherapy with gay men in the age of AIDS.* Washington, DC: American Psychiatric Press, 427–452.

Odets, W. (1995). *In the shadow of the epidemic: Being HIV-negative in the age of AIDS.* Durham, NC: Duke University Press.

Odets, W. (1996). Risk appraisals and HIV prevention. *FOCUS: A Guide to AIDS Research and Counseling, 11,* 1–4.

Ogden, G. (1999). *Women who love sex*, Cambridge, MA: Womanspirit Press.

O'Hara, S. (1995). Exit the rubberman. *Steam.*

O'Hara, S. (1997, July 8). Safety First? *The Advocate, 9.*

Osborne, D. (2002, October 11–17). A holistic approach to health: GMHC to fold multiple life issues with HIV prevention. *Gay City, 1,* 10.

Osborne, D. (October 7–13, 2004). Study finds meth–HIV link. *Gay City News.* http://www.gaycitynews.com/gcn_341/studyfindsmethhiv.html.

Ostrow, D., Beltran, E., Joseph, J., DiFrancisco, W., & the MACS/CCD Study Group. (1993). Recreational drugs and sexual behavior in the Chicago MACS/CCS cohort of homosexually active men. *Journal of Substance Abuse, 5,* 311–325.

Ostrow, D. (1999). Practical intervention issues. In D. Ostrow & S. Kalichman (Eds.), *Psychosocial and public health impacts of new HIV therapies.* New York: Kluwer Academic/Plenum Publishers.

Ostrow, D., & Shelby, D. (2000). Psychoanalytic and behavioral approaches to drug-related sexual risk-taking: A preliminary conceptual and clinical integration. *Journal of Gay and Lesbian Psychotherapy, 3,* 123–139.

Ostrow, D. E., Fox, K. J., Chimel, J. S., Silvestre, A., Visscher, B. R., Vanable, P. A., Jacobson, L. P., & Strathdee, S. A. (2002), Attitudes towards highly active antiretroviral therapy are associated with sexual risk taking among HIV-infected and uninfected homosexual men. *AIDS, 16,* 775–780.

Out Magazine. (1997, Summer). Drug users: Staying healthy on the street, 29–30.

Palacios-Jimenez, L., & Shernoff, M. (1986). *Facilitator's guide to eroticizing safer sex.* New York: Gay Men's Health Crisis.

Palmer, R., & Bor, R. (2001). The challenges to intimacy and sexual relationships for gay men in HIV serodiscordant relationships: A pilot study. *Journal of Marital and Family Therapy, 27,* 419 –431..

Parsons, J., & Halkitis, P. (2002). Sexual and drug using practices of HIV+ men who frequent public and commercial sex environments. *AIDS Care, 14,* 815–826.

Parsons, J., Halkitis, P., Wolitski, R., & Gomez, C. (2003). Correlates of sexual risk behaviors among HIV+ men who have sex with men. *AIDS Education and Prevention, 15,* 383–400.

Parsons, J., Wolitski, R., Purcell, D., Gomez, C., Schrimshaw, E., Halkitis, P., Hoff, C., & The SUMIT Team. (2004a, November 12).Use of harm reduction strategies in New York City and San Francisco. Presentation at the 5th National Harm Reduction Conference, New Orleans, LA.

Parsons, J. T., Bimbi, D., Grov, C. & Nanin, J. (2004b, November 12). Innovative approaches to harm reduction: The amazing things that 3-inch heels can do. Presentation at the 5th National Harm Reduction Conference, New Orleans, LA.

Parsons, J. T. (2005). HIV-positive gay and bisexual men. In S. C. Kalichman (Ed.). *Positive prevention: Reducing HIV transmission among people living with HIV/AIDS* (pp. 99–133). New York: Kluwer.

PATH (2005). www.pathinfo.org.

Patton, C. (1991). Visualizing safe sex: When pedagogy and pornography collide. In D. Fuss (Ed.), *Inside/out: Lesbian theories, gay theories.* New York: Routledge, 373–386.

Perel, E. (2003a, March 23). *Mating in captivity: rekindling eroticism in couples.* Psychotherapy Networker Symposium, Washington DC.

Perel, E. (2003b). Erotic intelligence. *Psychotherapy Networker, 27,* 24–31.

Perel, E. (2004, March 24). *Erotic intelligence: Reconciling sensuality and domesticity.* Psychotherapy Networker Symposium, Washington, DC.

Perel, E. (in press). *Mating in captivity: Reconciling eroticism and domesticity.* New York: Harper Collins.

Perez-Pena, R. (2003, August 9). Study finds many ignore warnings on sex practices. *New York Times,* B1, B4.

Peyser, M. (1997, September 29). A deadly dance. *Newsweek, 130,* 76–77.

Picciano, J., Roffman, R, Kalichman, S., Roger A., Rutledge, S., & Berghuis, J. (2001). A telephone-based brief intervention using motivational enhancement to facilitate HIV risk reduction among MSM: A pilot study. *AIDS and Behavior, 5,* 251–262.

Pinkerton, S., & Abramson, P. (1992). Is risky sex rational? *The Journal of Sex Research, 29,* 561–568.

Pinkerton, S., & Abramson, P. (1996). Occasional condom use and HIV risk reduction. *Journal of Acquired Immune Deficiency Syndrome, 13,* 456–460.

Pinkerton, S. D., & Holtgrave, D. (1999). Combination antiretroviral therapies for HIV: Some economic considerations. In D. G. Ostrow & S. C. Kalichman (Eds.), *Psychosocial and public health impacts of new HIV therapies.* New York: Kluwer Academic, 83–107.

Prieur, A. (1990). Norwegian gay men: Reasons for continued practice of unsafe sex. *AIDS Education and Prevention: An Interdisciplinary Journal, 2,* 109–115.

Prochaska, J., & DiClemente, C. (1982). Transtheoretical therapy: Towards a more integrative model of change. *Psychotherapy, Theory, Research, and Practice, 19,* 276–288.

Prochaska, J., DiClemente, C., & Narcross, J. (1992). In search of how people change. *American Psycholoigst, 47,* 1102–1114.

Purcell, D., Parsons, J., Halkitis, P., Mizuno, Y., & Woods, W. (2001). Substance use and sexual transmission risk history of HIV-positive men who have sex with men. *Journal of Substance Abuse, 13,* 185–200.

Quadland, M., & Shattls, W. (1987). AIDS, sexuality and sexual control. *The Journal of Homosexuality, 14,* 277–298.

Rawson, R., Gonzales, R., & Brethen, P. (2002). Treatment of methamphetamine use disorders: an update. *Journal of Substance Abuse Treatment, 23,* 145–150.

Reback, C. J. (1997). The social construction of a gay drug: Methamphetamine use among gay and bisexual males in Los Angeles. Report funded by the City of Los Angeles (Contract #93427).

Reback, C. J. & Grella, C. (1999). HIV risk behaviors of gay and bisexual male amphetamine users contacted through street outreach. *Journal of Drug Issues, 29,* 155–166.

Reid, D., Weatherburn, P., Hickson, F., Stephens, M., & Hammond, G. (2004) *On the move: Findings from the United Kingdom gay men's sex survey 2003.* Sigma Research. www.sigmaresearch.org.uk/downloads/report01.g.pdf.

Reiss, I. (1989). Society and sexuality: A sociological explanation. In K. McKinney & S. Sprecher (Eds.), *Human sexuality: The societal and interpersonal context.* Norwood, NJ: Ablex, 3–29.

Remien, R., Carballo-Dieguez, A., & Wagner, G. (1995). Intimacy and sexual risk behaviour in serodiscordant male couples. *AIDS Care, 7,* 429–438.

Remien, R. (1997). Couples of mixed HIV status: Challenges and strategies for intervention with couples. In L. Wicks (Ed.), *Psychotherapy and AIDS: The human dimension.* Washington, DC: Taylor & Francis, 165–180.

Remien, R. H., & Smith, R. A. (2000). HIV prevention in the era of HAART: Implications for providers. *The AIDS Reader, 10,* 247–251.

Remien, R. H., Wagner, G., Dolezal, C., and Carballo-Dieguez, A. (2001). Factors associated with HIV sexual risk behavior in male couples of mixed HIV status. *Journal of Psychology and Human Sexuality, 13,* 31–48.

Remien, R., Wagner, G., Dolezal, C., & Carballo-Dieguez, A. (2003). Levels and correlates of psychological distress in male couples of mixed HIV status. *AIDS Care, 15*, 525–538.

Remien, R., Halkitis, P., O'Leary, A., Wolitski, R., & Gomez, C. (2005). Risk perception, sexual risk and adherence among HIV-positive men on antiretroviral therapy. *AIDS and Behavior, 9*, 167-176.

Research and Decisions Corporation. (1985). *A Report on designing an effective AIDS prevention campaign strategy for San Francisco: Results from the second probability sample of an urban gay male community.* Prepared for the San Francisco AIDS Foundation.

Rezza, G., Andreoni, M., Dorrucci, M., Pezzotti, P., Monini, P., Zerboni, R. et al. (1999). Human herpesvirus 8 seropositivity and risk of Karposi's sarcoma and other acquired immunodeficiency syndrome–related diseases. *Journal of the National Cancer Institute, 91*, 1468–1474.

Rhodes, S. (2004). Hookups or health promotion? An exploratory study of a chat room–based HIV prevention intervention for men who have sex with men. *AIDS Education and Prevention, 16*, 315–327.

Richard, G. A., Morisky, D. E., Kyle, G. R., Kristal, A. R., Gerker, M. M., & Friedland, M. M. (1988). Sexual activities in bathhouses in Los Angeles County: Implications for AIDS prevention education. *The Journal of Sex Research, 25*, 169–180.

Ridge, D. T., Plummer, D. C., & Minichiello, V. (1994). Knowledge and practice of sexual safety in Melbourne gay men in the nineties. *Australian Journal of Public Health, 18*, 319–325.

Riley, N. (2005, February 24–March 2). The duties a super-virus imposes on our community. *Gay City News, 4*, 13.

Rofes, E. (1996). *Reviving the tribe.* Binghamton, NY: Harrington Park Press.

Rofes, E. (1997). The emerging sex panic targeting gay men. Speech given at the National Gay and Lesbian Task Force's Crating Change Conference, San Diego, CA. Downloaded from www.managingdesire.org/sexpanic/rofessexpanic.html.

Rofes, E. (1999). *Barebacking and the new AIDS hysteria: AIDS leaders defame gay men, misread data, and demand a crisis mentality. Is it any wonder gay men are tuning them out?* [Electronic version]. http://www.managingdesire.org/sexpanic/rofes499.html.

Rogers, G. et al. (2003). Depressive disorders and unprotected casual anal sex among Australian homosexually active men in primary care. *HIV Medicine, 4*, 271–275.

Roman, P., & Blum, T. (1997). *National Treatment Center Study.* Athens, GA: University of Georgia Institute of Behavioral Research.

Romanelli, F., Smith, K., & Pomeroy, C. (2003). Use of club drugs by HIV-seropositive and HIV-seronegative gay and bisexual men. *International AIDS Society, 11*, 25–32.

Rosengarten, M., Race, K., & Kippax, S. (2000). *"Touch wood, everything will be OK": Gay men's understandings of clinical markers in sexual practice.* Sydney: National Centre in HIV Social Research, University of New South Wales.

Rosenstock, I. (1974). Historical origins of the health belief model. *Health Education Monographs, 2*, 328–335.

Ross, M. (2002). The Internet as a medium for HIV prevention and counseling. *FOCUS: A Guide to AIDS Research and Counseling, 17*, 4–6.

Ross, M., & Kauth, M. (2002). Men who have sex with men, and the Internet: Emerging clinical issues and their management. In A. Cooper (Ed.). *Sex & The Internet: A Guide for Clinicians.* New York: Brunner-Routledge, 47–69.

Rotello, G. (1997). *Sexual ecology: AIDS and the destiny of gay men.* New York: Dutton.

Rothern-Borus, M. J., Lee, M., Zhou, S., O'Hara, P., Birnbaum, J. M., Swendeman, D. et al. (2001). Variations in health and risk behavior among youth living with HIV. *AIDS Education and Prevention, 13*, 42–54.

Routy, J. P., Brenner, B., Salomon, H., Quan, Y., Campos, A. F., Rouleau, D. et al. (2000). *Transmission of dual and triple-class drug resistant viral variants in primary/early HIV-1 infection (PHI) in Montreal.* Paper presented at the 7th Conference on Retroviruses and Opportunistic Infections, San Francisco.

Rowatt, W. C., Cunningham, M. R., & Druen, P. B. (1999). Lying to get a date: The effects of facial physical attractiveness on the willingness to deceive prospective dating partners. *Journal of Social and Personal Relations, 16*, 209–233.

Royce, R. A., Sena, A., Cates, W. Jr., & Cohen, M. S. (1997). Current concepts: Sexual transmission of HIV. *New England Journal of Medicine, 336*, 1072–1079.

Sadownick, D. (1996). *Sex between men.* San Francisco: Harper Collins.

Saghir, G. B., & Robins, E. (1973). *Male and female homosexuality: A comprehensive investigation.* Baltimore, MD: Williams & Wilkins.

Salyer, D. (1999). Along the latex highway: Getting real about barebacking [online]. http://www.thebody.com/asp/apr99/barebacking.html.

San Francisco Department of Public Health. (1996). *Oral sex: Using your head: For men who have sex with men.* San Francisco: SFDOPH.

Santora, M., & Altman, L. (2005, February 12). Rare and aggressive HIV reported in New York. *New York Times*, A1, B4.

Santora, M. (2005, March 30). Tests pending in cases tied to fierce HIV. *New York Times*, B1, B4.

Savage, D. (1999, March). The thrill of living dangerously. *Out Magazine*, 62, 64, 118.

Scarce, M. (1998). Back to barebacking [Electronic version]. *The New York Blade*. http://www.managingdesire.org/scarcebtb.html.

Scarce, M. (1999a). A ride on the wild side. *POZ Magazine*, online. http://www.poz.com/index.cfm?p=article&art_id=1787.

Scarce, M. (1999b). Safer barebacking considerations. *POZ Magazine*, online. http://www.poz.com/index.cfm?p=article&art_id=1786.

Schmidt, K., Fouchard, J., Krasnik, A., Zoffman, H., Jacobson, H., & Kreiner, S. (1992). Sexual behavior related to psychosocial factors in a population of Danish homosexual and bisexual men. *Social Sciences and Medicine, 34*, 1119–1127.

Schroeder, M., & Shidlo, A. (2001). Ethical issues in sexual orientation conversion therapies: An empirical study of consumers. *Journal of Gay and Lesbian Psychotherapy, 5,* 131–166.

Schroth, M. (1996). Scores on sensation seeking as predictor of sexual activities among homosexuals. *Perceptual and Motor Skills, 82*, 657–658.

Schwartz, D. (1995). Current psychoanalytic discourse on sexuality: Tripping over the body. In T. Domenici & R. Lesser (Eds.), *Disorienting sexualities.* New York: Routledge, 115–126.

Scragg, P., & Alcorn, R. (2002). Personality disorder and sexual health. In D. Miller & J. Green (Eds.), *The psychology of sexual health.* Oxford: Blackwell Science, 220–235.

Seal, D. W., & Agostinelli, G. (1994). Individual differences associated with high-risk sexual behavior: implications for intervention programmes. *AIDS Care, 6,* 393–397.

Seal, D. W., Kelly, J. A., Bloom, F. R., Stevenson, L. Y., Coley, B. I., Broyles, L. A. et al. (2000). HIV prevention with young men who have sex with men: What young men themselves say is needed. *AIDS Care, 12,* 5–26.

Seeley, S. (2002). CAMP Safe launches Internet-based prevention program. *Letters from Camp Rehoboth, 12,* 60.

Semple, S. J., Patterson, T. L., & Grant, I. (2002). Motivations associated with methamphetamine use among HIV+ men who have sex with men. *Journal of Substance Abuse Treatment, 22,* 149–156.

Sheon, N., & Plant, A. (1997). *Protease dis-inhibitors? The gay bareback phenomenon.* Retrieved from http://kali.ucsf.edu/social/social/spotlight/2098.3445.html.

Sherman, E. (2005). *Note from the margins: The gay analyst's subjectivity in the treatment setting.* Hillsdale, NJ: The Analytic Press.

Shernoff, M. (1988). Integrating AIDS prevention counseling into social work practice. *Social Casework, 6,* 334–339.

Shernoff, M., & Palacios-Jimenez, L. (1988). AIDS: Prevention is the only vaccine available: An AIDS prevention educational program. *Journal of Social Work & Human Sexuality, 6,* 135–150.

Shernoff, M., & Bloom, D.J. (1991). Designing effective AIDS prevention workshops for gay and bisexual men. *AIDS Education and Prevention, 3,* 31–46.

Shernoff, M. (1995). Male couples and their relationship styles. *The Journal of Gay & Lesbian Social Services, 2,* 43–58.

Shernoff, M., & Morin, J. (1999). Monogamy and gay men: When open relationships are a therapeutic option. *Family Therapy Networker, 23,* 63–71.

Shernoff, M. (2002). Body image, working out and therapy. *Journal of Gay and Lesbian Social Services, 14,* 89–94.

Shidlo, A., Schroeder, M., & Drescher, J. (2001). *Sexual conversion therapy: Ethical, clinical and research perspectives,* Binghamton, NY: Haworth Press.

Shidlo, A., & Schroeder, M. (2002). Changing sexual orientation: A consumer's report. *Professional Psychology: Research and Practice, 33,* 249–259.

Sigma Research. (2004). http://www.sigmaresearch.org.uk/about.html.

Signorile, M. (1994). Unsafe like me. *Out Magazine, 22–24,* 128.

Signorile, M. (1997). Bareback and reckless [Electronic version]. *Out Magazine.* http://www.signorile.com/col-bareback.html.

Signorile, M. (1997, October). In the company of men. *Out Magazine, 86,* 146–149.

Signorile, M. (1998). Sex panic! and paranoia [Electronic version]. *Out Magazine.* http://www.signorile.com/col-sexpanic.html.

Signorile, M. (1999). Don't fear the fear: When risk-taking seems sexy and being HIV-positive looks breezy and fun, maybe it's time to bring fear back into HIV prevention [Electronic version]. *The Advocate.* http://www.advocate.com/html/stories/0499A/0499_sig_sex.asp.

Signorile, M. (2001). The contradictory faces of Andrew Sullivan: An LGNY Exclusive [Electronic version]. *The Newspaper for Lesbian Gay New York, 159.* http://www.lgny.com/feature.html.

Silverstein, C. (1981). *Man to man: Gay couples in America,* New York: William Morrow.

Silverstein, C. (1996). History of treatment. In R. Cabaj, & T. Stein (Eds.), *Textbook of homosexuality & mental health.* Washington, DC: American Psychiatric Press, 3–16.

Silverstein, C. (1997). The origin of the gay psychotherapy movement. In M. Duberman (Ed.), *A queer world.* New York: New York University Press, 358–380.

Simao, P. (2003, July 29) *Rise of Internet fuels fears of AIDS resurgence.* Reuters News Service. http://reuters.com/newsArticle.jhtml?type=internetNews&storyID=3179188.

Simon, W., & Gagnon, J. (1967). Homosexuality: the development of a sociological perspective. *Journal of Health and Social Behavior, 8,* 177–185.

Socarides, C. W. (1978). *Homosexuality.* Northvale, NJ: Aronson.

Sonenschein, D. (1966). Homosexuality as a subject of anthropological inquiry. *Anthropological Quarterly, 39,* 73–82.

Sonenschein, D. (1968). The ethnography of male homosexual relationships. *Journal of Sex Research, 4,* 69–83.

Sontag, S. (1988). *AIDS and its metaphors.* New York: Picador.

Sorokin, E. (2003, January 24). Bug chaser AIDS story disputed. *The Washington Times,* retrieved from www.homosexissin.com/portal/'Bug%20chaser.htm.

Sowadsy, R. (1999). *Barebacking in the gay community.* http://www.thebody.com/sowadsky/barebacking.htm.

Specter, M. (2005, May 23). Higher risk: Crystal meth, the Internet and dangerous choices about AIDS. *The New Yorker,* 38–45.

Springer, E. (1991). Effective AIDS prevention with active drug users: The harm reduction model. In M. Shernoff (Ed.), *Counseling chemically dependent people with HIV illness.* Binghamton, NY: Harrington Park Press, 141–158.

Springer, E. (2004, May). Stages of change model and motivational interviewing. Handout given to students in one of the author's classes at Columbia University School of Social Work.

Stall, R., McKusick, L., Wiley, J., Coates, T., & Ostrow, D. (1986). Alcohol and drug use during sexual activity and compliance with safe sex guidelines for AIDS: Behavioral research project. *Health Education Quarterly, 13,* 359–371.

Stall, R., & Wiley, J. (1988). A comparison of alcohol and drug use patterns of homosexual and heterosexual men: The San Francisco Men's Health Study. *Drug and Alcohol Dependence, 22,* 63–73.

Stall, R., Ekstrand, M., Pollack, L., McKusick, L., & Coates, T. (1990). Relapse form safer sex: The next challenge for AIDS prevention efforts. *Journal of Acquired Immunodeficiency Syndrome & Human Retrovirology, 3,* 181–187.

Stall, R. D., Paul, J. P., Barrett, D. C., Crosby, G. M., & Bein, E. (1991). An outcome evaluation to measure changes in sexual risk taking among gay men undergoing substance use disorder treatment. *Journal of Studies of Alcohol, 60,* 837–845.

Stall, R. D., & Leigh, B. (1994). Understanding the relationship between drug or alcohol use and high-risk sexual activity for HIV transmission: Where do we go from here? *Addiction, 89,* 131–134.

Stein, D. (1978). Dr. Dan William: A physician to the gay community talks about hepatitis, V.D. control, and being an openly gay doctor. *Christopher Street, 2,* 10–23.

Stolte, I., deWit, J., van Eeden, A., Coutinho, R., & Dukers, N. (2004, July). *The perceived viral load level, and not the actual viral load, is a predictor for risky sex with steady partners among HIV-infected homosexual men.* Presentation at XV International AIDS Conference, Bangkok (WeOrC1334).

Strub, S. (1999). S.O.S. Safer Barebacking is in the grassroots, take charge of your own life tradition pioneered by Michael Callen. *POZ Magazine*, online. http://www.poz.com/index.cfm?p=article&art_id=1809.

Stulberg, I., & Smith, M. (1988). Psychosocial impact of the AIDS epidemic on the lives of gay men. *Social Work, 33*, 277–281.

Styrsky, S. (2005, February 24–March 2). Pushing gays to the margins. *Gay City News, 4*, 1, 6.

Suarez, T., Kelly, J. A., Pinkerton, S. D., Stevenson, Y. L., Hayat, M. J., Smith, M. D., & Ertl, T. (2001). The influence of a partner's HIV serostatus and viral load on perceptions of sexual risk behavior in a community sample of gay and bisexual men. *AIDS, 27*, 289–291.

Suarez, T., & Miller, J. (2001). Negotiating risks in context: A perspective on unprotected anal intercourse and barebacking among men who have sex with men — Where do we go from here? *Archives of Sexual Behavior, 30*, 287–300.

Sullivan, A. (1996, November 10). When plagues end. *New York Times Magazine*. Retrieved online at www.newyorktimes.com.

Sullivan, A. (1999). *Love undetectable: Notes on sex, friendship, and survival.* New York: Knopf Publishing Group.

Sullivan, A. (2001). Sexual McCarthyism: An article no one should have to write. www.Andrewsullivan.com.

Tashima, K., Alt, E., Harwell, J., Fiebich-Perez, D., & Flanigan, T. (2003). Internet sex-seeking leads to acute HIV infection: A report of two cases. *International Journal of STD & AIDS, 14*, 285–286.

Tatarsky, A. (Ed.). (2002). *Harm reduction psychotherapy. A new treatment for drug and alcohol problems.* New Jersey: Jason Aronson Inc.

Tewksbury, R. (2003). Bareback sex and the quest for HIV: Assessing the relationship in Internet personal advertisements of men who have sex with men. *Deviant Behavior, 24*, 467–482.

Thomas, S., & Ratigan, B. (2005). The psychodynamics of unsafe sex. In J. Hiller, H. Wood, & W. Bolton (Eds.), *Sex, mind and emotion: Innovation in theory and practice.* London: Karnac. In Press.

Tikkanen, R., & Ross, M. (2000). Looking for sexual compatibility: Experiences among Swedish men in visiting Internet gay chatrooms. *Cyberpsychology and Behavior, 3*, 605–616.

Tikkanen, R., & Ross, M. (2003). Technological tearoom trade: Characteristics of Swedish men visiting gay Internet chat rooms. *AIDS Education & Prevention, 15*, 122–132.

Tuller, D. (2001, October 16). Experts fear a risky recipe: Viagra, drugs and HIV. *New York Times*, http://query.nytimes.com/search/restricted/article?res=F70C1FFC355BOC758DDDA90994D9404482.

Tuller, D. (2004, October 26). Health officials put safer-sex message online. *New York Times*, F8.

Turner, W. (2001). ACT UP slams chat rooms–based surveillance as "dubious use of taxpayer dollars." Retrieved online http://www.glaa.org/archive/2001/actup2dohonstdgrant1029.shtml.

Ultimatebareback.com (2004). http://ubb1.ultimatebareback.com/index.asp.

Urbino, A., & Jones, K. (2004). Crystal methamphetamine, its analogues, and HIV infection: Medical and psychiatric aspects of a new epidemic. *Clinical Infectious Diseases, 38*, 890–894.

U.S. Public Health Service. (2001). Updated U.S. Public Health Service guidelines for the management of occupational exposures to HBV, HCV, and HIV and recommendations for postexposure prophylaxis. *Morbidity and Mortality Weekly Report, 50*, 1–52.

Valleroy, L. A., MacKellar, D. A., Karon, J. M., Rosen, D. H., McFarland, W., Sheehan, D. A. et al. (2000). HIV prevalence and associated risks in young men who have sex with men. *JAMA, 284*, 198–204.

Van de Ven, P., Campbell, D., Kippax, S., Knox, S., Prestage, G., French, J., Crawford, J. et al. (1998). Gay men who engage repeatedly in unprotected anal intercourse with casual partners: The Sydney Men and Sexual Health Study. *International Journal of STD and AIDS, 9*, 336–340.

Van de Ven, P., & Crawford, J. (1998a), Change in sexual practice among Australian men who have sex with men, 1992–1996. *AIDS, 12 (supplement B)*, S 66.

Van de Ven, P., Prestage, G., French, J., Knox, S., & Kippax, S. (1998b). Increase in unprotected anal intercourse with casual partners among Sydney gay men in 1996–98. *Australian and New Zealand Journal of Public Health, 22*, 814–818.

Van de Ven, P., French, J., Crawford, J., & Kippax, S. (1999). Sydney gay men's agreements about sex. In P. Aggleton, G. Hart, & P. Davies (Eds.). *Families and communities responding to AIDS*. London: University College London Press.

Van de Ven, P., Prestage, G., Knox, S., & Kippax, S. (2000). Gay men in Australia who do not have AIDS test results. *International Journal of STD and AIDS, 11*, 456–460.

Van de Ven, P., Rawstorne, P., Crawford, J., & Kippax, S. (2002). Increasing proportions of Australian gay and homosexually active men engage in unprotected anal intercourse with regular and with casual partners. *AIDS Care, 14*, 335–341.

Van de Ven, P., Kippax, S., Crawford, J., Rawstorne, P., Prestage, G., Grulich, A. et al. (2002b). In a minoirity of gay men, sexual risk practice indicates strategic positioning for perceived risk reduction rather than unbridled sex. *AIDS Care, 14*, 471–480.

Van de Ven, P., Mao, L., Fogarty, A., Rawstorne, P., Crawford, J., Prestage, P., Grulich, A., Kaldor, J., & Kippax, S. (2005). Undetectable viral load is associated with sexual risk taking in HIV-serodiscordant gay couples in Sydney. *AIDS, 19,* 179–184.

Vanable, P. A., Ostrow, D. G., McKirnan, D. J., Taywaditep, K. J., & Hope, B. A. (2000). Impact of combination therapies on HIV risk perceptions and sexual risk-taking among HIV-positive and HIV-negative gay and bisexual men. *Health Psychology, 19,* 134–145.

Vance, C. (Ed.). (1984). *Pleasure and danger: Exploring female sexuality.* Boston: Routledge & Kegan.

Vernazza, P., Troiani, L., Flepp, M., Cone, R., Schoci, J., Roth, F., Boggian, K., Cohen, M., Fiscus, S., & Eron, J. (2000). Potent antiretroviral treatment of HIV-infection results in suppression of the seminal shedding of HIV. The Swiss HIV Cohort Study. *AIDS, 14,* 117–121.

Vincke, J., Bolton, R., & DeVleeschouwer, P. (2001). The cognitive structure of the domain of safe and unsafe gay sexual behaviour in Belgium. *AIDS Care, 13,* 57–70.

Vittinghoff, E., Douglas, J., & Judson, F. (1999). Per-contact risk of human immunodeficiency virus transmission between male sexual partners. *American Journal of Epidemiology, 150,* 306–311.

Wagner, G., Remien, R., & Carballo-Dieguez, A. (1998). "Extramarital" sex: Is there an increased risk for HIV transmission? A study of male couples of mixed HIV status. *AIDS Education & Prevention, 10,* 245–256.

Wagner, G. J., Remien, R. H., & Carballo-Dieguez, A. (2000). Prevalence of extradyadic sex in male couples of mixed HIV status and its relationship to psychological distress and relationship quality. *Journal of Homosexuality, 39,* 31–46.

Wainberg, M. A., & Friedland, G. (1998). Public health implications of antiretroviral therapy and HIV drug resistance. *JAMA, 279,* 1977–1980.

Walker, D., & Roffman, R. (2004). Applying motivational enhancement therapy to HIV prevention and care. *FOCUS: A Guide to AIDS Research and Counseling, 19,* 1–4.

Warner, M. (1995). Why gay men are having risky sex. *The Village Voice,* 32–37.

Weatherburn, P., Davies, P., Hickson, F., Hunt, A., McManus, R., & Coxon, A. (1993). No connection between alcohol use and unsafe sex among gay and bisexual men. *AIDS, 7,* 115–119.

Weatherburn, P., Hickson, F., & Reid, D. (2003). *Net benefits: Gay men's use of the Internet and other settings where HIV prevention occurs.* Sigma Research, London. Retrieved off the Internet http://www.sigmaresearch.org.uk/downloads/report03b.

Weinberg, G. (1983). *Society and the healthy homosexual.* New York: St. Martin's Press.

Weinberg, M., & Williams, C. (1974). *Male homosexuals: Their problems and adaptations.* London: Oxford University Press.

Weinberger, L. E., & Millham, J. (1979). Attitudinal homophobia and support of traditional sex roles. *Journal of Homosexuality, 4,* 237–246.

West, D. (1987). *Sexual crimes and confrontations: A study of victims and offenders.* Aldershot, England: Gower Publishing Co.

White, E. (1983). Sexual culture. *Vanity Fair.* Republished in D. Bergman (Ed.), *The burning library: Essays.* New York: Vintage Books, 1995, 57–67.

Whitfield, C. (1996, November). Crystal and the gay men of L.A. *Sexvibe, 13,* 16–32.

Wiley, D. J., Visscher, B. R., Grosser, S., Hoover, D. R., Day, R., Gange, S. et al. (2000). Evidence that anoreceptive intercourse with ejaculate exposure is associated with rapid CD4 loss. *AIDS, 14,* 707–715.

Wilton, L. (2001). Perceived health risks and psychosocial factors as predictors of sexual risk-taking within HIV-positive gay male seroconcordant couples. *Dissertation Abstracts International: Section B: the Sciences and Engineering, 61,* 3867.

Wolitski, R. J., Valdiserri, R. O., Denning, P. H., & Levine, W. C. (2001). Are we headed for a resurgence in the HIV epidemic among men who have sex with men? *American Journal of Public Health, 91,* 883–888.

Wolitski, R., & Branson, B. (2002). "Gray area behaviors" and partner selection strategies: Working toward a comprehensive approach to reducing the sexual transmission of HIV. In A. O'Leary (Ed.), *Beyond condoms: Alternative approaches to HIV prevention.* New York: Kluwer Academic 173–198.

Wolitski, R., Parsons, J., & Gomez, C. (2004). Prevention with HIV-seropositive men who have sex with men: Findings from the seropositive urban men's study (SUMS) and the seropositive urban men's intervention trial (SUMIT). *Journal of Acquired Immune Deficiency Syndrome, 37, Supplement 2,* S101–S109.

Wolitski, R. (2005). Listening to gay and bisexual men living with HIV: Implications of the seropositive Urban Men's Study for Psychology and Public Health. In P. Halkitis, C. Gomez, & R. Wolitski (Eds.), *HIV+ sex: The psychological and interpersonal dynamics of HIV-seropositive gay and bisexual men's relationships.* Washington, DC: American Psychological Assn., 233–254.

Wolitski, R., & Bailey, C. (2005). It takes two to tango: HIV-positive gay and bisexual men's beliefs about their responsibility to protect others from HIV infection. In P. Halkitis, C. Gomez, & R. Wolitski (Eds.), *HIV+ sex: The psychological and interpersonal dynamics of HIV-seropositive gay and bisexual men's relationships.* Washington, DC: American Psychological Assn., 147–162.

World Health Organization. (2002). Department of Reproductive Health and Research, Gender and Reproductive Rights. http://www.who.int/reproductive-health/gender/sexual_health.html.

Woody, G. E., Donnekk, D., Seage, G. R., Metzger, D., Marmor, M., Koblin, B. A. et al. (1999). Noninjection substance use correlates with risky sex among men having sex with men: Data from HIVNET. *Drug and Alcohol Dependence, 53,* 197–205.

Xiridou, M., Geskus, R., de Wit, J., Coutinho, R., & Kretzschmar, M. (2003). The contribution of steady and casual partnerships to the incidence of HIV infection among homosexual men in Amsterdam. *AIDS, 17,* 1029–1038.

Yep, F., Lovaas, K., & Pagonis, A. (2002). The case of riding bareback: Sexual practices and the paradoxes of identity in the era of AIDS. *Journal of Homosexuality, 42,* 1–14.

Yerly, S., Jost, S., Monnat, M., Telenti, A., Cavassini, M., Chave, J., Kaiser, L., Burgisser, P., Perris, L., & Swiss HIV Cohort Study. (2004). HIV-1 co/superinfection in intravenous drug users. *AIDS, 18,* 1413–1421.

Yoshida, T. (1997). Use and misuse of amphetamine: An international overview. In H. Kell (Ed.), *Amphetamine misuse.* Amsterdam: Harwood Academic Publishers, 1–16.

Young, I. (November/December 1997, February/March 1997). The AIDS cult and its seroconverts. *Continuum.* www.virusmyth.net/aids/data/iycultsero.htm

Zucker, K. J. (1996). Sexism and heterosexism in the diagnostic interview for borderline patients? *American Journal of Psychiatry, 153,* 966.

Zuckerman, M. (1993). Impulsive sensation seeking and its behavioural, psychological, and biochemical correlates. *Neuropsychobiology, 28,* 30–36.

Zuckerman, M. (1994). *Behavioral expressions and biosocial bases of sensation seeking.* Cambridge, England: Cambridge University Press.

Index

That which we know or perceive
but for which there are no
words for —

There may be words for it
in a language other than our
own

Worth reading Article about
Spelke's work with infants
in the New Yorker
9/4/06 by
Margaret Talbot